Clinical Governance and Best Value

(

For Churchill Livingstone:

Senior Commissioning Editor: Susan Young
Project Development Manager: Katrina Mather
Project Manager: Pat Miller
Designer: Judith Wright
Illustration Manager: Bruce Hogarth

Clinical Governance and Best Value

Meeting the Modernisation Agenda

Edited by

Sharon Pickering MSc BA(Hons) BSc(Hons) PGDip(HSSM) DipN(Lond) RGN
Head of Education and Training,
Trent NHS Workforce Development Confederation, UK

Jeanette Thompson MA BSc(Hons) RNMH PGDipMan DipHSSM CertEd DipN(Lond)
Lecturer in Learning Disabilities, Department of Health Sciences,
University of York, York, UK

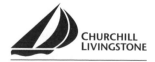

CHURCHILL
LIVINGSTONE

EDINBURGH LONDON NEW YORK OXFORD PHILADELPHIA ST LOUIS SYDNEY TORONTO 2003

CHURCHILL LIVINGSTONE
An imprint of Elsevier Science Limited

First published 2003

ISBN 0 443 07167 5

British Library Cataloguing in Publication Data
A catalogue record for this book is available from the British Library

Library of Congress Cataloging in Publication Data
A catalog record for this book is available from the Library of Congress

Note
Medical knowledge is constantly changing. As new information
becomes available, changes in treatment, procedures, equipment and
the use of drugs become necessary. The editors/contributors and the
publishers have taken care to ensure that the information given in this
text is accurate and up to date. However, readers are strongly advised
to confirm that the information, especially with regard to drug usage,
complies with the latest legislation and standards of practice.

 your source for books,
journals and multimedia
in the health sciences

www.elsevierhealth.com

The
publisher's
policy is to use
**paper manufactured
from sustainable forests**

Printed in China

Contents

Contributors

Andy Alaszewski BA PhD HonMFPHM
Professor of Health Studies, Director,
Centre for Health Services Studies, University
of Kent at Canterbury, Canterbury, UK

Amanda Ashton MSc BA(Hons) DPNS RN(G)
Director for Nursing, Research and
Development, Leicester City West Primary Care
Trust and Senior Research Fellow, Division of
Primary Care, De Montfort University,
Leicester, UK

Melissa C Brouwers PhD MA BSc
Associate Director – Program in Evidence-based
care, Cancer Care Ontario, Assistant Professor
Faculty of Medicine, McMaster University
Health Sciences Center, Ontario, Canada

Helen Chin RN MSc
Programme Associate, Centre for the
Development of Nursing Policy and Practice,
School of Healthcare Studies, University of
Leeds, Leeds, UK

Jane Clayton BA(Hons) RGN MSc PhD
Research Fellow, Sheffield Teaching Hospitals
NHS Trust, Sheffield, UK

Brian Footitt OBE
Director of Nursing Development, South Tees
Hospitals NHS Trust, James Cook University
Hospital, Middlesbrough, Cleveland, UK

Christina Funnell BA (Spec Hons in Soc Admin)
Organising Secretary of the Health Coalition
Initiative, Consumer Health Information Centre,
London, UK

Kate Gerrish PhD MSc BN
Professor of Nursing Practice Development,
School of Nursing and Midwifery, University of
Sheffield, Sheffield, UK

Phil Glanfield BA MA MBA CQSW
Director, Rapid Response Unit, National Clinical
Governance Support Team, NHS Modernisation
Agency, UK

Ian D Graham PhD MA BA DEC
Senior Social Scientist and Associate Director,
Clinical Epidemiology Program, Ottawa Health
Research Institute, Canadian Institutes of Health
Research New Investigator, Associate Professor
of Medicine and Epidemiology and Community
Medicine, University of Ottawa, Ottawa, Canada

Margaret B Harrison PhD MHA BN RN
Associate Professor, School of Nursing, Faculty
of Health Sciences, Queen's University,
Kingston, Ontario, Canada

Rob McSherry MSc BSc(Hons) DipN(Lond) RGN PGG RT
Principal Lecturer, Practice Development,
School of Health, University of Teeside,
Middlesbrough, UK

Alan Maynard BA BPhil FMedSci Hon FFPHM
Director, York Health Policy Group Department of Health Sciences, University of York, York, UK

Elaine Morris RN RM RHV BSc(Hons) MBA
Project Consultant, Middlesbrough Primary Care Trust, Cleveland, UK

Sue Merrylees CertEd MA RNMH
Head of Nursing Studies, Department of Nursing and Applied Health Studies, University of Hull, Hull, UK

Sharon Pickering MSc BA(Hons) BSc(Hons) PGDip(HSSM) DipN(Lond) RGN
Head of Education and Training, Trent NHS Workforce Development Confederation

Paul Ramcharan BSc PhD
Reader in Cognitive Disabilities, Department of Mental Health and Learning Disabilities, School of Nursing and Midwifery, University of Sheffield, Sheffield, UK

Marc Saunders BSc(Hons) MA RNMH DPSN
General Manager, North Warwickshire PCT, Kidderminster, UK

Shirley Taylor MA BSC(Hons) DipN CertEd RGN
Principal Lecturer, Research, School of Health, University of Teeside, Middlesbrough, UK

Carl Thompson RN BA DPhil
Research Fellow, Centre for Evidence-Based Nursing, Department of Health Sciences, York, UK

Jeanette Thompson MA BSc(Hons) RNMH PGDipMan DipHSSM CertEd DipN(Lond)
Lecturer in Learning Disabilities, Department of Health Sciences, University of York, York, UK

Preface

We chose to write this book because of our experiences in trying to implement best practice in a variety of settings. This experience provided us with a variety of insights as to what the important issues were and where people frequently experienced difficulties. As such, we have used this to inform the chapters within this text and the way in which each section within the book is structured. We hope that this text will prove an all round resource for people embarking upon the implementation of best practice.

This book is essentially a practice-based text that is aimed at providing all practitioners in both health and social care with the opportunity to reflect upon their practice, consider approaches to developing their practice and identify ways of implementing high quality care and support. As such, many of the chapters contain activities that are designed to assist in this process and some contain useful resources and web sites for further guidance.

The value base upon which this book is founded essentially places the user of the service at the centre of all developments and consequently advocates that these people are actively involved in all aspects of service development, delivery and evaluation. Fundamental to this is the use of appropriate positive and valuing terminology. It is for this reason that the term patient is only used when necessary rather than as a catch all term for anyone in receipt of welfare services.

This text has been a product of many hours of effort from a variety of people. We have all learnt from writing this book and we hope that you find it a useful resource in your quest to deliver high quality care.

2003

Jeanette Thompson
Sharon Pickering

Political context of care delivery

SECTION CONTENTS

This section explores the current context in which health and social care is delivered. It focuses upon the political drivers and the structures and systems that have been put in place to support the achievement of the modernisation agenda within welfare services. In addition, it considers some specific aspects of the modernisation agenda, particularly the area of service user and patient involvement in the development, delivery and evaluation of welfare services. This is addressed from the perspective of people who use mental health and learning disability services and those people using acute and rehabilitative services who have a chronic health condition. In addition, and perhaps unusually, this section includes a chapter that focuses upon the economic influences and techniques that can be used to inform decision-making processes in times of limited resources and demands for increasing quality.

1

Clinical governance and best value: a toolkit for quality

Jane Clayton

KEY ISSUES

◆ Defining quality

◆ Systems and structures to support quality improvement

◆ Measuring and managing quality

◆ User satisfaction and value for money

INTRODUCTION

If everyone involved in the health and social care arena, including patients, clients, service users, practitioners, managers and commissioners, is to feel confident that those who provide services are 'doing the right thing right', they need to engage with the idea of continuous quality improvement. In addressing this issue, professionals and providers alike will be addressing one of the central themes within the modernisation agenda, as is outlined within policy documents such as *A First Class Service: Quality in the new NHS* (Department of Health 1998a).

This chapter will consider what is meant by the term quality, and how quality can be achieved in practice using structures and systems that support continuous quality improvement. In addition, it will explore how quality is measured and managed, particularly in terms of user satisfaction and value for money. Finally, this chapter will examine how practitioners can take control of the systems that underpin quality improvement and the role of leadership within this. Consequently, the aim of this chapter is to demonstrate the relationship between quality, best value and clinical governance. Other strands of the modernisation agenda will be addressed throughout the remaining chapters of this text; these include service user involvement, individual and organisational change, leadership, accountability, risk management, audit, finding and implementing best practice, and some structured approaches to care delivery.

DEFINING QUALITY

In everyday terms *quality* is defined as 'the degree or extent of excellence of something, a high standard' (Chambers 1996). So what is continuous quality improvement? *Continuous* means unbroken like a circle and *improvement* means to get better than it is. Hence continuous quality improvement describes the never-ending pursuit to raise standards in health and social care.

Dale et al. (1997, p. 3) suggest that while '... many people say that they know what is meant by quality ... it is in fact ... quite difficult for many people to grasp and understand'. Over the last decade this concept has been used in a variety of ways, to describe and define some of the fundamental elements and structures of provision in health and social care. However, it is not an absolute concept and is subjective in its nature and is, therefore, difficult to measure. In addition, quality means different things to different people:

- For patients and service users quality represents the care they receive in terms of their quality of life.

- For staff quality is a measure of the care they deliver.
- For any organisation quality is reflected in the service they provide.

The following case study illustrates the different perspectives outlined above.

Case study

'Reducing waiting lists' in the NHS has been identified as a target for quality improvement by the government, in the hope that the lists of those people waiting for operations would become shorter. This was intended to ensure that people waiting for surgery would have their operation sooner than had become the 'norm' and that this would be an improvement for them. However, if the shorter lists meant that some people were put on to different lists, which meant they waited even longer than before for their operation, that would not be seen as an improvement by them. If the new targets also meant longer working hours for some practitioners and longer times on hospital trolleys for those admitted as emergencies, this would not be seen as an improvement by them. From the organisational perspective they may be able to satisfy government targets for waiting lists, but would they be meeting targets for 'improving working lives' and the expectations within the NHS Plan around meeting patient or service user needs?

As a progression from this situation and in an attempt to meet the quality demands of more groups most stakeholders have moved to use 'time' as a way of measuring the effective access to services. In terms of numbers and patient/client satisfaction, both recognised measures of quality, this new target is already seen as an improvement by many people.

Activity 1.1

Think about a practice-related quality issue within your service. Talk to a service user, another member of the staff team and a service manager about their view of the issue. What are the common themes from each of your discussions and what are the differences?

When talking with these people you may have noticed how they had different perspectives on the issue in question, much as in the case study above. You may well have been focused upon the quality of care delivered, whilst your manager may have been concerned about the efficient use of resources and the targets that the service has to meet. Meanwhile, the person using the service may have been much more interested in what the effect of the treatment or intervention may have on them personally and what it means for their quality of life. Because these view points were different it does not mean that any one of them was wrong or irrelevant. What it does mean is that we need to find ways of meeting all the different agendas in a way that is meaningful for all concerned.

MAKING QUALITY VISIBLE IN HEALTH AND SOCIAL CARE

When major reforms of health and social services were introduced in 1990 in the NHS and Community Care Act 'the government put quality on the agenda for the first time' (Øvretveit 1992, p. xi). The reforms were based on two white papers: *Working for Patients* (Department of Health 1989a), with its focus on the NHS, and *Caring for People* (Department of Health 1989b), which addressed care in the community. Initially the NHS received most attention and quality issues were influenced by those already used in business and industry where a market economy approach prevailed. This resulted in the notion of setting up an 'internal market' in the health service represented by initiatives like:

- the purchaser–provider split
- the introduction of GP fundholding
- greater involvement of the private healthcare sector
- more rigorous monitoring of services
- regarding the patient/client as a 'consumer'.

Activity 1.2

What is the continuing impact of this culture upon the welfare services of today?

The NHS was urged to engage with the principles of supply and demand where 'quality' would be acknowledged much more explicitly than ever before both by the provider and the 'customer' or 'consumer'. In the event, quality tended to become associated with audit, quality assurance and total quality management, which for practitioners often felt more like sticks than carrots or as ways to identify problems and apportion blame rather than means to encourage improvement. The stretched financial resources of the health service resulted in a preoccupation by government and managers alike with cost, and what they described as a need to provide 'value for money'.

By 1993 the delayed community care plans, which local authorities were required to produce by the reforms, had been introduced by most social services departments and once again funding was a key issue. The new initiatives this time included:

- the introduction of care management
- enabling people to remain longer in their own homes
- ensuring support for carers

- making clear the lines of responsibility and accountability
- promoting more involvement of the independent sector
- involving service users in their care.

Once again the emphasis on quality was acknowledged in an economic context since one of the main issues was the need to transfer the costs of residential care for older people from an already overstretched social security budget to local authorities and to service users themselves. Collaboration and co-operation between agencies was encouraged, joint planning was to become the basis for a 'seamless service' and local authorities were required to establish inspection and registration units to monitor the standards of care, all in order to improve the quality of provision. However, the focus remained that of ensuring 'value for (taxpayers') money' and the promotion of a 'mixed economy' of welfare (Leathard 2000). Consequently, in the provision of both health and social care, the use of the term 'value for money' became a quasi-economic idea relating to quality.

The next major quality initiatives in health and social care came about with a change in government in 1997 as part of a new 'modernisation agenda'. The NHS Bill (1999) would enact those modernising measures for health services requiring legislation set out in three white papers for England, Scotland and Wales. The government proposals for Northern Ireland were set out in a consultative document. These papers reflected the differing structures of the four countries and the moves towards devolution in Britain. They included:

- *The new NHS, Modern and Dependable* (Department of Health 1998b) in England
- *Designed to Care* (Secretary of State for Scotland 1997) in Scotland
- *Putting Patients First* (Secretary of State for Wales 1998) in Wales

- *Fit for the Future* (Department of Health for Northern Ireland 1998) in Northern Ireland.

The NHS Bill (1999) had been raising the standards in the quality of care at its core. The government's quality strategy was presented in a consultation paper: *A First Class Service: Quality in the new NHS* (Department of Health 1998a) that set out a package of proposals 'to support the delivery of more consistent and higher quality care to patients'. A quality framework was proposed through which:

- standards of service would be set at national level
- responsibility for their delivery would lie at local level
- consistent monitoring of these arrangements was put in place.

The NHS Bill also introduced measures to promote partnership in order to facilitate less bureaucratic and more efficient ways of providing services by:

- requiring NHS organisations to co-operate with each other and with local authorities through health improvement programmes (HImPs) and joint investment plans (JIPs)
- introducing more flexible arrangements for joint working between health and social services set out in *Partnerships in Action* (Department of Health 1998c) (partnership consultation document).

Finally, the NHS Bill acknowledged a shift from what had appeared to be a preoccupation with cost at the expense of quality by proposing to abolish GP fundholding and replace it with Primary Care Trusts (PCTs). This has resulted in some fundamental organisational changes at local level, with the newly formed organisations being expected to work within the quality programme set out above.

The modernising measures for social services were set out in a white paper: *Modernising Social Services* (Secretary of State for Health 1998), which would introduce 'modern and dependable social services to match the modern and dependable NHS' (NHS Confederation 1998a). The aim was to:

- protect vulnerable people, for example children, people with mental health problems, older people and those with learning difficulties
- support welfare reform and social inclusion by promoting independence. The Social Exclusion Unit was established in 1998 and 'pathfinder' districts of deprivation were identified as targets for a programme to reduce poverty and inequality
- raise standards of care to ensure the delivery of top-quality services.

Legislation was promised that would make it easier for health and social services to work together, to pool budgets, delegate the lead for commissioning services and integrate provision (Department of Health 1998c). This became a reality with the inception of the health flexibilities outlined in *The NHS Bill* (1999). In addition, improvements to training and performance reviews following the same lines as the Health Service were included in the quality strategy for Social Services.

Activity 1.3

What partnerships do you need to establish both within or outwith your organisation in order to meet the clinical governance and best practice agenda more effectively?

You may have thought about the partnerships you have with other professionals; this will vary depending upon the nature of the organisation you work within, as will the complexity of managing those relationships. In addition to professionals such as social workers, doctors or therapists, you may have considered the departments that support your service and in particular the clinical

governance and best value agenda. These may include audit, information management, education and training, and research or best practice departments. External to your organisation you may have thought about the need to establish links with your local university, libraries or national organisations such as professional bodies, Royal Colleges and service user groups or forums.

STRUCTURES THAT CURRENTLY SUPPORT CONTINUOUS QUALITY IMPROVEMENT

Clear, common, national standards are being set for service provision and treatment, and guidance on developing best clinical practice is now provided through:

- National Service Frameworks (NSFs). (Those for cancer services, mental health, coronary heart disease and the care of older people were among the first to be published.)
- the National Institute for Clinical Excellence (NICE) which acts as a nationwide appraisal body for new and existing treatments and disseminates consistent advice on what works and what does not.

NICE influences quality by:

1. assessing the clinical and cost effectiveness of new healthcare developments
2. issuing guidance on whether and how treatments should be made available, for example, the drug Tamoxifen used in the treatment of breast cancer
3. producing and disseminating guidelines, based on the available evidence of clinical and cost effectiveness, for example, the guidelines on the management of pressure damage (Royal College of Nursing 2000)
4. providing associated clinical audit methodologies and information on best practice.

A similar body, the Social Care Institute for Excellence, has been set up to support quality in social care services.

Ensuring that the impact of these standards reach patients and service users is a key thrust within the modernisation agenda. This is further reinforced through patient and public involvement in both professional self-regulation, life-long learning and continuing professional development initiatives.

Mechanisms that monitor these standards and systems to ensure continuous quality improvement include:

- the Commission for Health Improvement (CHI)
- National Performance Framework
- a National User and Patient Survey
- National Care Standards Commission
- Social Care Institute for Excellence.

MEASURING AND MANAGING QUALITY

It is to be expected that if quality is essentially a subjective concept the requirements for practitioners to contribute to a continuous quality improvement ethic might involve processes of implementation and management that are both difficult to identify and to measure. Examples of the way practitioners can engage with these processes is by examining:

- the role of satisfaction and value for money in quality improvement measures
- the way transformational and innovative leadership can help them to evolve the systems which underpin continuous improvement.

SATISFACTION AND VALUE FOR MONEY IN QUALITY IMPROVEMENT

One of the main aims of this book is to examine the importance of 'doing the right thing right'

from the service user or patient perspective. An effective way of doing this is to ask how satisfied people are with the services they receive.

Activity 1.4

How do you know whether the people who you provide a service to are satisfied with that service?

What strategies do you use to ensure the information you receive is reliable, valid or genuine?

How do you use the information you receive to improve service delivery in your area of work?

Satisfaction

Satisfaction, like quality, involves a subjective response that reflects people's hopes, expectations, values and beliefs both as individuals and as members of society; and takes account of what they know and understand, their past experiences and lifestyles (Carr-Hill 1995).

Patient or user satisfaction surveys serve different functions when used as a measure of quality of service provision in health and social care. It is important to be sure that those asking and those asked about satisfaction are both clear about the purpose of the survey and use common criteria as measures of satisfaction. If patients or service users are asked about satisfaction with regard to their preferences about the range and type of services they would like, it is important that they know the following:

- what is available
- what can be afforded
- the difference between the range of options
- whether they are responding from their own individual perspective or from a more collective service user perspective.

Activity 1.5

How does your organisation help people who use the service understand what is available, what can be afforded and the difference between the range of options?

You may have identified a number of approaches to achieve this level of understanding. The important thing to consider when examining each approach is whether they help the user to identify what they genuinely need from the service or whether they simply help them to choose what is already provided. If these approaches guide the user into stating the services they genuinely need are those already provided, we are simply reinforcing the status quo. Under these circumstances we are highly unlikely to achieve any real change in order to genuinely meet the needs of those in receipt of services. However, this has to be balanced with the very real fear that asking people what they truly want could raise expectations to a level that welfare services are unable to meet.

If service users are asked about their satisfaction with services as a way of quantifying or scoring the quality of the care they receive, it is important to provide some measures of that care and to be clear what aspects of the service are being reviewed.

Activity 1.6

What areas does the satisfaction survey used in your department focus on? You may find the following categories useful:

- resource based issues
- information needs
- organisational issues
- effectiveness agendas.

You may consider some of the following issues:

- The environment – Was the ward clean and comfortable? The food – Was there enough to eat and was it hot? (All things that depend on the availability and use of resources.)
- Aspects such as their treatment or management, or the interpersonal skills of staff – Did they get or feel better? Were the staff kind and did they listen? (All the things that are influenced by the processes of care or 'practice'.)
- The provision of information – Were they told enough about what was happening to them?
- The access to, availability of, convenience of and timeliness of the service – Was it too far to travel? Was their appointment in the middle of their working day? (All elements of the organisational aspects of service provision.)
- The effectiveness of interventions and the way this is viewed in terms of quality of life – Can they do the things that they want to do as a result of the service they have received? Did they feel they got value for money?

Used in this way measures of satisfaction may be a means of demonstrating individual accountability and corporate responsibility. This is an area now explicitly required as part of the modernisation agenda; the accountability of providers to those who purchase and commission services, of the individual practitioners to their professional bodies and of organisations who answer to government.

The new National Performance Framework (NHS Confederation 1998b) covers health improvement; fair access to services; effective delivery of appropriate health care; efficiency and value for money; patient, service user and carer experience; and health outcomes.

Activity 1.7

Think about how you can measure satisfaction within the service you work in.

Satisfaction questionnaires have become accepted tools with which service providers try to measure patient/user satisfaction. They are often supported by instruments that measure particular aspects of quality of life such as: physiological, psychological, social/emotional well-being, e.g. the Hospital Anxiety and Depression Scale (HADS) or the Nottingham Health Profile, and, more recently, by gathering opinions through the use of focus groups.

The patient and service user responses to these measures of satisfaction are used as:

- performance indicators to measure service efficiency
- quality indicators for service providers and those who commission or purchase services
- outcome measures of service effectiveness
- policy prompts to involve patients and service users in their care
- part of the evidence base which underpins practice.

There is much debate about the use of patient/user satisfaction, some of which revolves around the various definitions of what satisfaction involves both as a theoretical concept and in practical terms (Carr-Hill 1992, 1995, Williams 1994, Avis et al. 1995).

Questions surround the validity and reliability of patient and user satisfaction measures, the dimensions of satisfaction and their relevance to patients and users when evaluating their experiences of service provision and care. Carr-Hill (1995) argues it may be more appropriate to consider sources of dissatisfaction and use complaints in a positive way to improve service provision. A study of dissatisfaction with health care (Coyle 1999) found that, based on a similar understanding of satisfaction, patients and service users have recently shown a greater willingness to complain. Some people are more ready to complain than others, for example women compared with

men, and relatives or carers more often than patients and service users.

Coyle (1999) identified the particular 'ingredients' of many complaints. These included:

- aspects of a practitioner's professional integrity, both interpersonal and practical behaviours expressed by service users as 'not caring'
- justifying complaints by citing other experts and accepted sources or by making comparison
- lay carers identifying with the professional roles
- demonstrating health awareness and awareness of the appropriate use of services
- showing concern for others in society 'I wouldn't like it to happen to anyone else'
- acknowledging both their own contribution to the problem and external factors, and recognising the contribution of the global state of welfare services.

In general, respondents in this study felt they had not been treated equally and had received 'poor quality care' (Coyle 1999, p. 729). This was expressed in comments about the 'uncaring or unsympathetic attitude' of practitioners and questions about their competency with suggestions of 'lack of knowledge or expertise'. In addition, Coyle found gender and cultural differences in people who complain. Although women represented the largest group of those to complain, this was not the case for women from ethnic minorities. Women from this group complained less because they felt that their intelligence was undermined by the service if English was not their first language.

One of the main concerns was that professional providers did not acknowledge the competencies of individuals as lay care providers. Another concern, which was demonstrated by Coyle (1999), was that some people are reluctant to complain and are often prepared to accept poor quality care in order to avoid doing so, which poses real questions about the validity of satisfaction surveys. However, these findings do still offer practitioners a starting point from which to strive for quality improvement from the patients' and service users' point of view. Mangan (1995) suggests that 'instead of feeling powerless and frustrated by patient/service user complaints, practitioners and providers of services' should turn them to their benefit as a way of 'adding weight to the real dissatisfaction they themselves feel about the services they deliver' and hence provide 'opportunities to make improvements'.

Williams (1994, p. 509) suggests that 'to be of any practical use we must know what people mean when they say they are satisfied with a particular aspect of a service' and in order 'to make any relevant changes in service provision we must know why they believe what they do and how they arrived at that view'. Williams also questions the use of an expectation-fulfillment model to measure satisfaction. Avis et al. (1995, p. 320) suggest that it presupposes a positive attitude to care and claim that 'if we wish to understand the views of service users and patients we must discover what rights and obligations they sense they have, because their evaluations may not be embodied in expressions of satisfaction'.

In a recent study of the criteria used by healthcare professionals, managers and patients to evaluate the quality of care (Attree 2001) there was a general consensus on the criteria identified by all three groups. However, there were also some significant differences in emphasis. Participants' perceptions of quality care and factors that increased or reduced care quality were identified in three categories; these included care resources, care processes and care outcomes.

Care resources incorporated the human, environmental, physical/material, and financial factors that might affect the quality of care, and suggestions for the need of more staff, time and equipment came from all three groups of participants.

Managers focussed on the importance of resource control and management whilst practitioners, patients and clients stressed the lack of resources to meet needs and standards of care.

Care process criteria involved the nature of practice and the nature of practitioners; 'what they do and how they do it' (Attree 2001, p. 72). Staff and users of the service cited poor communication and information sharing as areas for quality improvement. Whilst the nature of practice is usually the subject of regular audit and review, the nature of practitioners is less exposed to scrutiny except in satisfaction surveys. This is because it is considered more difficult to demonstrate and evaluate empirically. However, it is of considerable importance to patients/clients in terms of the quality of care they receive.

The **outcomes of care** relate to 'what good is being done', if any, for the person in terms of the way they feel. Improvements in their health or social status and 'going or being at home' were included as outcome measures in the study. Practitioners and managers tended to focus on the second and third of these measures. These were typically interpreted as length of stay, bed blocking or inappropriate admission. The patient or service user was more interested in the first and second criteria. Attree (2001, p. 77) suggests that by including consensual criteria in the evaluation of quality, the multiple perspectives of all the stakeholders involved in the provision, delivery and receipt of health and social care can be represented, and can therefore subsequently influence the quality of welfare services.

Duff et al. (1996) examine the 'value of working with patients and service users to bring about quality improvements', in particular 'involving them in making decisions about their care' (p. 63). They believe that when working to improve care it is important to 'understand all the judgement criteria used by patients and service users. This means giving people both a voice and a choice' (p. 64) as well as involving users at all stages of the care processes and giving them information on which to base their choice. It is also important to ensure that individuals understand the implications and likely impact or consequences of all the available options, thereby giving them the confidence to make choices. Subsequently, when measuring performance it is important to be clear whose outcome measures have been used, those of the professionals or those of the patient or service user. Ideally a combination of both is necessary to ensure quality from everyone's point of view. Finally, the study suggests that it is vital to make explicit that patients and service users have been listened to and their suggestions acted upon in order to encourage their continued participation and involvement in the process.

Abbott et al. (2001) explored user involvement in their study focusing upon people in receipt of care packages in the community. From this study two important issues became apparent. These included the degree of satisfaction with 'good quality (comprehensive) information' and consistency or 'continuity of contact with professionals and/or services'. (p. 80).

Value for money

As noted above, quality and effectiveness have different meanings for different groups of people, in the same way value for money can also have a variety of meanings. Economic terms like cost utility, cost effectiveness and cost benefit are often used interchangeably as measures of value for money, which is in fact a quality concept providing a subjective description of 'worth' in financial terms. Value for money is a measure of what an individual or organisation is prepared to spend for what is available and what they expect for what they pay (see Box 1.1).

These measures may produce quite different monetary amounts depending on whose point of view they represent, for example; if someone gives up their job to care for a young child or

---

Box 1.1

If cost = value in £s as a monetary amount then:

- cost effectiveness = 'impact' measured or evaluated in £s
- cost benefit = 'worth' measured or evaluated in £s
- cost utility = satisfaction measured or evaluated in £s
- opportunity cost = 'sacrifice' measured or evaluated in £s

---

older parent the opportunity cost to them may be much greater through the loss of salary than the saving in residential care costs or child minding fees. It may be a cost benefit to the local authority and health services but how do we really measure the satisfaction of the child who has mum or dad at home or the older person who is supported to live in their own home?

Since many health and social services have been provided free at the point of delivery in the United Kingdom, value for money is often thought to be a difficult concept for the stakeholders to engage with. In other parts of the world where care has traditionally been 'paid for' either directly by patients and service users or through insurance schemes, it is already used as a measure of satisfaction. The following points encapsulate some of the differing perspectives on value for money:

- For patients and service users, value for money represents their quality of life in terms of the costs (to everyone) of the care they receive and might have to pay for.
- For the 'providers' of services, both organisations and individual practitioners, value for money represents the cost and quality of care they deliver.
- For purchasers and commissioners of services value for money represents the cost and quality of the service they receive.

A measure of quality that is sometimes used to try to bridge the gap for providers in understanding quality of life from the patients' or service users' point of view is the quality-adjusted life years (QALYs). It is used to assess the outcome of an initiative, intervention or treatment in terms of additional life years and the quality of life during these years. A patient or service user makes use of this concept when they say 'if I could have 5 more years as good as I am now' to describe their hopes or expectations about an intervention. This helps in decision making in terms of cost utility and is a concept that is further discussed in Chapter 2.

TRANSFORMATIONAL AND INNOVATIVE LEADERSHIP AND THEIR CONTRIBUTION TO THE MODERNISATION AGENDA

Practitioners may find it difficult to improve their own practice without support and commitment from the organisation that provides the service they deliver. Developing practice in this way requires continuous evaluation and skills in introducing innovation and change (Brown et al. 1997). To encourage individual workers to be committed to a continuous quality improvement ethic they need to feel they have some control over the systems of care delivery as well as feeling that they are involved in creating, adopting, adapting or replacing those systems. In this way they will be acknowledged as being both professionally accountable, responsible and directly engaged in the on going evaluation of their work, all of which reflects the political requirements for quality, best value and clinical governance. In addition, it is important to remember that 'quality of care for staff and for patients go hand in hand' (NHS Confederation 1998c) and one of the success criteria set out by government in securing a 'quality workforce' involves 'job satisfaction through empowerment and involvement in decision making' (p. 2).

Activity 1.8

What strategies might you use to empower staff and facilitate their engagement in practice development?

Strategies for empowering team members:

- The ability to determine the way care is delivered at a local level and influence the structure and functions of welfare services more strategically.

- Understanding that control involves professional accountability, personal competence, skill and knowledge, responsibility for the direct delivery or overseeing of care provision, ongoing evaluation of the quality of their provision and ability to make any improvements deemed necessary.

- Recognising change as a normal part of any service provision as an acknowledgement of dynamic development to be embraced not as a threat or an unnecessary chore.

Change in relation to quality improvement involves collaboration and participation with service users and other stakeholders. In addition, it is important to ensure that any new regimes or initiatives can be clearly justified and that they are not carried out purely for their own sake. This requires individual practitioners to adopt leadership characteristics and respond enthusiastically to challenges: inspire confidence. Managers also need to develop an environment that encourages and supports innovation and therefore ensures quality improvement becomes a continuous process. This requires everyone to play a part in decision-making and quality-improvement activities, an approach that has been described as a 'collaboration and involvement model of quality improvement' (Brown et al. 1997, p. 36). Brown et al.'s (1997) model provides practitioners with the principles and tools of quality improvement. These principles include the ability to motivate staff, to provide reflective and critical evaluation skills, and to allow them to decide how quality is to be improved.

LEADERSHIP

The characteristics of leadership that any individual might demonstrate include:

- effective communication skills
- the respect and support of others
- the ability to demonstrate a range of skills as a role model
- confidence and the acknowledgement of their own responsibility
- accountability and creativity.

These attributes are typical of innovative leaders and this style has been defined as 'transformational'.

Transformational leaders are seen to be considerate and supportive, intellectually stimulating, creative, empathetic, charismatic, inspirational and to lead without authority. Such leaders encourage new ideas from others as well as producing them. In addition, they are receptive to unconventional approaches to problem solving and change (Wedderburn-Tate 1999). Transformational leadership is more about attitudes and attributes that are not easily measured, and are not easily taught. Leadership is viewed as 'the process of guiding, teaching, motivating and directing the activities of others towards attaining goals' (Ellis & Hartley 2000, p. 5) functions that are part of every practitioner's responsibility when providing or delivering services.

Leadership skills are required and can be developed as characteristics by any individual. Leadership style is demonstrated in the way the activities of others are planned, organised encouraged and directed.

Activity 1.9

What does innovative leadership involve? You might find it helpful to think about people who have inspired you.

'Innovators take a good idea, test it out and produce a benefit' from using it (Calpin-Davies 2001, p. 22). Innovation is the capacity to profit from new ways of thinking and differs from creativity which actually generates new ideas but may not consider their specific application. Innovation flourishes where managerial control is replaced by influential leadership.

This type of control is often demonstrated in the healthcare arena where quality of care can be seen to range from being vibrant and innovative to being entrenched in routine and ritual. It is possible to have such wide variations within one organisation. The determining factor is often personal characteristics, particularly those of the leaders (Cook 2001). Innovative leaders make explicit the characteristics of their particular style and usually make good change agents as distinct from managers. Practitioners need to be able to develop and adapt their own leadership styles to reflect the diverse range in the needs of patients and service users for whom they aspire to provide high-quality services and care (Wedderburn-Tate 1999).

CONCLUSION

This chapter has explored the various meanings of quality within welfare services and explored these in the context of clinical governance and best value. In addition, it has considered the different ways of exploring alternative methodologies for measuring quality. It has also considered the macro level with regard to quality improvement that includes the national institutions responsible for this. The chapter has also identified practical strategies for managing the quality agenda.

APPENDIX: DEFINITIONS

Continuous quality improvement: preventive problem solving that results in exemplary service. It is prevention orientated, proactive, cross-functional (wide not narrow), raises standards, leadership leading and empowering, productive (not just busy), experiments and takes risks, sees quality and problem solving as the responsibility of everyone (not just those in authority), takes an organisational perspective (not us/them) and involves new optimism (not cynicism) and sees the employee as a customer not as expendable (Tomey 2000, p. 387).

Cost benefit: measures the 'worthwhileness' of a particular initiative, intervention or treatment by weighing the benefits against the financial costs. It is used to assist decisions about resource allocation.

Cost effectiveness: is a measure of how to meet a particular need or provide a service at least financial cost.

Cost utility: measures the relative economic value of different outcomes produced by a specific initiative, intervention or treatment. It is used to make choices between initiatives etc., but does not help to justify decisions about them for their own sake.

Critical thinking: involves higher order reasoning and evaluation and demonstrates insight, intuition and empathy.

Decision making: choosing a particular course of action.

Ethic: a moral system or set of principles particular to a certain person, community or group.

Followership: not always agreeing with the leader but taking their point of view into account when brainstorming alternatives. Maintains independent and critical thinking.

Innovative leadership: leading in an unconventional way in a fluid and ever-changing environment.

Leadership: showing or marking the way, guiding the course of things involves influence with an emphasis on effectiveness.

Management: activity that involves planning, organising and directing and implies authority with an emphasis on control.

Opportunity cost: involves sacrifice to obtain effect or benefit by using resources in a particular way. It estimates or calculates the monetary value of the sacrifice when resources are not available for the best alternative use.

Policy: a governing plan adopted by an organisation for accomplishing goals and achievements or 'the way we do it here'.

Problem solving: a systematic process which analyses a difficult situation.

Procedure: chronological sequence of steps within a process.

Protocols: locally agreed ways of working.

Strategy: a particular long-term plan for success.

Transactional leadership: offers a contract for mutual benefits that has contingent rewards by identifying the needs of followers and provides rewards to meet those needs in exchange for expected performance. The leader is a caretaker who sets goals, focuses on day-to-day operations and uses management by exception (Tomey 2000, p. 145) It is conforming, explicit and orderly in achieving its tasks (Broome 1998).

Transformational leadership: a style that works on ideas and visions and builds common commitment (Broome 1998). Promotes employee development, attends to needs and motives of followers, inspires through optimism, influences change in perception, provides intellectual stimulation and encourages follower creativity (Tomey 2000).

REFERENCES

Abbott S, Johnson L, Lewis H 2001 Participation in arranging continuing health care packages: experiences and aspirations of service users. Journal of Nursing Management 9: 79–85.

Attree M 2001 A study of the criteria used by healthcare professionals, managers and patients to represent and evaluate quality care. Journal of Nursing Management 9: 67–78.

Avis M, Bond M, Arthur A 1995 Satisfying solutions? A review of some unresolved issues in the measurement of patient satisfaction. Journal of Advanced Nursing 22: 316–322.

Broome A 1998 Managing change, 2nd edn. Macmillan, London.

Brown J, Kitson A, McKnight TJ 1997 Challenges in caring. Nelson Thomes Ltd, Cheltenham.

Calpin-Davies P 2001 Innovate and prosper. Nursing Management 7(10): 22–23.

Carr-Hill R 1992 The measurement of patient satisfaction. Journal of Public Health Medicine 14: 236–249.

Carr-Hill R 1995 Measures of user satisfaction. In: Wilson G (ed) Community care: asking the users. Chapman & Hall, London.

Chambers 21st century dictionary 1996 Chambers, Edinburgh.

Cook M 2001 Clinical leadership that works. Nursing Management 7(10): 24–28.

Coyle J 1999 Understanding dissatisfied users: developing a framework for comprehending criticisms of health care work. Journal of Advanced Nursing 30(3): 723–731.

Dale B, Cooper C, Wilkinson A 1997 Managing quality and human resources: a guide to continuous quality improvement. Blackwell, Oxford.

Department of Health 1989a Working for patients: the Health Service. Caring for the 1990s. Cm 555. HMSO, London.

Department of Health 1989b Caring for people: community care in the next decade and beyond. Caring for the 1990s. HMSO, London.

Department of Health 1998a A first class service: Quality in the new NHS. DoH, London.

Department of Health 1998b The new NHS, modern and dependable: a national framework for assessing performance. DoH, London.

Department of Health 1998c Partnerships in action; new opportunities for joint working between health and social services. DoH, London.

Department of Health for Northern Ireland 1998 Fit for the future. Department of Health, Belfast.

Duff L, Kelson M, Marriott S et al 1996 Involving patients and users of services in quality improvement: what are the benefits? Journal of Clinical Effectiveness 1(2): 63–67.

Ellis J, Hartley C 2000 Managing and coordinating nursing care, 3rd edn. Lippincott, Philadelphia.

Leathard A 2000 Health care provision; past present and into the 21st century, 2nd edn. Stanley Thornes, Cheltenham.

Mangan P 1995 Complaints can improve care. Nursing Times 91(41): 32.

NHS Confederation 1998a Update: Modernising Social Services. Issue 25.

NHS Confederation 1998b Briefing: a national framework for assessing performance. Issue 11.

NHS Confederation 1998c Briefing: working together: securing a quality workforce for the NHS. Issue 20.

NHS Confederation 1999 Update: the NHS Bill. Issue 7.

NHS Executive 1998 In the public interest: developing a strategy for public participation in the NHS. NHSE, Leeds.

Øvretveit J 1992 Health service quality; an introduction to quality methods for health services. Blackwell, Oxford.

Royal College of Nursing 2000 Pressure ulcer risk assessment and prevention: clinical practice guidelines. Royal College of Nursing, London.

Secretary of State for Health 1998 Modernising social services: promoting independence, improving protection, raising standards. Cm 4169. The Stationery Office, London.

Secretary of State for Scotland 1997 Designed to care: renewing the National Health in Scotland. Cm3811. The Stationery Office, Edinburgh.

Secretary of State for Wales 1998 NHS Wales: putting patients first. Cm3841. The Stationery Office, Cardiff.

Tomey AM 2000 Guide to nursing management and leadership, 6th edn. Mosby, St. Louis.

Wedderburn-Tate C 1999 Leadership in nursing. Churchill Livingstone, Edinburgh.

Williams B 1994 Patient satisfaction: a valid concept. Social Science Medicine 38(4): 504–516.

2

An economic approach to clinical governance

Alan Maynard

KEY ISSUES

- The goal of health care is to improve patient/client outcomes, i.e. enhance the length and quality of life of people.

- Clinical governance is a system whose purpose is to improve quality, or patient/client outcomes.

- Contemporary policy in the 'new NHS' focuses on spending and activity rather than outcomes.

- Data are available to inform governance, but are often ignored. An example of this is Hospital Episode Statistics (HES).

- Data that could be collected, e.g. functional quality of life, are usually not collected systematically.

- The challenges in clinical governance are to identify cost effective interventions and to create incentives for practitioners to translate such evidence into changes in behaviour.

- The need for better evaluation of outcomes and activity-outcome relationships (e.g. do nurse and doctor staffing levels affect the outcomes of care?)

◆ Incentive systems are essential *elements* of clinical governance, which are ignored at the risk of wasting scarce resource and damaging the health of individuals.

INTRODUCTION

Everyone is now in favour of increasing investment in 'clinical governance'. Whilst this phrase was unknown 5 years ago, it is now the focus of much trumpeting by the health care 'tribes' as they jostle for a share of this new healthcare feast! Thus nurses want more money to measure better the incidence and prevalence of hospital-acquired infections. These largely avoidable infections cost the NHS over £1 billion each year, as well as imposing much suffering on patients/clients and their carers.

The 'medical profession', better known as doctors, have only recently admitted the scale of error. Whilst overseas this discovery has focused on the measurement of population error rates sometimes in excess of 10% of hospital admissions, in Britain such failures have focused on the failures of individual practitioners. Thus, the Bristol inquiry has demonstrated not only that individual doctors used damaging techniques, but also that the system in which they worked was incapable of managing manifest failure. The private sector demonstrated in the Ledward case, that they, like the NHS, were incapable of detecting error and protecting their subscribers from its effects. Such poor consumer protection was also demonstrated in primary care by the serial killer, Harold Shipman. He was the most popular practitioner in Hyde, Manchester, with people queuing to get onto his list and be exposed to considerable risk of premature death.

The government's reaction to these problems has been an epidemic of new regulatory controls. Whilst the Royal Colleges, for no good reason, have been left largely untouched in this flurry of government reaction, the General Medical Council has been obliged to reform at long last and will be reformed further. The Commission for Health Improvement (CHI) has been created to inspect hospital and primary care performance. Chief Executives of Trusts are now responsible not only for financial balance but also for 'quality'. A new agency has been created to retrain doctors found to be deficient in their practices and after much delay annual consultant appraisals are being put in place and the GMC will institute 5-yearly re-validations of all doctors. The NHS Plan includes provision for a 'super' agency, which will regulate the regulators.

In retrospect, it is remarkable that such controls were not instituted decades ago. After the creation of the NHS, there appeared to be a social contract in which the government took care of funding and the medical professions were trusted by society to manage quality. Whilst Thatcher's internal market reforms broke this contract and sought to manage practitioners more, her government made little attempt to measure and manage the clinical quality of care. Their funding and management of 'medical audit' was captured and neutered by the medical profession, at considerable expense to the taxpayer and with little benefit to the individual.

Should then, the long delayed attention to quality and clinical governance be welcomed? The answer is both yes and no. It is essential to focus attention on how the processes of care affect the outcome, in terms of health status, for both the person and their carers. After all, the purpose of the NHS and all healthcare systems is to improve health and not merely keep employees in a job! However, the current epidemic of 'initiatives' within clinical governance could be said to be unfocused, ill coordinated and poorly managed.

There are a number of key issues which need to be resolved if investments in clinical governance are to be productive in terms of improving the quality of health care. Firstly, the goals of clinical governance need to be clearly defined. Of particular relevance is the need to consider whether goals are related to the processes of care, e.g. clean hospitals and polite practitioners, or to the outcomes for patients/clients, in terms of increased length and quality of life? Or is governance about both process and outcome, and if so, how are these aspects of the care process prioritised?

The second issue, after having identified the policy goals, is what are the competing intervention options and, subsequently, what is the evidence base regarding their cost effectiveness? Both of these areas are essential in the decision-making process. Also important is an analysis of risk and its appropriate management. 'Clinical risks' are many and can be managed in a variety of ways. As resources are finite, it is necessary to ration them and target them carefully to interventions, which give the greatest benefit (in terms of process and/or outcome) at least cost. Such prioritisation and the use of the evidence base are not always apparent in the management of clinical governance.

CLINICAL GOVERNANCE: WHAT IS THE PROBLEM?

This section considers the history of quality and performance management, the politics of outcome measures and, finally, the need to define the problem. Essentially it focuses upon the following points:

- The attempts to measure 'success' and 'failure' in healthcare systems during previous decades, many of which have proved limited both in the UK and the USA.
- The focus on inputs and processes/activity, rather than outcomes (Campbell 1969).

- The issue of 'medical errors' which have only recently been 'discovered'. This has led to much greater focus on avoidable mortality and morbidity and how both the level and variations in errors can be better managed.
- The measurement and management of outcomes in terms of avoidable mortality and morbidity.

A retrospect on quality and performance management

The reluctance of decision makers in healthcare systems to measure (and reward) success in terms of patient/client outcomes has been a characteristic of the sector for thousands of years. The ancient Babylonians recognised the need for 'success' criteria and (vicious) reward systems in the governance of surgeons. Thus in the Laws of Hammurabi (BC1792) it was stated:

If a surgeon has made a deep incision in the body of a man with a lancet of bronze and saves the man's life, or has opened an abscess in the eye of a man and has saved his eye, he shall take 10 shekels of silver.

If a surgeon has made a deep incision in the body of a man with his lancet of bronze and so destroys the man's eye, they shall cut off his forehand

The ancients were concerned not only with the performance management of success in terms of outcomes, but also questioned the nature and causes of medical specialisation:

The practice of medicine they split into separate parts, each doctor being responsible for the treatment of only one disease. There are, in consequence, innumerable doctors, some specialising in the diseases of the eye, others of the head, others of the teeth, others of the stomach and so on: whilst others, again, deal with the sort of troubles which cannot be localised (Herodotus 1954).

The questioning of medical practice and practitioners was not confined to the ancient world. Francis Clifton who was physician to King George 1st of England argued for outcome measurements over 250 years ago:

In order therefore to procure this valuable collection, I humbly propose, first of all, that three or four persons should be employed in hospitals (and that without in any ways interfering with the gentlemen now concerned), to set down the cases of patients there from day to day, candidly and judiciously, without any regard to private opinions or public systems, and at the year's end publish these facts just as they are, leaving everyone to make the best use he can for himself (Lancet 1841).

This British 'tradition' of performance management continued in the 19th century. The editor of the Lancet in 1841 re-iterated the advocacy of Clifton:

All public institutions must be compelled to keep case notes and registers, on a uniform plan. Annual abstracts of results must be published. The annual medical report must embrace hospitals, lying-in hospitals, dispensaries, lunatic asylums and prisons.

Florence Nightingale (Nightingale 1863) reflected not only her experiences in the Crimea but also current health policy debate when she argued:

I am fain to sum up with an urgent appeal for adopting this or some uniform system of publishing the statistical records of hospitals. There is a growing conviction that in all hospitals, even in those which are best conducted, there is a great and unnecessary waste of life ....

In attempting to arrive at the truth, I have applied everywhere for information, but in scarcely an instance have I been able to obtain hospital records fit for any purpose of comparison. If they could be obtained, they would enable us to decide many questions beside the ones alluded to. They would show subscribers how their money was being spent, what amount of good was really being done with it, or whether the money was doing mischief rather than good.

Nightingale reiterated the outcome measures set out in the current legislation (e.g. the 1842 Lunacy Act), which required measurement of success in terms of whether people were dead, relieved or unrelieved. This three-fold measure was used in all psychiatric hospitals and some acute hospitals (e.g. St Thomas's) until the creation of the NHS in 1948.

The British were not alone in such advocacy of performance management in relation to outcomes. An American physician, Codman, wrote in 1914:

We must formulate some method of hospital reporting showing as nearly as possible what are the results of treatments obtained at different institutions. This report must be made out and published for each hospital in a uniform manner so that comparison is possible. With such a report as a starting point, those interested can begin to ask questions as to management and efficiency.

It is remarkable that despite centuries of advocacy of measurement and management of outcomes so little use is made of such data and healthcare managers and policy makers worldwide remain largely ignorant of causes in variation of mortality or 'success' in minimising it. Why is this so? Surely it is subtler than Sir Humphrey Appleby's comments in the BBC-TV series 'Yes, Minister': 'it is folly to increase your knowledge at the expense of your authority'! But, as ever with Sir Humphrey, there is a chilling element of reality, as professionals everywhere hate to be 'confused' and undermined by facts!

The politics of outcome measurement

The Thatcher reforms of the NHS in 1991 led to radical restructuring and the creation of trading or exchange relations between purchasers and providers. One of the primary foci of these reforms was the secondary (hospital) sector. General practice fund holding was almost a casual 'add-on' to the reforms.

In both the primary and secondary sectors, the purchaser–provider split involved contracting. The primary focus of this was activity (volumes of people treated and waiting list issues) rather than outcomes or quality (whether, and by how much, health status was improved). The political imperative at the time was the problem of waiting times and the Conservative government sought to deal with this issue by unevaluated structural changes and increased resourcing of the NHS. In doing this issues of outcomes and quality were addressed indirectly by processes that were divorced from clinical management. Particularly as there was little evidence that audit processes informed contract design and management. Thus the 'internal market' tended to focus on volumes and prices, and ignore quality in terms of process (customer satisfaction) and outcomes (improvements in the length and quality of life).

The Blair government inherited and developed this focus on 're-disorganisation' of structural organisation and renewed emphasis on activity. One of its electoral 'pledges' was to reduce waiting lists by 100 000. The architect of this policy goal was never identified and only when in office did the new government recognise that such objectives required not only management of the supply of care, but also control of the demand for hospital care, in particular the management of GP referrals.

The current 'solution' for the activity problem within the NHS is to spend more. This has two limitations. Firstly, rapid increases in purchasing power when capacity is constrained are likely to cause cost inflation. Thus spending more when the supply of doctors, nurses and private nursing home beds is relatively fixed, merely leads to increased pay and higher private sector prices. As a consequence, increased spending has little effect on capacity and the volume of care, but makes the owners of labour skills and private facilities richer.

The second problem with the 'funding solution' is that the focus of policy is still on activity rather than the quality of outcomes. It is remarkable how the political focus for over 20 years has been on inputs (spending) and activity (waiting times), with the neglect of measuring and managing levels and changes in terms of individual and population health. The recent problems arising from the practice of individual consultants and GPs, such as Ledward and Shipman, does not appear to have shifted this focus. The government initiative in 2001, to measure quality in hospitals consists of patient satisfaction questionnaires that were completed by 500 patients in all Trusts. Politicians and bureaucrats still fail to recognise that patients can be 'satisfied' with services of deplorable quality, as can be seen with a level of satisfaction demonstrated by the patients of the GP, Harold Shipman.

This restricted and unfortunate perception of quality as being about process alone is unfortunate and a major challenge for those involved in clinical governance. Can managerial perceptions and governance structures be shifted away from concerns of process and activity in isolation from a need for a primary focus on outcomes? One major obstacle to such a consideration of this issue is the political reluctance to create performance management structures that focus on patient/client outcomes.

Defining the problems

The current increase in interest in performance in relation to outcomes is the result of the medical errors debate. The US Institute of Medicine published a book called *To Err is Human* (Kohn et al.

1999). This Shakespearian title recognised the fact that doctors, nurses and other medical practitioners are human and will make errors, which maim and kill people. Whilst accepting this premis the policy challenge is to identify measures that allow us to learn from mistakes and ensure control systems are in place that identify and effectively manage 'clusters' of adverse events.

The Institute of Medicine extrapolated the results of two large studies; the first in Utah and Colorado, and the second in New York. This study found that adverse events occurred in 2.9 and 3.7% of hospitalisations respectively. Using the Utah and Colorado data and grossing this to the USA, the authors concluded that 44 000 Americans die each year as a result of errors. Using the New York rates, the figure may be as high as 98 000. With the lower estimate, medical errors are the eighth leading cause of death with more people dying because of such events than die from AIDS (16 516), breast cancer (42 297) or motor vehicle accidents (43 458). In addition, it would seem that in the USA more people die from medication errors (7000) than die from work-place injuries and these errors kill annually more than twice the number who died in the attack on the World Trade Center in New York. Whilst there is considerable effort made to measure and reduce work place injuries, there is relative silence about injuries in the medical market place, public and private. This silence and inaction is remarkable not just in the USA, but also throughout the rest of the world.

Errors can take place in both the planning and the execution of a task. They can occur in diagnosis, treatment, rehabilitation and social care. They may involve the delivery of the wrong medication, the wrong provision of the wrong dose of a drug, the wrong location of surgery or general failures, which produce hospital-acquired infections. An Australian group measured medical errors and concluded that the rate there might be over 15% of admissions (Runciman et al. 2000). Their criteria were very detailed and when the Utah and

Colorado criteria were applied to this data set, the error rate was slightly in excess of 10%, i.e. one in ten hospital admissions were associated with errors. In Britain the quantity and quality of data about medical errors is limited. A retrospective study in one English hospital detected an error rate of 10.8% (Vincent et al. 2001). In most political and policy announcements, it is generally asserted that the error rate is about 10%.

Such errors result in mortality and morbidity for individuals. The effects of such morbidity on functional status (i.e. physical, social and psychological well-being) have never been measured systematically in any healthcare system. Furthermore, the benefits of reducing such errors in terms of increased length and quality of life for people who use services, may be quite limited. Hayward and colleagues found that many 'victims' of medical errors would not have lived much beyond 3 months even in the absence of mistakes (Hayward et al. 2001). Elderly people and those with chronic illnesses are most likely to consume intensive and complex care and, therefore, to experience errors.

POLICIES FOR CHANGE

The failure to measure and manage outcomes has potentially damaged the health of many people. This poor management, by non-clinical managers and health professionals, has taken place despite the collection and availability of routine NHS data about processes, activity and outcomes (mortality).

The availability of 'routine' data

Each year every NHS Trust in England returns Hospital Episode Statistics (HES) data to the Department of Health. Similar data collection takes place elsewhere in the UK. In principle this HES data can be used to investigate and manage central aspects of the demand for hospital care (by GPs) and its supply by consultants. For instance, the following questions can be investigated using HES data:

- Which GPs refer to the hospital, and what are the variations in referral rates?
- By using postcodes and mapping social deprivation data at the ward level (using census data), the social characteristics of individuals referred to the hospital can be analysed.
- The activity rate of consultants in terms of finished consultant episodes (FCEs), adjusted for case mix by health-related group (HRG) can be determined, and the large variations in activity monitored and managed.
- Activity – outcome relationships can be investigated as the HES data include a measure of mortality, e.g.:
  - Is the mortality rate for weekend emergency admissions higher than for emergency admissions during the working week? A Canadian study (Bell & Redelmeier 2001) demonstrated that weekend admissions had high mortality rates. Such a finding could be verified or refuted using HES data and is a central element of clinical governance. Analysis of mortality during bank holidays is also essential for the management of quality and governance.
  - There is evidence of a relationship between volume (activity) and 30-day mortality rates, in areas such as vascular surgery and upper gastrointestinal work (NHS Centre for Reviews and Dissemination 1996). HES data can be used to determine whether surgeons do the necessary minimum level of interventions to ensure mortality risks for people are minimised.

Mortality data are produced as part of HES but have been routinely ignored by managers and professionals. Kind used this data to measure age and sex adjusted mortality rates by health authority in 1987 (Kind 1987). He demonstrated significant variations in performance but NHS managers have continued to ignore this information.

More recently, a private organisation called Dr Foster published standardised mortality rates for all hospitals in the United Kingdom and the Republic of Ireland (Good Hospital Guide 2001). This material built on Jarman's work and concluded that the major explanation of variations in hospital mortality rates is levels of staffing (Jarman et al. 1999). Even if this explanation is valid in part or in whole, why does staffing vary so much when needs weighted capitation formulae (such as RAWP) have supposedly equalised the financial capacity of different purchasers?

In addition to HES, other data are collected with varying degrees of rigour and compatibility. For instance, data on hospital-acquired infections are collected, as is material on 'adverse events'. The latter is collected with varying degrees of effectiveness, and increasingly 'nil' and low returns are being seen as evidence either of lying and/or administrative incompetence. Adverse events include medical errors and as already stated we might expect rates of 5–10% of admissions to fall into this category, if reporting systems are of good quality. Casual empiricism shows that rates vary enormously, e.g. a District Hospital in Yorkshire reports 7000 adverse events whilst a Teaching Hospital in the South reports 4000. With 'medical scandals' (e.g. Bristol and Shipman) adverse incidents are being reported more accurately, but the fear of 'naming and shaming' remains an obstacle to accurate reporting.

Augmenting the information base

Some improvements in the information flow to inform clinical governance are urgently required.

- **The integration of public (NHS) and private activity data**: NHS consultants, especially in surgery, carry out a considerable number of procedures in the private sector. For public and private purchasers to appreciate fully the nature of, for instance, volume–mortality relationships for individual consultants they need integrated public and private data.

Private purchasers (insurers) want access to NHS data to ensure 'consumer protection' for their beneficiaries. The NHS wants access to private sector activity data to inform consultant appraisal (mandatory since April 2001), performance management and 5-yearly revalidation of fitness to practice by the General Medical Council. With this situation it is remarkable the data are not already integrated.

- **Improving the quality of activity and outcome data**: the Department of Health have invested in improving the quality of HES data for surgical activity in particular. However, the scope for improving the quality of reporting activity and outcome and for developing its scope is considerable.

The quality of medical data in HES is poor. There is evidence that conditions like gastric bleeds are under-reported. Many physicians complain about the quality of the HES but they, like their surgical colleagues, determine its quality by their lack of rigour in reporting their activities. For instance, the HES surgical data attributes activity to a named consultant. However, the consultant, his registrar or the senior house officer, with or without supervision, may do the procedure. New 'fields' will be developed in HES to identify who does what, with or without supervision.

Perhaps the best way to improve the quality of the HES data is to use it routinely in consultant appraisal, GMC revalidation, performance management and all other aspects of clinical governance. Used in this way it will provide a sharp incentive for practitioners to report activity *and* outcomes more accurately and in a timely fashion. However, such efforts will have to be supplemented by better training and staffing within information departments. 'Economising' techniques in such departments whereby, for instance, deaths are pooled for irregular reporting rather than when they happen, distorts an information base, which is essential for management.

Quality of life

Whilst the HES reports mortality in hospital, most people leave hospital alive, thankfully! The current fashion of measuring quality in terms of satisfaction (process) is grossly incomplete: 'the operation was a success, but the patient died'. Mortality outcome data need to be complemented with data about the functional status of all individuals.

In an ideal world, generic quality of life measures would be the basis of this record. Such quality of life measures are short and completed by individuals who are asked to assess their physical, psychological and social well-being, including absence or presence of pain. Every time they use the healthcare system a quality of life measurement could identify the person's current and previous functional status. Such an approach would enable, for instance, measurement of a persons' health status at a GP visit, before the hip replacement procedure and 3 and 6 months after the operation. This means that recovery functional status could be charted and variations in consultants' success in terms of changes in health status can be identified.

The questions used in EQ5D (the EuroQol) instrument to measure health status are set out in Box 2.1. This instrument has been used in hundreds of clinical trials and appears to be valid and consistent in its measurement. The questions are supplemented by a 'thermometer' scale from 100 (best imaginable health state) to 0 (worst imaginable health state) upon which respondents are required to value 'their own health today'. Also respondents are required to give personal details, such as their age, sex, postcode and educational qualifications, which can be used in the analysis of population data.

Box 2.1   Describing your own health today

By placing a tick in one box in each group below, please indicate which statements best describe your own health state today.

Mobility
I have no problems in walking about ☐
I have some problems in walking about ☐
I am confined to bed ☐

Self-care
I have no problems with self-care ☐
I have some problems washing or dressing myself ☐
I am unable to wash or dress myself ☐

Usual activities
(e.g. work, study, housework, family or leisure activities)
I have no problems with performing
   my usual activities ☐
I have some problems with performing
   my usual activities ☐
I am unable to perform my usual activities ☐

Pain/discomfort
I have no pain or discomfort ☐
I have moderate pain or discomfort ☐
I have extreme pain or discomfort ☐

Anxiety/depression
I am not anxious or depressed ☐
I am moderately anxious or depressed ☐
I am extremely anxious or depressed ☐

Source: EuroQol Group

For more details contact:
Frank de Charro, EuroQol Group Business Manager,
Centre for Health Policy and Law, Erasmus University,
Rotterdam, PO Box 1738, 300DR Rotterdam,
The Netherlands

Tel: +31 10 408 2364
Fax: +31 10 452 5303
Email: deCharro@gbr.frg.eur.nl

An alternative quality of life instrument is SF36 (short form 36) (Brooks et al. 1990). This was devised and used in a large randomised trial of different health insurance plans in the USA (the Rand Insurance experiment). There is a shorter version (SF12), with fewer questions than the EQ5D. However, it does not use the thermometer aspect of EQ5D and cannot be reduced to a single score for the health status of the population (as EQ5D allows). Both instruments are available in many languages and in variants of English (e.g. Australian, American and English!).

SF36 is being evaluated by the private insurer, the British United Provident Association (BUPA). They offer SF36 to all their insurees before a surgical procedure, and then seek their responses to the same instrument 3 months after the intervention. The preliminary results show considerable variations in success, in measures of physical, social and psychiatric functioning, and variations in the success of consultants in restoring individual functioning. Such results, if validated, would be invaluable guides to people when choosing consultants. It would also be invaluable to BUPA in determining who they wish to use to provide care to their subscribers.

Why is it that these instruments exist, are well validated in clinical trials but not piloted to measure population quality of life over time? Such measures could be invaluable guides to decision making by people who use services, practitioners and policy makers. They could show how patients progress, in terms of functional capacity, over the course of illness episodes.

POLICY OPTIONS

Most contemporary discussions of clinical governance begin with the definition from Donaldson and Scally (Scally & Donaldson 1998), that has been repeated in numerous government publications but remains at best circular and at worst unhelpful and ambiguous. They defined clinical governance as 'a framework through which NHS organisations are accountable for continuously improving the quality of their services and safeguarding high standards of care by creating an environment in which excellence in clinical care will flourish'. This definition is vague and is often used as rhetoric rather than the basis for the efficient use of resources to improve the health of the population.

Two key words in this definition are 'quality' and 'excellence', both of which are not clearly defined either in pronouncements about clinical governance or in its development. Whilst everyone, in particular service users, would agree that the purpose of health care is to improve health, this is not measured routinely. Recently, the government has published mortality data. Such data have been available for decades in the service; it is part of HES, however, managers have ignored it. The usual excuse for this is that the HES are inaccurate. Why we allow clinicians to record data about their practices inaccurately and why we allow managers to send this inaccurate data to the Department of Health is curious, stupid and wasteful. Where the data are collected and checked carefully, they reveal much about practice, which can be questioned and subsequently better managed. As data such as HES are a centrally set 'performance indicator' for Trusts, it is likely that *its* accuracy will improve.

Some policy options

There are a range of policy options, which those managing the process of clinical governance can investigate and prioritise:

- HES
  The HES data exist and all Primary Care Trusts (PCTs) and Trusts should invest in collecting these data in a way that is reliable and 'cleaned' (i.e. checked and error rates reduced). These data can then be used routinely to monitor and manage clinical activity and mortality. Generally, mortality rates by specialism and consultant may be low. As a consequence time series (annual data pooled over 5 to 10 years) analysis is required.

  However, all such analysis must be undertaken with great care. Administrative data, such as HES, are crude and simple manipulation of them may not take account of case severity.

Could unmeasured differences in the severity of disease account for higher weekend mortality rates (Bell & Redelmeier 2001, Halm & Chassin 2001)? However these crude data are the starting point for all management processes.

- Staffing issues
  When weekend mortality rates for emergency admissions are higher (Bell & Redelmeier 2001) and some hospitals have higher standardised mortality rates than others (Good Hospital Guide 2001), what are the explanations of these differences? One explanation offered by some researchers (Jarman et al. 1999) is nurse and doctor staffing levels. Bell and Redelmeier (2001) focused on three procedures (ruptured abdominal aortic aneurysm, acute epiglottis and pulmonary embolism) in their identification of higher weekend mortality rates. A crucial element in the management of these conditions is speed of diagnosis. Is this dependent or independent of staffing levels? Currently, we do not know the answer to this question.

  Many investigations relating to staffing or staff mix in the context of hospital outcomes have focused upon nursing, however, the results are mixed. For instance Needleman and colleagues found some evidence that nurse staffing levels are related to outcomes *and are* potentially sensitive to nursing levels, but they are wary of the quality of the data. Other American evidence (Wunderlich et al. 1996), *clearly* links nurse staffing to outcomes. There appear to be no UK studies. Why? Is opinion preferred to analysis of the link between nurse staffing levels and patient *outcomes* in this country?

- Measuring quality of survival
  Whilst health measures like SF36 and EQ5D have been available and used in clinical trials for several decades, there is little investment in routine measurement of the functional status of individuals at the population level. This may be changing in continental Europe where one Scandinavian country is discussing the

population use of EQ5D. The insurer, BUPA, is using SF36. However, no NHS purchaser or provider is piloting such measures. The scope for piloting is great and the potential benefits to be derived from the successful application of such instruments are considerable.

- Primary care and general practice
  Primary care and general practice can in some respects be seen as largely a 'data-free' environment making clinical governance a considerable challenge for practitioners and for their employing bodies. Questions include: What do GPs do? There is no national data set which reveals, like the HES in the hospital sector, processes and activities in primary care. Simple manipulation of the HES and the General Household Survey, which includes some GP data in its questionnaire, reveals that activity per doctor in primary and secondary care appears to have been constant for decades (Bloor & Maynard 2001). Thus apparently constant 're-disorganisation' of the NHS, in terms of changes in its organisational structure, has had little observable effect on doctors' volumes of care! Given there has been no measurement of outcomes, the impact of reform on 'quality' and 'excellence' is unknown. Why aren't such 'experiments' evaluated (Campbell 1969)?

  Electronic prescribing offers the prospect of adding diagnostic categories to the prescription together with patient/client linkages. This will facilitate the time series analysis of utilisation by diagnostic and age groups as well as adherence to the guidelines of the National Institute for Clinical Excellence (NICE) and the Scottish Intercollegiate Guidelines Network (SIGN) (Cookson et al. 2001).

  Hospital referral data from HES can be used to compare GP referral rates and variations. In time this can be linked to NICE guidelines to manage practitioners better and ensure appropriate treatment, which is clinically, and cost, effective.

The clinical governance challenge in primary care is even sharper than that in the hospital sector. The 'corner shop' culture of primary care and the independent contractor status of GPs have not engendered systematic data collection and thorough audit. Investments in this sector need careful piloting and evaluation rather than optimistic funding of evidence-free interventions.

- Incorporating quality measurement in NHS management
  Discussion of 'quality' and 'clinical governance' remains process/activity orientated because Chief Executives are rewarded (and dismissed!) for failure to meet process targets. Outcome is measured poorly and only weakly incorporated within management structures. Until politicians shift the 'goal posts', managers will ignore data (such as HES) and prosper (job-wise) by inappropriate management practices. As a consequence contracting will continue to focus on the numbers of procedures. A decision by a PCT to buy 400 hip replacements without consideration, measurement and management of mortality and QoL is in principle incompetent and immoral as it potentially wastes resources and puts people's health (and lives) at risk.

  The reform of professional regulation could oblige practitioners to measure and evaluate their practice. Thus for doctors the General Medical Council could oblige all practitioners to report their activity and outcome data as part of revalidation procedures. This would necessitate the integration of NHS and private sector activity and outcome data so that as full a picture as is possible could be gathered for each practitioner. Individual Trusts have been obliged to carry out annual consultant appraisals since April 2001. These should involve the use of HES activity and outcome data so that practitioners are aware of their relative performance.

Reform of the remuneration systems is planned both for GPs and for hospital consultants. These new pay systems can be used to enhance quality control by performance management. A nice example of this was the 1990 GP contract. The architects of this payment system recognised that several cost effective preventive procedures were not implemented even though GPs were paid fee per item of service to deliver them. In order to enhance take up of immunisation, vaccination and cervical cytology, a system of graduated fees per item of service was introduced, with higher fees paid the larger the percentage of eligible people on the GPs list who took up the interventions. More recently (2000), fees were introduced for influenza vaccination. Prior to such fees, many GPs delivered this cost effective intervention to only 30% of eligible patients/clients. After the introduction of payments, the take up rate for older people and those with chronic illnesses rose to 80%.

Such mechanisms have significant but limited application. If payments are targeted at inappropriate activities resources can be wasted. For instance, the 1990 GP contract offered payments for health promotion clinics and for the annual screening of those over 75 years old. The latter has no evidence base in terms of clinical or cost effectiveness. The former, health promotion clinics, were so ill defined initially that one Sheffield GP had to be paid for playing Jane Fonda workout videos (Bloor & Maynard 2001)!

Simply relating activity to payment can thus generate inefficiency. Therefore, if consultants were offered pay related to performance in an effort to reduce waiting times, the effects on quality are ambiguous. If payments were merely related to numbers, clinicians may do minor rather than major procedures. If payments were related to case-severity, a complicated fee schedule would be required. Such a schedule would inevitably be 'gamed' by unscrupulous practitioners. Such gaming is evident in the private sector where the insurers invest significantly to ensure that procedures claimed have been delivered: the policing of cheating can be expensive (Maynard & Bloor 2001)!

The generally used definition of clinical governance can lead to the failure to focus on outcomes. In particular, the continued failure to use existing data (HES activity and mortality outcome information), an absence of systematic experimentation with quality of life measures and the lack of recognition of the advantages and limitations of using contract and payment systems in incentivising the processes of clinical governance. Such deficiencies are evident in current policies in clinical governance and can be mitigated by the use of explicit allocation procedures to determine how scarce resources can be best invested.

PRIORITISING INVESTMENT IN CLINICAL GOVERNANCE

Life is always risky!

Misguided optimism, fuelled by media sensationalism, encourages members of society to believe that risk can be eradicated from our lives. This is nonsense. All activities have risks associated with them, e.g. attending a cricket or a football match can result in physical and psychological damage. School teachers facing litigation when children die on school trips or are damaged in the play ground are reacting by banning such activities: the benefits of banning them have to be set against the benefit losses to children. A heart transplant is risky and people die whilst having wisdom teeth removed and hernias repaired. Your dentist and podiatrist may not sterilise her instruments and give you hepatitis. Your child may pull the kettle over and scald himself seriously.

There is an optimal level of risk in all these activities, and it is generally not zero. It is too expensive to take away all risks and, as a consequence it is efficient and unavoidable that all risks are not eradicated. Consumers should be aware of the risks of mountain climbing, travelling by car (3400 die each year in car crashes), travelling by rail (much safer than road travel), and using fireworks. Only where there is evidence that investment reduces risk efficiently (e.g. speed cameras to reduce road traffic deaths) should scarce resources be spent. Resources used inefficiently to reduce risks could be used alternatively to reduce risks efficiently or to produce effective care: the opportunity cost or the value investments foregone should not be ignored when clinical governance programmes are designed.

Unfortunately, in the area of clinical governance there is a tendency to act vigorously without recourse to the existing evidence base and its development by systematic experimentation. This 'drunken sailor' syndrome has considerable opportunity costs and is evident in both measurement and management activities.

The first point to emphasize is that the benefits of remedying many errors may be minor, as the person may have died anyway. Thus an American study (Hayward et al. 2001) found that almost one-quarter of active care deaths could be rated as possibly preventable by optimal care, with 6% rated as probably or definitely preventable. However, the reviewers of these cases estimated that only 0.5% of people who died would have lived 3 months or more in good cognitive health if optimal care had been given. This result means that in these study hospitals, optimal care delivery would result in 1 person in 10 000 living 3 or more months in good cognitive health. Such results need replication in the UK but demonstrate for the USA that investment in error reduction may yield a very modest benefit (Hayward & Hofer 2001). Perhaps before rushing into clinical governance, it would be wiser to define the problem more clearly and target investments carefully.

Targeting investments in clinical governance

Such targeting of clinical governance investments is difficult because of the dominance of the clinical effectiveness model and the paucity of the evidence base. Any query about 'what works' is difficult to answer. The scope for clinical governance investment is broad and ill defined. It may be as simple as improving sign posting throughout an organisation or encouraging staff to wash their hands in order to better control infections. Conversely, it may be as complex as using quality-adjusted life years (QALYs) to inform service delivery. Unfortunately, the knowledge base about how best to inform clinical teams about risks and alter their behaviour over long periods is not well defined. Furthermore, and unfortunately, the evidence that is available is often ignored (Pittet et al. 2000).

Let us assume that intervention A produces 5 QALYs and intervention B produces 10 QALYs. B is clinically superior to A. But what if intervention A costs £5000, and intervention B costs £20 000? In this case A produces a QALY at the cost of £1000, and B produces a QALY at the cost of £2000. Alternatively B produces 5 more QALYs at an additional cost of £15 000, i.e. the incremental cost of producing a QALY by investing in B is £3000 per QALY. Thus, if the total budget available is £500 000, investment in A would produce 500 QALYs, whilst investment in B would produce only 250 QALYs. Whilst B is clinically superior to A, A is more cost effective. If the social goal is the maximisation of population health from a finite budget, resources should be allocated in relation to cost effectiveness and not mere clinical effectiveness. What is clinically effective may not be cost effective, but those interventions which are cost effective, are always clinically effective (Maynard 1997). Choices about which clinical governance programmes to adopt must be determined by evidence of cost effectiveness if scarce resources are to produce the maximum possible gain in population health from a limited budget.

The Cochrane Collaboration, which reviews the evidence base of interventions, has tended to emphasise the issue of clinical effectiveness. However, the medical researcher after whom the collaboration is named was quite clear about the need to consider both costs and benefits to individuals when making investments in health care (Cochrane 1972).

> *Allocations of funds and facilities are nearly always based on the opinions of senior consultants, but, more and more, requests for additional facilities will have to be based on detailed argument with 'hard evidence' as to the gain to be expected from the patient's angle and the cost. Few could possibly object to this.*

Given that it is essential to use evidence about costs *and* benefits when investing in clinical governance, it is remarkable how this lesson is ignored and the designers of risk reducing regulations avoid this evidence base to create inefficient regulations. This is the current problem with clinical governance: policy designed in isolation from economics-based medicine.

An example of this is the work of Tammy Tengs and her colleagues nearly a decade ago (Tengs 2000). This study sought estimates for the cost effectiveness of over 500 interventions. It found data on costs and effectiveness for only 185 interventions and then contrasted the current pattern of investment in these areas with the 'optimal' pattern given the economic evidence base. They found little relationship between investment implementation and cost effectiveness and concluded that if resource allocation had been based on economic evidence more than half a million more life years would have been produced. Tengs concluded that because we fail to base healthcare investments on cost effectiveness data 'we sacrifice many lives each year'.

The inefficient use of resources typified by the continuing reluctance to implement economics-based medicine, creates avoidable mortality and morbidity. Such inefficiency wastes resources and is unethical because it potentially deprives people of care from which they may benefit. Whilst such arguments have been made for decades by economists, policy makers and clinicians continue to abuse the trust put in them by society by refusing to base their choices on information relating to cost and effectiveness.

A recent Department of Health publication (2001) setting out the policy and the research agenda for clinical governance continues to ignore the relevance of the economics evidence base and the need to develop it further by funding appropriate research. In part, this document is a product of the continuing dominance of the medical profession in forming policy in an area where past practices have been demonstrably inadequate.

CONCLUSIONS

The central issue in clinical governance is the enhancement of patient/client outcomes (health status) at least cost. Most discussions of clinical governance are fragmented and linked to political obsessions with inputs (spending) and processes of care (activities such as volumes and wasting time). Despite advocating performance management processes that relate to individual outcomes all healthcare systems appear to remain reluctant to measure changes in length and quality of life following healthcare interventions.

Much routine data in the NHS are ignored. For instance HES have been collected for decades but are not used to manage activity and outcomes. There is a nice choice of policy options on clinical governance or quality enhancement. These involve not only investment in the quantity and quality of basic data needed to manage the system, but also in the appraisal of methods to incorporate these data into routine NHS management. For example, the knowledge base on hand hygiene to reduce hospital-acquired infections is good but often ignored (Pittet et al. 2000).

The central policy challenge is to make managers and professionals interested in and focus on the measurement and management of outcomes in their everyday work. Progress towards this goal can be made in the contracting processes between purchasers and providers, by shifting the focus from volume to outcomes, and by improving incentives for practitioners to translate evidence into practice.

However, such a process is not without its problems. Thus, when Dr Foster published hospital mortality rates in cardio-thoracic surgery, one Midlands Trust responded by changing patient entry criteria for care (taking the 'easier', fitter patients) and reduced throughput to give more attention to patients. This no doubt improved their 'performance', but it also excluded sick patients from care because they were 'too risky'. Similar effects have been detected in New York and Pennsylvania where the authors of a study concluded that health report cards can fail patients. In particular, they noted 'For sicker patients, doctors and hospitals avoided performing cardiac surgical treatments of all types. These changes were particularly harmful, leading sicker patients to have substantially higher frequencies of heart failure and repeated heart attacks and ultimately higher costs of care' (Dranove et al. 2001).

Finally, it is important to recognise always that much everyday activity is based on custom and trust. When trust breaks down the cost of policing people's behaviours can become very costly and is often very difficult. The challenge is to sustain and develop trust by open and simple systems of accountability and professional surveillance. The 18th century political economist Adam Smith, often cited by Reagan and Thatcher as the architect of 'free enterprise', argued convincingly that competitive markets (self interest and greed) were not the primary determinants of exchange.

Those general rules of conduct when they have been fixed in our mind by habitual reflection, are of great use in correcting the misrepresentations of self-love concerning what is fit and proper to be done in our particular situation ... The regard of those general rules of conduct, is what is properly called a sense of duty, a principle of greatest consequence in human life, and thereby principle by which the bulk of mankind are capable of directing their actions (Smith 1790, Chapter v, para 1, pp. 160–162).

Interest in clinical governance has erupted because individual practitioners have betrayed the public's trust. In responding to this with investments to improve quality, the baby (trust and professional self regulation) should not be thrown out with the bath water and all those interested in efficiency and the consumer's welfare should adopt a focus on outcomes for the individual patient and the cost effectiveness of competing methods of improving healthcare quality.

REFERENCES

Bell CM, Redelmeier DA 2001 Mortality among patients admitted to hospitals on weekends as compared to weekdays. New England Journal of Medicine 345(9): 663–668.

Bloor K, Maynard A 2001 Workforce productivity and incentive structures in the UK National Health Service. Journal of Health Service Research and Policy 6(2): 105–113.

Brooks RG, Jedtag S, Lundgren B, Persson U, Bjork S 1990 EuroQol: health related quality of life measurement. Health Policy 18: 37–48.

Campbell DT 1969 Reform as experiments. American Psychologist 24(4): 409–429.

Cochrane AL 1972 Effectiveness and efficiency: random reflections on health services, Nuffield Provincial Hospitals Trust, London.

Codman EA 1914 The product of a hospital. Surgery, Gynaecology and Obstetrics 18: 491–496.

Cookson R, McDaid D, Maynard A 2001 Wrong SIGN, NICE mess: is national guidance distorting allocation of resources? British Medical Journal 323:743–745.

Department of Health 2001 Building a safer NHS for patients: implementing an organisation with a memory. DoH, London.

Dranove D, Kessler D, McClellen M, Satterthwaite M 2001 Is more information better? The effects of 'report cards' on health care providers. National Bureau for Economic Research (NBER), Working Paper 8697, New York.

Good Hospital Guide for Britain and Ireland, part 1, Sunday Times, 14 January 2001.

Good Hospital Guide for Britain and Ireland, part 2, Sunday Times, 21 January 2001.

Halm EA, Chassin MR 2001 Why do hospital death rates vary? New England Journal of Medicine 345(9): 692–694.

Hayward RA, Hofer TP 2001 Estimating hospital deaths due to medical errors: preventability is in the eye of the reviewer. Journal of the American Medical Association 286(4): 415–420.

Herodotus 1954 The histories. Penguin Books, London.

Jarman B, Gault S, Alves B, Hider A, Dolan S, Cook A 1999 Explaining differences in English hospital death rates using routinely collected data. British Medical Journal 318: 1515–1520.

Kind P 1987 Hospital death – the missing link; measuring outcomes in hospital activity data. Discussion paper 44. Centre for Health Economics, University of York.

Kohn LT, Corrigan JM, Donaldson MS (eds) 1999 To err is human: building a safer health system. Institute of Medicine, National Academy Press, Washington DC.

Maynard A 1997 Evidence based medicine: an incomplete method for informing treatment choices. Lancet 349: 126–128.

Maynard A, Bloor K 2001 Reforming the contract of UK consultants. British Medical Journal 322: 541–543.

Needleman J, Buerhaus PI, Mattke S, Steward M, Zelevinsky K. Nurse staffing and patient outcomes in hospitals, final report, Health Resources and Service Administration. (http://bhpr.hrsa.gov/dn/staffstudy.htm)

NHS Centre for Reviews and Dissemination 1996 Hospital volume and health care outcomes, costs and access. Effective Health Care. Bulletin 2, 8. Churchill Livingstone – Royal Society of Medicine, Edinburgh.

Nightingale F 1863 An essay on hospitals, 3rd edn. Longmans Green, London.

Patrick DL, Ericksson P 1993 Health status and health policy: allocating resources to health care. Oxford University Press, New York.

Pittet D, Hugonnet S, Harbarth S, Mourouja P, Sauven V, Touveneau S, Perneger TV and members of the infection control team 2000 Effectiveness of a hospital wide programme to improve compliance with hand hygiene. Lancet 356: 1307–1312.

Runciman WB, Moller J. Iatrogenic injury in Australia, Australian Patient Safety Foundation. http://www.apsf.net.au

Scally G, Donaldson LJ 1998 Clinical governance and the drive for quality improvement in the new NHS. British Medical Journal 317: 61–65.

Smith A 1790/1976 A theory of moral sentiments. Oxford University Press, London and Oxford.

Tengs TO 2000 Dying too soon: how cost effectiveness analysis can save lives. In: Jones L (ed) Safe enough? Managing risk and regulation. The Frazer Institute, Vancouver, Canada.

Vincent C, Neale G, Wooloshynowych M 2001 Adverse events in British hospitals: preliminary retrospective record review. British Medical Journal 322: 517–519.

Wunderlich GS, Sloan FA, Davis CK 1996 Nurse staffing in hospitals and nursing homes: is it adequate? National Academy Press, Washington DC.

3

Clinical governance and best value: the user perspective

Paul Ramcharan

KEY ISSUES

- ◆ The contribution of service users to the clinical governance agenda

- ◆ Identifying ways to gain real involvement from service users

- ◆ Supporting an independent voice within the clinical governance agenda

- ◆ The role of advocacy in supporting service user contributions

- ◆ The importance of management support

- ◆ The impact of professional decision making upon quality of care and quality of support.

INTRODUCTION

The clinical governance agenda is associated most closely with the term 'quality' (Department of Health 1998a). One could be mistaken when reading the burgeoning literature on clinical governance that it means nothing less than re-inventing the health service and healthcare practice. As a 'fortunate term', quality is easily adopted by individuals as a feature of any studies, actions, plans or practice that they undertake as professional workers.

In discussing the origins and foundations of clinical governance, members of the National Clinical Governance Support Team place the patient–professional partnership at the pinnacle of their 'temple model'. The seven pillars holding the temple up are the elements of clinical governance: clinical effectiveness, risk management, communication effectiveness, resource effectiveness, strategic effectiveness, learning effectiveness and patient experience. The authors argue that:

> At the centre of clinical governance must be a real partnership between patients and professionals. It is the patients who can best tell it 'as it really is' and professionals need to develop the mechanisms and skills to listen to patients with authentic curiosity … Only when we can see 'through the patient's eyes' can we be confident that we are building into organisations and systems deliverables which are really meaningful for patients …
> (Nicholls et al. 2001, p. 174).

In addition, officially published and recognised advice suggests in regard to policy that:

> If a best value review is to be genuinely 'whole systems', then it will need to consider the NHS for people who have a learning disability. It will thus need to pay attention to clinical governance, which in many ways can be seen as the NHS equivalent of best value
> (Poxton et al. 2001).

However, what does this actually mean in practice and how can this be accomplished? Swage (2000) identifies a substantial range of activities that constitute clinical governance. These include: clear lines of accountability and responsibility, a comprehensive programme of quality-improvement activities and clear policies aimed at managing risk, and remedies for poor professional performance (Swage 2000, pp. 5–6).

Within Swage's model the user perspective comes a poor second to issues of professional interest and service management. Her discussion on the user perspective on quality identifies the growth of consumerist principles within health as having led to user and community views being expressed in and through community health councils, complaints procedures, the patients' charter, advocacy, other user-led groups and in a limited way in service planning.

Swage tells us that studies of patient/client views indicate that they want helpful information and to exercise choice. The view of those who use services is best garnered through questionnaires, surveys, satisfaction audits, focus groups, patient/client participation groups, through consultation on plans and through newsletters. Other writers suggest, in relation to capturing the user perspective, the merits of satisfaction tools (Poulton 1998) or rapid appraisal (Murray et al. 1994), whilst policy has highlighted the importance of a national patient and user survey (Department of Health 1998a, Department of Health 2001, p. 92). The merits of these approaches in relation to 'one-stop' users of health services in reflecting upon their experiences seems apt, allowing largely retrospective analysis by users of the care and services they have received.

However, this largely 'one-stop' approach to securing quality is insufficient in relation to people who have a learning disability and certainly not the limit to what is intended in relation to quality services for people who have a learning disability in present policy. First and foremost, people who have a learning disability and other related groups (e.g. those with mental health problems or older people) are likely to have an enduring relationship with health and social-care support services. Moreover, such services do not only look after health needs, but provide support in relation to education, employment and day services, housing, leisure and promoting independence to name but a few. The outcomes relating to these areas of life experience are likely to define the person's quality of life and are ones in which their needs and wishes are paramount and should be pervasive over time. The white paper *Valuing People* (Department of Health 2001) suggests this is to be organised at an individual level through person-centred planning. In summary, this involves, supporting people in taking control of their own lives and life spheres through listening and working towards individual achievements, giving them the capacity to meet their own stated wishes.

This relates to a second point, i.e. that the user perspective has a much longer and well-established history in relation to people who have a learning disability. A century separates formal accepted policy in the provision of services to people who have a learning disability from theories based upon eugenics and institutionalisation to those based upon 'rights, independence, choice and inclusion' (Department of Health 2001). There has been a growing commitment to deinstitutionalisation in the post-war years, recognising that people who have a learning disability should lead normal lives (Nirje 1969, Bank-Mikkelson 1980) and, later, the impact of normalisation (Wolfensberger 1972, Wolfensberger & Glenn 1973). This has consolidated the move towards policies reflecting ideals of individuality, choice and valued social roles within wider society. Thus, *Better Services for the Mentally Handicapped* (Department of Health 1971) promoted the idea of normal lives to the extent that 'handicaps permit'. The publication of *An Ordinary Life* (King's Fund 1980) and a number of innovative attempts at service delivery (Felce et al. 1998, pp. 10–14) culminated, in the 1980s, in the first comprehensive national strategy in Wales for the provision of services to people who have a learning disability. The All Wales Strategy (AWS) presaged many of the changes mooted in *Valuing People* (Department of Health 2001) with an emphasis on individual and strategic planning and the provision

of quality services. Its relevance will, therefore, be further detailed in the main sections of this chapter along with a local example in a learning disability hospital in Wales to ask what might be learned from the Welsh experience. Much policy has also emerged since the end of the first phase of the All Wales Strategy in the early 1990s some of which has been influenced by the experience in Wales.

Policy has, more systematically over time, emphasised the centrality of the user perspective within the provision of services. For example, policy has exhorted involvement and participation as the key to a person-centred service (NHS Executive 1992, p. 3, Department of Health 2001, p. 49) to individual, essential lifestyle- or person centred-planning (Welsh Office 1983, p. 7, NHS Executive 1998, p. 4, Department of Health 2001, p. 45), in service planning and in terms of having a say in services received (Welsh Office 1983, Department of Health 1990, p. 27, Department of Health 1998a, p. 39).

Over the past 20 years or so the user perspective (Ramcharan & Grant 2001) has also featured more in research through life histories (Deacon 1982, Lundgren 1993, Atkinson et al. 1997) and as participant researchers (March et al. 1997, Minkes et al. 1995, Williams 1999). The advocacy movement, self-advocacy in particular, has grown substantially (Crawley 1988, Ramcharan et al. 1996) as have publications by the self-advocacy groups themselves (Change 1997, Liverpool and Manchester People First 1996, Speak Up Self Advocacy 1998, Walsall Women's Group 1999, People First 1993, 1994, 1997, 1998). People who have a learning disability have, therefore, become involved not only within services, but also in themselves by setting the agenda through having their voices heard at all levels of policy, theory and service provision.

In the recent past learning disability policy had already recognised that it is possible to establish the views of most people who have a learning disability (NHS Executive 1998, p. 3) and that it is also possible to promote their participation (Department of Health 1990, p. 25) and to develop partnerships (NHS Executive 1996).

Activity 3.1

Think about the people that you provide a service to and consider the ways in which you can ascertain their real views about the service they receive.

What criteria would you use to assess whether you have established a genuine partnership with the people who you provide a service to?

Valuing People identifies the new framework for quality in learning disability services (Department of Health 2001); this interfaces with the clinical governance agenda outlined in *A First Class Service* (Department of Health 1998a), both of which can be seen as the key to delivering high quality services in relation to a wide range of life spheres. In addition the white paper asserts that:

> *The government expects people who have a learning disability and their carers to be fully involved in planning, monitoring and reviewing services; and also in evaluating the quality of services they receive under the new Quality Framework for Social Care (Department of Health 2001, p. 92).*

The white paper represents perhaps the acceptance that user involvement is to be regarded as 'an expectation' as well as 'good' practice (Department of Health 1998b, Department of Health 1995). Indeed, users were involved in the Commissioning Group, produced their own report (People First London et al. 2000) and were employed together with others in reviewing research proposals for the Department of Health research initiative accompanying its launch (Grant & Ramcharan 2002). Moreover, *Valuing People* is backed up with additional funding for advocacy, and calls for participation in the new Partnership Boards (Department of Health 2001, p. 106, p. 108), the Learning Disability Task Force (Department of Health 2001, p. 112) and in planning, monitoring and reviewing services (Department of Health 2001, p. 92).

Pougher (1997) has argued that quality services can best be achieved with, 'a clear set of values … a framework for meeting these objectives … and a range of relevant tools' (1997, p. 71). From the above review it might be argued that the perspective of people who have a learning disability has been at the forefront of developing new ideas about the value base that should underlie policy and provision. However, there remains little evidence in the literature about different frameworks or tools in terms of their outcomes. What is clear from the cursory consideration of the user perspective outlined above, is that simplistic retrospective and one-off user satisfaction surveys would be wholly insufficient in developing and implementing a user perspective from a clinical governance perspective for people who have a learning disability, or any other group of people who have an enduring relationship with service providers. There is a need to go, not only well beyond Swage's recommendations for the use of retrospective means of assessing services, but also even beyond the 'authentic curiosity' suggested as necessary by the National Clinical Governance Support Team.

What evidence might inform the clinical governance agenda about how best to optimise the user perspective as a foundational element in improving service quality? Rather than write a chapter immersed in the theory relating to clinical governance I felt this was an opportune time to recount two related 'stories' about the user perspective. The first of these stories is set in Wales, a land with a recent history of innovative provision of quality services for people who have a learning disability. The second story is largely about the wish of staff within a learning disability hospital in Wales to improve the lives of the people who lived there, and the relevance of a small piece of research (*Fostering a Culture of Civil Rights*, Ramcharan 1998), aimed at supporting this. Reflecting upon the 'values', 'frameworks' and 'tools' (Pougher 1998) for improving service quality and the relative success of different strategies the text will be interspersed with activities that are designed to support you to engage with the agenda of introducing quality and service user involvement in the clinical governance agenda.

THE ALL WALES STRATEGY

Implemented in 1983 the All Wales Strategy (AWS) forms the backdrop for the first of these stories. The AWS for the development of services for mentally handicapped people (Welsh Office 1983) set out a national strategy supported from the centre by the Welsh Office. It was founded upon stated value-based principles and funded through additional ring fenced monies.

Central to the AWS were the ideas of planning at two levels. Individual programme planning (IPP) for each person with learning disabilities: this meant 'all professionals concerned with the individual meeting at regular (6 monthly) intervals, together with the client and family, to plan short- and long-term aims for the person' (Felce 1998). The user perspective was not only meant to be central to the identification of individual needs and planning, but was to facilitate involvement in developing service priorities, planning, implementing, evaluating and overseeing the management of new services. In addition, county planning groups for the eight Welsh counties were to include representatives from the statutory sector, voluntary sector, parents and representatives of people who have a learning disability. The idea was that since all individual needs would have been individually assessed it would be possible to decide, within budgetary constraints, the service priorities to implement and then monitor

these new value-based services. The voice of service users and their perspective was seen as an essential part of this strategic planning and service implementation.

Valuing People shows striking similarities to the AWS in having a joint service planning arrangement organised through the new Partnership Boards and an emphasis on person-centred planning, each to be organised with the direct input of people who have a learning disability and family carers. What then might *Valuing People* learn from the AWS experience?

Activity 3.2

The voice of people who have a learning disability should be heard at individual, service and strategic planning levels. This should also be the case for all people who use services.

Think about the group of people you work with. What structures, processes and systems exist to help you hear the voice of those people?

From the perspective of learning disability services you may have considered things such as user engagement projects, involvement in Partnership Boards and person-centred planning. For other services you may have thought about Patient Advocacy and Liaison services (PALS), citizens' juries, patient councils, focus groups, integrated care pathways among others.

Despite the intention in Wales to involve people who have a learning disability on county and local groups (Felce et al. 1998, pp. 73–91) they were reported in 1986 to be '…conspicuous by their absence' (SCOVO 1986, p. 7), and in 1987 that 'there has been little direct involvement in planning services by mentally handicapped people', (Welsh Office 1987, p. 22). With guidance and exhortation from the Welsh Office, the representation of people who have a learning disability increased in county and local groups up to 1991.

During this period the number of self-advocacy groups from which representatives had largely been drawn also grew from a base of zero at the start of the AWS period to 30 in 1991, and to 58 by 1994 (Ramcharan et al. 1996).

Activity 3.3

A strong independent voice is vital in supporting the participation of people who have a learning disability and others as well.

Does an independent advocacy movement exist locally? How might you and your organisation be involved in supporting the development of such an independent voice?

In most of the eight Welsh counties there was now representation of people who have a learning disability on local and county planning to a greater or lesser degree. An independent sub-group on consumer involvement advising the Welsh Office had also provided a list of involvement optimising strategies and this has been further elaborated recently by the Head of the Implementation Support Team for Valuing People (Greig 2001).

Activity 3.4

How many of the following strategies for optimising user involvement are in place in your organisation?

☐ Pre-preparation for meetings

☐ Preliminary work on meeting agendas

☐ Accessible format agenda and summaries circulated well before meetings

☐ Independent support at meetings

☐ Several forums or sub-groups

☐ Provision of transport to meetings

☐ Appointment of participation officers

☐ Quality action and monitoring groups

During the AWS years, questions remained about how much say people who have a learning disability actually had in planning forums, despite best efforts. Professionals and others seemed to have a disproportionately strong voice in such groups. A review of the proportion of contributions made in such groups by professionals, parents, voluntary sector representatives and people who have a learning disability indicated that for people who have a learning disability 'consumer involvement takes the form of physical presence, but falls a long way short of participation' (Welsh Office 1989).

Moreover, as the All Wales Advocacy Project (AWAP) on consumer involvement reported, far too much emphasis had been placed on service planning at the expense of the management and review of services. Yet 'people are more likely to seek involvement and participation when the stake they have is greater, and where the topics of discussion have an immediacy to their lives' (Felce et al. 1998, p. 90). In this light, the perspective and voice of people who have a learning disability was more likely to be heard when they were involved in the management and evaluation of service quality (Whittaker et al. 1990, Whittaker 1997, McIntosh & Whittaker 1998) than in relation to strategic planning and issues of funding.

Activity 3.5

People who have a learning disability are more likely to want to become involved in managing and evaluating their own services, because of the direct relevance to their personal experience. Anecdotal evidence suggests that this is the case for other people who use NHS and social care services.

Think about the areas you identified in Activity 3.2. How much does the focus of these activities relate to the service users' direct experience? In those situations where it does not, how much do you think this affects the motivation and contribution of people who use the service? You might find it useful to discuss this with people who use your service.

The limited success up to 1991 described above was soon to be sorely challenged. The implementation of the NHS and Community Care Act (NHSCCA) became a priority for the Welsh Office. The idea of the IPP for all was to be superseded by the need to prioritise those most in need (Department of Health 1989), the new guidance for the re-launched AWS was not as strong in relation to involvement (Welsh Office 1996) and ultimately the ring-fenced funds for the provision of services was taken back into the revenue support grant.

The new care planning arrangements under the NHSCCA meant that in seeking funds for services, people who have a learning disability would have to vie for funds with other social care specialties such as services for older people and those with mental health problems. The local and county planning groups became less relevant. Moreover, Welsh local government reorganisation in 1996 meant that the eight counties became 22 unitary authorities. This effectively undermined over a decade of effort at building a county- and locality-based system of participation and involvement for people who have a learning disability. It highlighted the need for a well-funded user voice existing independent of services so that their input could outlive transitory policies or demographic change.

The period of the AWS up to 1991 generated substantial change. Given its common policy with England prior to 1983 it is possible to show the achievements of the AWS after the 1983 policy watershed. For example, family-based respite per million of the Welsh population was nine compared to 5.8 in England in 1993. Short-term care was largely in ordinary housing and non-hospital settings in Wales, but still largely in hospitals in England. The average size of residence for people living independently in Wales in the local statutory sector was just over four and for the independent sector just over three. This compared with an average size of 13 in England with none catering for four or less people despite the growing acceptance that small provision was more desirable from the perspective of the person who has a learning disability. The provision of value-based services during the AWS period changed substantially the structure and availability of services and, ultimately, had an effect on the quality of the services provided.

The Fostering a Culture of Civil Rights research

This research forms the basis of story two and offers one approach to how the clinical governance agenda can be realised in practice, particularly in relation to people who have an enduring relationship with welfare services. It can be argued that many of the changes during the AWS period were achieved through a system of information exchange, consultation, involvement and participation in which people who have a learning disability played some part. This was the case not only in the community and in relation to social provision but, also, in relation to health.

Within the hospital that is the focus for this second story an advocacy group had been in operation since 1989. Having started as a citizen advocacy project it had widened its interests over time to include: self-advocacy groups supported within and outside of the hospital, a user council made up of people living within the hospital, an evaluation of service quality for a period of time, professional advocacy through visits to villas, and representation for individuals in their case reviews and during their resettlement. The management in the hospital had, at all times, been supportive of these efforts and in seeking to maximise the relevance of the user perspective to the hospital's work.

Activity 3.6

Managers and service workers have to be fully committed and supportive if the user voice is to be heard. This is not always easy, but it is essential.

Think about what a full commitment to and support of a user voice means in practice. Does your organisation meet these criteria? How might this be improved?

In 1994 I was approached by the unit general manager who was interested in examining ways to maximise the quality of life of people living in the hospital. The interest stretched along a continuum between the prevention of abuse in its various forms on the one hand, to promoting and protecting rights on the other. A small-scale piece of research was undertaken and the final report entitled *Fostering a Culture of Civil Rights* (FCCR) was later published. The research was undertaken prior to the government clarifying its position on clinical governance. However, since the publication of this report its recommendations have been incorporated by the hospital as a significant strand of the clinical governance framework that they are presently struggling to implement.

The collection of data for the FCCR study was undertaken in a number of ways. The extent to which residents could speak and act on their own behalf marks not only the limit to which on their own they can secure these rights, but also the degree to which staff and others need to advocate on their behalf (Ramcharan 1995, p. 234).

A *communication questionnaire* was, therefore, completed by key workers for 136 individuals (response rate 94%). Questions were asked about how people communicated basic needs and preferences, initiated communication, made requests, understood labels, responded to questions, asked questions, made comments, and showed pleasure or displeasure. A basic scale of continence, mobility and challenging behaviour as well as self-care ability was also rated for each person.

After analysis of the communication questionnaire a sub-sample of 20 respondents representative in terms of communication ability, and other characteristics, were chosen and time was spent with them. A questionnaire guide relating to daily routine, food, involvement in decision making, relationships, ownership, holidays and personal money was used to talk with people about these aspects of their lives. A good proportion of the respondents were able to talk about their lives and experiences in these areas and their appraisals about the service they received. Conversely, there was also a substantial group for whom observation was necessary to examine the types of life they experienced and the advocacy decisions being taken on their behalf.

In summary, it might be argued that the research examined as far as was possible the 'user perspective of the care they received'. However, in the absence of users to speak or act for themselves, the outcomes and quality of care will be represented by the decisions and actions others pursue on their behalf. In research terms it was, therefore, essential to undertake observation of the decisions made and outcomes produced.

Activity 3.7

Where people cannot speak or act on their own behalf your actions will affect their quality of care and, more importantly, their quality of life.

Identify all those decisions and actions you take for or on behalf of service users. What impact do these decisions have on the quality of life experienced by the person? Would they agree with your assessment of the situation? You might find it useful to discuss this with the person themself or someone that is important to the person you are providing support for.

With this in mind two further questionnaires were sent to staff. One was constructed to see how staff viewed their advocacy role and that of the hospital's advocacy project as well as constraints in securing a good quality of life for people (response rate $n = 54$, 49%). The second questionnaire related to issues of physical or psychological abuse between people who have a learning disability and staff and clients. Staff were asked why, if they had witnessed such events, they had not acted and what could be done to improve things. The results of the latter work are not reported here.

Summary of FCCR findings and recommendations

The FCCR research found that there are groups within the hospital whose quality of life was lower than others. These included: those less able to communicate, those with higher self-care needs, and those not allowed or unable to move off the villas unaccompanied.

Their quality of life was substantially reduced. They had fewer day services, were less likely to get off the villa during the day, go on trips outside of the hospital or go on holiday. Given such reduced movement, it was also not surprising that this group did not have the same breadth of relationships as other residents, nor indeed the same positive interactions on the villa.

Activity 3.8

A quality service is marked by the equitable distribution of resources and equal outcomes. Those least able to have their voice heard are likely to be the most disadvantaged where there is inequity in provision. Measuring equitable distribution may address the 'postcode lottery' within any service as part of a clinical governance strategy.

How would you measure inequitable distribution of service provision?

How might you address inequitable provision within your service?

This meant that there were major implications in relation to the rights to 'freedom of movement' and 'freedom of association'. If people could not move around on their own nor attend social, educational or other events then their rights to such freedom remained theoretical unless staff or others were in a position to ensure their movement and association with others. Observation of the comparative experience of individuals living within the hospital demonstrated the effect of the above findings further. For example, those left on the villas during the day were most likely to have higher support needs and lower communicational ability. Yet staff treated villa time during the day as 'dead time', prioritising administration or other domestic work whilst clients slept on chairs, watched the TV or, in a handful of cases, simply rocked in boredom.

It was, therefore, recommended that a *'minimum standards package'* should be operationalised in relation to the spread of support services received, e.g. day services, leisure, trips out and so forth. It was also recommended that these minimum standards should become part of a written 'Duty of Care document' and be considered at an individual level for residents in their multidisciplinary review meetings, or as would now be termed their person-centred planning (PCP) meeting.

Activity 3.9

Minimum standards are one way of levelling the outcome for all users of a service.

Does your organisation already use a standards package? If yes, are these standards agreed with users of the service, and what impact do they have? If no, what sort of standards would improve the quality of your service provision? What do you need to do to implement these?

It will be noted that people who relied upon others to take decisions for them because they could not communicate their wishes and needs were likely to be receiving less services. In this sense the actions of others are 'a surrogate user perspective'. Where the voice of users cannot be heard, then decisions about how to improve quality should be based on principles of the equity of service provision and equity in the outcomes of care and in relation to other freedoms (e.g. of association and movement). Minimum standards are also likely to be a useful 'surrogate measure' of outcome. It is in this sense that the user perspective is intimately tied to advocacy and substitute decision making for those unable to speak and act for themselves.

Recommendations were made on the basis of these findings: the appointment of a peripatetic activities organiser for villas during the day; high staff levels, although seldom experienced, should not be seen simply as a resource for trips out with a small number or only one resident, but as an opportunity for improving villa time and, finally, prompting the advocacy project and user council to address the needs of those requiring higher levels of support (not least because staff felt the advocacy project was providing services for the more able). It was also suggested that there was a need to seek to maximise the social contacts for residents by developing meaningful and sustainable social networks: not seeing trips off the hospital grounds as 'one-off enjoyment', but using clubs where relationships might be struck up; providing dances, cinema, sports within the hospital (many of which had been stopped on the grounds that they somehow infringed the principles of normalisation); and, thinking of new ways of involving the community in the hospital.

Activity 3.10

At the heart of our sense of self and leading a fulfilled life lies the love, support, nurturance, and reciprocity of our relationships. Measuring outcomes is insufficient without fostering and supporting relationships.

What strategies might you employ to support the people with whom you work to develop and maintain meaningful relationships within the service setting and the community?

The emphasis in relation to the FCCR study as outlined so far has been on the 'surrogate' user perspective of staff advocates. One of the vital reasons why this is so important is that the voice of people who have a learning disability is often the voice of those more able to speak for themselves. The proposals so far made have a universal applicability to quality across the ability range of all users and sit largely within Pougher's (1998) 'framework for meeting objectives' category.

But how can the user's voice be heard at an individual level and rights be protected on this individual basis? One of the recommendations of the study was to implement a policy of 'non-negotiables' (Smull & Burke Harrison 1992). Non-negotiables are those aspects of people's lives which they expect as a matter of course. These might be simple things (such as tea made a certain way, eating non-meat products if a vegetarian) or more complex issues such as moving into a new residence as soon as possible or going on holiday yearly. Even for those unable to communicate verbally it would be possible through staff who knew the person well, to establish such non-negotiables. It would be the responsibility of staff likely to be in contact with the individual to know their non-negotiables intimately. Used as part of an individual review process it would be possible, over time, to build up a substantial number of such non-negotiables. These would act as a 'will for living' or a statement of 'personal rights' expressed from the point of view of each user. In doing this, broad level statements about rights could be personalised and infringements made a serious matter. Such an approach personalises the quality of care reflecting most closely the perspective of each individual user.

Activity 3.11

How might you individualise rights for each person with whom you work?

FCCR AND THE CLINICAL GOVERNANCE AGENDA

The FCCR work reported briefly above, and by no means comprehensively, led to a number of working groups with representation from management, staff and residents that have continued to date. These groups were based on partnership arrangements between management, care staff and clients so that they could each claim ownership of their decisions. The FCCR work was given its own logo (a butterfly) and was reported regularly in the hospital's newsletter.

With the opportunity to write this chapter I arranged to visit the hospital again. On my return visit I undertook several tasks: I read through the documentation provided in relation to the hospital's implementation of a clinical governance strategy; I met with the hospital's Unit General Manager and the clinical governance lead to review the FCCR implementation and the new clinical governance strategy; I attended a meeting of the User Involvement Task Group; I visited and talked with the charge nurse of each villa about the FCCR project and about the implementation of the new clinical governance policy within the hospital; and I met a number of residents, many involved in the original FCCR study.

In terms of the ability of the user perspective being heard within the hospital in relation to clinical governance there had, since my previous work, been a number of significant changes. Resident numbers had reduced from 154 to 107 and the advocacy project was not being given as much funding. The project was originally funded largely by the counties and later unitary authorities to which residents would be resettled. Unitary authorities were now seeing their advocacy funding as being more of a priority *outside* of the hospital because of the fall in resident numbers. This meant there was no longer any self-advocacy groups operating in the hospital but, rather, several in the community supported by staff from the hospital advocacy service. The advocacy staff were attending six multidisciplinary case reviews per week but, unlike in previous days, were not able to spend time preparing for each case prior to the meeting. This, together with a reduced number of visits to the villas, led charge nurses on some villas to assert that the advocacy service was not as available as it had been before.

In addition, one of the recommendations of the FCCR project had been in relation to the user's council having more of a say in the management and services in the hospital. However, those being resettled were described as being 'the more able'. This meant that only three members of the user group remained with two of these people moving out at the end of the year. Repeated attempts to recruit more people had been unsuccessful. Therefore, one of the major forums through which the users would have a voice in relation to the quality services was unavoidably rendered impotent.

There had also been a number of changes that had grown out of the FCCR study. A questionnaire issued by the hospital showed that 86% of staff were aware of the aims of the FCCR study and that 63% had looked at the report. Fifty-nine per cent had attended meetings on the standing conference on rights. Of those who had attended meetings, the majority (65%) felt the standards agreed were useful. All staff expressed the view they were more aware of rights.

Immediately after the study a steering group was set up for implementation and four sub-groups relating to: **the communication of residents and advocacy,** practice issues, policy issues, and management, training and research (Box 3.1a, b). These groups were comprised of a broad range of staff, managers, residents and advocacy representatives. On the recommendation of the FCCR study many areas of good practice already happening were catalogued as a basis for working on new developments, i.e. building on the evidence available and working to collect any more of relevance.

Later, the standing conference on rights, which comprised staff from across the hospital and to which all staff were invited, was instituted. In this forum the discussion about resident rights and the implementation of the FCCR study have continued to date. Areas considered drawn largely from the FCCR report are outlined below (Box 3.1a, b), though it is not possible in such a short paper to do justice to the breadth of work that was involved.

Activity 3.12

Improving quality involves systematic review of what is presently happening in your organisation. It involves hearing all relevant voices and drawing on present good practice and other evidence to set targets for change.

Has your service organised a systematic review of quality? What are the key areas that require a review in order to ensure the provision of a quality service? Have service users been involved throughout the process of seeking to plan and implement change?

My meetings with the charge nurses on each of the eleven remaining villas on my return visit also provided an upbeat assessment of the effect of the FCCR study and the subsequent work undertaken in the hospital. The most positive

---

Box 3.1a Range of issues discussed in FCCR groups

Management, training and research:
- How do we measure how well we work with residents?

Policy:
- Knowledge of policy
- Policies that seem to 'choke' each other
- Policies are often hard to understand and cumbersome
- Involvement in drawing up policy
- Training in need for policy and its use
- Blanket use of policies
- Policies that are needed

Advocacy, communication and practice:
- Holidays
- Handovers
- Personal monies
- Equality of opportunity and experience*
- Extending day timetable to include evening and weekend structured activites
- Evening activity freedom of association issue
- Recognising examples of good practice
- Staff stress
- Health
- Cusp of abuse
- Freedom of movement and association of residents
- Documentation of activities of daily living
- Consent
- Privacy
- Confidentiality
- Complaints
- Where rights are not clearly detailed in policy, inadvertent abuse can easily take place
- Involvement of residents in making decisions on the villa
- Staff undertake a substantial amount of substitute decision making
- Key working relationships
- Relationships
- Communication with residents
- Choice and decision making.

* This item is further outlined in **Box 3.1b**.

Box 3.1b   Extract from hospital document outlining the work of the FCCR group considering equality of opportunity and experience

Each area was considered in a standardised way to establish the issue, outline constraints, list good practice, provide recommendations and identify the agents who would lead implementation of any change. This very much reflects the view that:

> Clinical governance is not about reinventing quality from scratch. It is much more about improving and co-ordinating many existing strands of activity ... reviewing the whole system to identify priorities, identifying priorities where action can make a difference and focusing on improving processes to achieve consistent performance (Poxton et al. 2001).

Issues discussed	Constraints	Good practice	Recommendations	Who might do this work?
Equality of opportunity and experience. FCCR findings that those with least skills and least self-help skills have least day services, relationships, holidays, choices.	Many people do not see that there is no equality of opportunity and experience for the least able, and sometimes we look at simple explanations without looking at how we can create opportunities. The constraints in resources, staff, etc., to provide for the least able. Service does not often know what the least able people would wish (dead time). Still a feeling that care is task orientated.	Has been a big change in care plans in focusing on individuals. Individualised outings, activities, etc. Referrals to day service are now individualised and priority is given to the least able. Staff work creatively and innovatively to individualise activities. Some villas record uptake of activities, in particular day services and in some cases minimum standards for leaving the villa.	Minimum standards as part of the 'duty of care document'. Service-wide monitoring of equality of opportunity and minimum standards. Residents' diaries to be considered for a record of their activities. Day services to review all timetable and to produce a report that addresses inequality. MDR to focus on quality of life issues with more attention to likes/dislikes and unidentified needs.	Senior nurse monitoring group. Day services. Senior nurse monitoring group. Charge nurses, primary nurses, professional advocacy group.

feelings were expressed in relation to the effect of the implementation of the non-negotiables in the multidisciplinary case reviews. Typical responses were:

- 'They are used a lot and ... play an important role.'
- 'It seems to humanise the review.'
- 'Somebody's non-negotiable is his ball – removal would be abuse.'

- 'We review them and think about them virtually every day.'
- 'At first I didn't realise its significance. It's part of our culture now. It has changed the lives of residents and changed the attitudes of staff.'
- 'Non-negotiables are coming up as a standard item and staff feel involved.'
- 'There's now lots of choice offering what the client says.'

Additionally, the day services had implemented changes to ensure that all people had a chance to use day services each week. This had meant a redistribution of resources that has benefited people who would otherwise have had fewer chances of leaving their villas during the day. One charge nurse related that they had worked at the hospital for 26 years and more change had taken place in the last 2 years than in all the years preceding put together.

We have established in relating the above story the ways in which change was organised within one hospital in ways designed to establish the voice of users at the heart of their strategy for generating quality services. In August 2000, the NHS Trust incorporating the learning disability services launched a drive to develop and implement a clinical governance strategy. Findings from the meetings with service managers were translated within the hospital into:

- The appointment of a clinical governance lead manager
- A clinical governance newsletter
- Training for staff on what constituted clinical governance
- Setting up a series of task groups, these related to: dysphagia, autism, abuse, behaviour management, alternatives to seclusion, medical records and case notes, medication prescribing, multidisciplinary review, ethics, library, care pathway, epilepsy and *user involvement*.

As part of my visit to the hospital I was invited to attend the User Involvement Task Group. As described earlier the work of the advocacy project had been reduced and the user council was on the verge of folding. The user involvement sub-group was, therefore, having great difficulties in involving individuals in the meetings and had major reservations about the ways in which the views of users might be incorporated both into the task group and in terms of change within the hospital.

In terms of task group involvement there were thoughts registered at the meeting about the possibility of bringing in people who had previously lived in the hospital to advise or represent others within the hospital or, alternatively members of local self-advocacy groups within the community. There are some ways in which this stretches the notion of representation and yet there are good examples of cases in which the merit of non-users of services prove discerning in their judgements about service quality (Whittaker et al. 1990, Whittaker 1997, McIntosh & Whittaker 1998).

But the issue of representation within the task group meetings was complemented by the issue of how to hear the user perspective in terms of service delivery and quality. One of the discussions here surrounded the continued role of the advocacy service, of developing involvement of users in villa meetings and in passing judgements about their services. But it was also suggested that the idea of the non-negotiable clearly linked individual rights to quality outcomes. In this sense it was possible to 'hear' the user voice and to be able to establish a baseline against which standards of individual care could be measured over time. This would go hand in hand with standards packages relating to the equitable distribution of differing services and the experiences described earlier.

There was a general acceptance by the group that, in terms of user involvement in clinical governance, no single solution exists. Rather there is best practice given the circumstances. And it is in this sense that following the evidence base as it exists at any one point in time lies at the heart of any clinical governance strategy.

CONCLUSIONS

The evidence base established through relating the above two stories, though by no means exhaustive, suggests the following. Producing quality services for people who have a learning disability, and others who have an enduring relationship with welfare services, requires substantially more than is indicated in the broader clinical governance literature in relation to the user perspective. The overarching values that Pougher (1998) argues should guide the actions of staff should come not only from the rights agenda, but also from people who have a learning disability themselves. In terms of the framework and tools for accomplishing quality services to which Pougher (1998) alludes, the perspective of people who have a learning disability can be heard through a graded range of strategies from consultation, involvement, participation and, ultimately, ownership by users themselves and each approach has its place dependent upon the issue being addressed. For people who have a learning disability who can and do become involved, major lessons have been outlined about how best to optimise their involvement. These include having the right support, transport, payment and recognition for their participation. It involves service personnel and managers being open-minded and listening to the voice of people who have a learning disability. It will be about providing prior consideration of minutes for meetings, support in the meetings and meetings held using plain language. Participation in developing the framework within which quality services are produced will benefit from an independent user voice such as from the self-advocacy movement. At an individual level the voice of the user can be made central by establishing individual rights and, where necessary, having an independent advocate available to speak on the person's behalf. Lastly, it must be recognised that there are higher level values such as equity of provision across services (i.e. overcoming the postcode lottery) which are central to ensuring quality and the outcomes between individuals and groups.

However, although these may contribute to our knowledge of how best to make the user perspective central to improving quality, there are several cautionary lessons to be taken from the stories outlined above. Firstly, any substantial policy change is likely to affect and undermine efforts at developing a user input in the development of quality services. In the above stories, the policy shift to the NHSCC Act, local government reorganisation and a 'watering down' of the AWS undermined huge efforts over a decade to provide a participatory framework for people who have a learning disability in Wales. Within the hospital, the lack of funding for independent advocacy has reduced the opportunities for people who have a learning disability being supported to have a voice within the hospital. Demographic changes within the hospital because of resettlement have greatly reduced the numbers of people who are willing and able to contribute to the users' council. In short, arrangements for advocacy and support need to be planned independently and to be organised in such a way as to be able to outlast or to survive major policy or other changes. This is one of the important challenges faced in the implementation of *Valuing People* which has committed only £1.3 million per annum over 3 years for the development of advocacy.

Another issue is what legitimacy and power is accorded the user perspective and voice within the clinical governance framework? Is it to be seen as **the** voice that determines the direction of change and the outcomes to which services should work? Is it considered to be a voice to be listened to whilst the decisions about action remain with the professionals? Is it a voice seen as exerting pressure for change? In short, what weight does the voice carry as an **evidence base** and what validity is attributed to this voice? Whilst answers remain to be clarified for these questions it is clear that if the notion of evidence is too weighted to the scientific at the expense of perceived outcomes by users there is a danger that their voice will be stifled. So too will it be stifled by professionals who cannot learn to work in partnership with people who have a learning disability. It is hoped that some of the thinking outlined in this chapter will provide the grounds upon which such meaningful partnerships might be built.

ACKNOWLEDGEMENTS

The author wishes to acknowledge the support of the publishers in part funding a visit to the hospital where this research was undertaken for the purposes of writing this paper, and the management staff and residents of the hospital who gave of their time so freely.

REFERENCES

Atkinson D, Jackson M, Walmsley J 1997 (eds) Forgotten lives: exploring the history of learning disability. BILD Publications, Kidderminster.

AWAP 1991 Consumer involvement and the all Wales strategy: report to the all Wales advisory panel from the consumer involvement sub-group. Welsh Office, Cardiff.

Bank-Mikkelson N 1980 'Denmark'. In: Flynn RJ, Nitsch KE (eds) Normalization, social integration and community services. Pro-Ed, Austin, Texas.

Change 1997 More access please. Change, London.

Crawley B 1988 The growing voice: a survey of self advocacy groups in adult training centres and hospitals in Britain. Values into Action, London.

Davies K 1990 Some issues around consumer participation in service planning and management. In: Ramcharan P, McGrath M, Grant G (eds) Individual planning and the all Wales strategy in the light of the community care white paper. Bangor: Centre of Social Policy Research and Development. University of Wales, Bangor.

Deacon JJ 1982 Tongue tied: fifty years of friendship in a subnormality hospital. Royal Society for Mentally Handicapped Children and Adults, London.

Department of Health 1989 Caring for people – community care in the next decade and beyond, CM849. HMSO, London.

Department of Health 1995 Consumers and research in the NHS. Department of Health, Leeds.

Department of Health 1998a A first class service: quality in the new NHS. HMSO, London.

Department of Health 1998b Modernising social services – promoting independence, improving protection, raising standards. HMSO, London.

Department of Health 2000 A quality strategy for social care: a consultation document. HMSO, London.

Department of Health 2001 Valuing People: A new strategy for learning disability for the 21st century, CM5086. HMSO, London.

Felce D, Grant G, Todd S, Ramcharan P, Beyer S, McGrath M, Perry J, Shearn J, Kilsby M, Lowe K 1998 Towards a full life: researching policy innovation for people who have a learning disability. Butterworth Heinemann, London.

Grant G, Ramcharan P 2002 Researching Valuing People. Tizard Learning Disability Review 7(3):27–33.

Greig R 2001 Partnership boards – discussion paper. Policy_Forum@Maelstrom.st.johns.edu. Friday 5th October.

Liverpool and Manchester People First 1996 Our plan for planning. People First, Manchester.

Lundgren K 1993 Ake's book. Bokforlaget Libris, Orebo, Sweden.

McIntosh B, Whittaker A 1998 Days of change: a practical guide to developing better day opportunities with people with learning difficulties. King's Fund, London.

March J, Steingold B, Justice S 1997 Follow the yellow brick road! People with learning difficulties as co-researchers. British Journal of Learning Disabilities 25: 77–79.

Minkes J, Townsley R, Weston C, Williams C 1995 Having a voice. Involving people with learning difficulties in research. British Journal of Learning Disabilities 23(3): 94–98.

Murray SA, Tapson J, Turnbull L, McCallum J, Little A 1994 Listening to local voices: adapting rapid appraisal to access health and social needs in general practice. British Medical Journal 308: 698–700.

NHS Executive 1992 Health services for people who have a learning disability (mental handicap). HSG (92)42, 26th October.

NHS Executive 1996 Patient partnership: building a collaborative strategy. Department of Health, Leeds.

NHS Executive 1998 Signposts for success – in commissioning and providing health services for people who have a learning disability. HMSO, London.

Nirje B 1969 The normalization principle and its human management implications. In: Kugel R, Wolfensberger W (eds) Changing patterns in residential services for the mentally retarded. Presidential Committee on Mental Retardation, Washington DC.

People First 1993 Oi! It's my assessment – why not listen to me? People First, London.

People First 1994 Helping you get the services you want: a guide for people with learning difficulties to help them through their assessment and get the services they want. People First, London.

People First 1997 Access first. A guide on how to give written information to people with learning difficulties. People First, London.

People First 1998 Access first: directory. People First, London.

People First London, Change, Speaking Up in Cambridge and Royal MENCAP 2000 Nothing about us without us – the learning disability strategy: the user group report. Department of Health, London.

Pougher JD 1997 Providing quality care. In: Gates B (ed.) Learning Disabilities. Churchill Livingstone, Edinburgh.

Poulton B 1998 Shaping care with patients and carers: user satisfaction tools. Nurse Researcher 5(3): 33–42.

Poxton R, Greig R, Giraud-Saunders A 2001 Best value reviews of learning disability services for adults: a framework for applying person-centred principles. Department of Health and Community Care Development Centre, Institute for Applied Health and Social Policy, London.

Ramcharan P 1995 Citizen advocacy and people who have a learning disability in Wales. In: Jack R (ed) Empowerment in community care. Chapman Hall, London.

Ramcharan P 1998 Fostering a culture of civil rights. A report to the Gwynedd Community Trust, Learning Disability Services. CSPRD, University of Wales, Bangor.

Ramcharan P and the combined representatives of self advocacy groups for people who have a learning disability in the Trent NHSE region 2001 Workforce planning: giving us the best in the future by hearing our voice. South Yorkshire Training and Education Consortium, Sheffield.

Ramcharan P, Grant G 2001 Views and experiences of people with intellectual disabilities and their families: the user perspective. Journal of Applied Research in Intellectual Disabilities 14: 348–363.

Ramcharan P, Whittell B, Thomas B, White J 1996 The growing voice in Wales: people with a learning difficulty and self advocacy in Wales. CSPRD, University of Wales, Bangor.

Smull A, Burke Harrison S 1992 Supporting people with severe reputations in the community. Alexandria, Virginia.

Speak Up Self Advocacy 1998 Its my IPP. Pavilion Publishing, Brighton.

Standing Conference of Voluntary Organisations for People with a Mental Handicap in Wales (SCOVO) 1986 Evidence from Welsh voluntary organisations for the Welsh Office AWS three year review. SCOVO, Cardiff.

Swage T 2000 Clinical governance in health care practice. Butterworth Heinemann, Oxford.

Todd S, Felce D, Beyer S 1997 Stakeholder perspectives on the course of the All Wales Strategy. Welsh Centre for Learning Disabilities Applied Research Unit, University of Wales College of Medicine, Cardiff.

Walsall Women's Group 1999 No means no. Pavilion, Brighton.

Welsh Office 1983 The all Wales strategy for the development of services for mentally handicapped people. Welsh Offfice, Cardiff.

Welsh Office 1987 The all Wales strategy for the development of services for mentally handicapped people: review of progress since March 1983. Welsh Office, Cardiff.

Welsh Office 1989 Still a small voice: consumer involvement in the all Wales strategy. Welsh Office, Cardiff.

Welsh Office 1991 The review of the all Wales strategy: a view from the users. Welsh Office, Cardiff.

Welsh Office 1996 The Welsh mental handicap strategy: guidance 1994. Welsh Office, Cardiff.

Whittaker A, Gardner G, Kershaw J 1990 Service evaluation by people with learning difficulties. King's Fund, London.

Whittaker A 1997 Looking at our services: service evaluation by people with learning difficulties. King's Fund, London.

Williams V 1991 Researching together. British Journal of Learning Disabilities 27: 48–51.

Wolfensberger W 1972 The principle of normalization in human services. National Institute on Mental Retardation, Toronto.

Wolfensberger W, Glenn S 1973 Program analysis of service systems. National Institute on Mental Retardation, Toronto.

4

Service user and professional partnerships in the modernisation agenda

Christina Funnell

KEY ISSUES

◆ Changing the culture

◆ The impact of language

◆ Communication and culture change

◆ Partnerships with patients and clients

◆ Partnerships with user representative groups.

INTRODUCTION

I am writing this chapter using 20 years' experience of working with patients, carers and users of health and welfare services. Most of that time my work has focused around the needs of people who have a chronic long-term disease. As such, this chapter will use experiences from the secondary care sector. The issues discussed within this chapter do, however, have relevance for all other sectors.

One of the core concepts of clinical governance is that the patient or client should be at the centre of their healthcare experience. In the paternalistic health service it would have been claimed that this was the case, but in fact the disease or the condition was the major focus of the treatment, and care was built on a narrow medical model with the doctor making all the decisions. In welfare services of the 21st century this paternalistic approach is no longer acceptable. The current expectation is that the individual will be central to their care experience and this means that they are actively engaged in all parts of their care journey and in all stages of the decision-making process. The need for placing the user at the heart of the clinical governance and best value agenda is illustrated in the following quote:

> When acute disease was the primary cause of illness, patients were generally inexperienced and passive recipients of medical care. Now that chronic disease has become the principal medical problem, the patient must become a co-partner in the process (Holman & Lorig 2000).

It is the intention of this chapter to consider the role of patients/clients in achieving the aims of the clinical governance agenda. It will achieve this through exploring the culture of welfare services, both historical and contemporary, and by considering the need to change this culture. In doing this the chapter will address the language used within these services and how this impacts upon the patient's experience and the relationship between clients/patients and practitioners. The chapter will also consider the role of communication in culture change and the importance of partnerships with both service users and representative or voluntary organisations.

POLICY AND CONSUMER INVOLVEMENT

The implementation of the clinical governance agenda can be seen as the most fundamental challenge facing the health service, healthcare professionals, patients and carers that has occurred in the history of the NHS. As such, it has necessitated changes in service delivery, particularly in relation to planning, delivery and evaluation and

the role of the consumer in each part of this process. One of the key structures for achieving this is the National Service Framework (NSF) Programme. These initiatives clearly seek to ensure that the voice of the consumer or patient is heard.

This need to shift from a professional to a client/patient-centred focus is further illustrated by the findings of research by Jenkins, Fallowfield and Saul on the information needs of patients with cancer (2001). In that study they report:

- 87% of cancer patients wanted all possible information, both good and bad news
- 94% wanted to know what all the possible treatments were
- 97% wanted to know what all the possible side-effects of treatment were.

Interestingly, this is a significant increase on a previous, oft-quoted study by Meredith et al. (1996) which found:

- 79% wanted all possible information
- 86% wanted to know what all the possible treatments were
- 97% wanted to know what all the possible side-effects of treatment were.

Therefore, the success of the clinical governance agenda will be overtly influenced by the culture of welfare services. Cultural change is, therefore, the central tenet of the clinical governance agenda. Whilst this is challenging for all professionals, it is particularly challenging for nurses as they are frequently caught between the doctor and the patient. As such, the mediation role undertaken by nurses can have a crucial impact on the effectiveness of many clinical activities and, subsequently, any clinical governance initiatives. Managing this agenda will be a testing process for all concerned, but one worth the effort as it offers possibilities to define new and valued roles for team members and leaders in the change process.

CHANGING THE CULTURE

The NHS Plan (Department of Health 2000a) and the Department of Health report of an expert group on learning from adverse events in the NHS, *An Organisation with a Memory* (Department of Health 2000b) are important documents in laying out the proposals for the new look NHS. Since then there have been a whole series of reports, proposals and publications developing the detail and focus of the changes, both structural and cultural. Two aspects will have particularly far-reaching effects for the health- and social-care professions. First is the creation of major new national bodies with powers to ensure that standards of care delivery are raised. These include;

- The National Institute for Clinical Excellence
- Commission for Health Improvement
- Social Care Institute for Excellence
- The Modernisation Agency
- National Clinical Assessment Authority
- National Patient Safety Agency
- Regulatory bodies for Health and Social Care, e.g. Nursing and Midwifery Council (NMC), Council for Health Professions (CHP) and General Social Care Council (GSCC).

The second aspect is the involvement of lay people, patients and voluntary health organisations in discussions, consultations and the delivery of the NHS Plan, as well as the mandatory inclusion of lay people as members of the executive boards and governing bodies.

Activity 4.1

Write a list of people who you think make up the team where you work. Discuss this with your work colleagues. Did you include patients/clients and carers as part of the team? If not, why not?

Alongside the above developments has been the creation of PALS (Patient Advice and Liaison Services) in every NHS and Primary Care Trust, and the commission for patient and public involvement in health, with patient forums within strategic health authorities, local authorities and Primary Care NHS Trusts. It is also proposed that there be an independent complaints advocacy service. For the voluntary health organisations and 'patient groups' finding enough people with the appropriate skills, expertise and time to participate in all these bodies at a national, regional and local level is a challenge. But it will also be a challenge for health professionals and managers, who will increasingly have to work in a different way, as the old ways of doing things – from decision making to implementation – will not stand the test of time in this more open and transparent environment.

Throughout government policy there has been a constant emphasis on the need to 'change the culture'. The building blocks for clinical governance are identified as:

- changing the culture
- sharing information with other colleagues as well as with patients and their carers
- clear professional leadership.

The culture of an organisation exists at various levels. Within this chapter we are concerned with individual healthcare professionals and how they can adapt their attitudes and behaviour to continue to be fit for purpose and fit for practice in the rapidly changing environment of welfare services. A fundamental aspect in changing this culture is consideration of the language we use.

LANGUAGE: PATIENT OR PERSON

The language used to describe people and events indicates the sorts of models, values and beliefs that are subconsciously held by the speaker. Thus, in nearly every meeting I have attended in over

20 years of working with and for patients and their carers, there has been a debate about how to describe the people receiving the service.

The paternalistic view of the patient has, as its base, the person who is seen as a clinically interesting condition, that comes into the hospital, sits in a bed, has things done to it, and then walks out well and full of grateful thanks to the doctor for 'the cure' and the nurse for 'the care'. This approach places the disease, rather than quality of life, at the forefront of the interchange between the person and the professional and focuses upon medical care. As such, this may have narrowed thinking and resulted in systems that have inhibited a full and open interchange between both these groups of people. It has also created a focus to the healthcare relationship that places the doctor at the centre of the process rather than one in which the treatment of the patient is built around the strengths and expertise of the multidisciplinary team as well as the needs, wants and lifestyle of the person involved.

Activity 4.2

What does the term quality of life mean to you? Talk to a person who uses your service about how their condition or disease impacts on their life. How do they manage to attain what they see as a good quality of life? Thinking about how you defined quality of life at the beginning of this activity, what assumptions might you have made about the quality of life of the person you talked to?

We all know how much our physical, material, social and psychological well-being interact as important influences on how we are able to live our lives. It is just the same for people who have a chronic disease, except they have less control over the physical impact of the disease. It is important

that we strive to ensure that no matter what disease or disability people are living with they are able to achieve their full quality of life. The description of how they perceive that quality of life, and the different values they may place on certain aspects of their lives are important to them, and may be very different from the values defined by the healthcare professional. Respecting the values placed by the individual on what they regard as important to achieving their quality of life is the most important element of achieving a person-centred service. In achieving this it is important to consider how your construct of the physical well-being of a person who is deemed to be 'ill' may lead you to believe that their quality of life is less than your own. For the person receiving services the outcome of such belief systems may be further complicated by the interface between a person's physical well-being and their opportunities for paid employment and subsequently for their social and psychological health.

The medical, technical and pharmaceutical breakthroughs that have occurred during the last 10 years have resulted in the patient profile changing dramatically. Many people with rare and long-term conditions that may have previously been either fatal or disabling, are now leading full and reasonably active lives. These people have as a consequence of their situation become expert on their health needs, their condition and its management, and its impact on their lives, and on the lives of their families and their carers. This is, in part, as a consequence of living with their condition 24 hours a day, 7 days a week, 52 weeks a year. In addition, the increasing access to information both on the internet and in other formats, along with increased longevity and reduced morbidity, has resulted in greater expectations by patients and their carers about the control they have over their lives and what they need from healthcare professionals. In short, their use of health services, and their relationships with health professionals will be radically different to that of patients with acute conditions, or those attending either A&E departments, or GP surgeries.

Within the current context of healthcare delivery the use of the word consumer to describe people using health services has its attractions. However, this word can also be criticised as the consumer movement tends to operate on the principle that their view is the only one that should be considered. Within a healthcare context it would seem to be just as inappropriate to consider the consumer or patient view in isolation from professional expertise as the current situation in which the professional view predominates. In health care the view that the customer is always right can be seen as threatening and potentially confrontational. In addition, for people with long-term conditions the description 'people with ...' or 'people who have ...' may be more accurate, and is for many individuals preferable to the description '... sufferer' which they perceive to be totally demeaning and unacceptable both in relation to the assumptions implicit about their situation, as well as its focus upon the medical model of care.

Overall, the use of either word indicates implicit values and assumptions that may then start to influence the responses of both the healthcare professionals and the consumer or patient within any interactions. Essentially, I suggest that the word patient could be used for people actively engaged in treatment and care, for example, a consultation or a stay in hospital. The word consumer could be used when planning and evaluating services, or when trying to envisage what it feels like to undertake the patient journey in a particular healthcare setting.

Case example

This discussion took place on the UKCC (now the Nursing and Midwifery Council) Higher Level Practice Working Group (UKCC Working Group 2001). It was an important discussion because we

were trying to set a higher level standard which could be transferable across all specialities as well as all settings. For clarity of thought the group decided on:

- **Communities** – a set of people who are united through a common geographical location, a common aspect or common interest.
- **Group** – describes a number of people together who might be considered to be a unit such as the families, partners, friends, significant others or carers of an individual; or a collection of individuals who come together out of a common interest (a patient support group for instance). The interests and needs of groups are not necessarily the same as those of individuals within the groups (such as the differences in need between patients and their carers).
- **Individual** – any person who is the focus of the activity, most often patients and clients.

Therefore, using the phrase 'people who have ...' for example, eczema, diabetes or asthma, is more helpful. It starts from the premise that we are talking about a whole person; someone who is also a wife, mother, daughter, etc. or husband, father, son, etc. as well as individuals who have skills and interests, social concerns, beliefs, problems and emotional difficulties, etc. In addition, this approach goes a long way to acknowledging that people also have pressures, concerns, deadlines to meet, demands on their time, and are part of a family, with work and social interests, networks and communities around them. In short, patients or consumers are people who just happen to have a part of their body that is not working, and is causing problems in living out their daily life.

For many people who live with chronic conditions every day of their lives, going to see the doctor can often be a last resort. When that point is reached, to then have to face delays and waits, and be treated as just a condition or someone in a bed, can be the cause of much distress. Couple that indifference and lack of attention to a situation where only poor-quality information, or no information at all is available, and it perhaps becomes more understandable if the outcome is more and more frequently anger and outrage, and of course complaints.

Clearly for people who suddenly have a heart attack or stroke, or who are injured in an accident, the decision to seek health care is taken for them by circumstances. But they will still be the sum of all their parts, now having to deal with one more thing – sometimes a life changing event. It is important for healthcare professionals to keep in mind the impact that the first engagement with the health service can have. How this is handled can have significant consequences for the individual. Most people make few visits to the GP let alone the hospital, so it can be a sharp learning curve to suddenly have to understand and work out what is happening, what it all means and where everything is, particularly when the healthcare professionals are using technical language and jargon.

Activity 4.3

Talk to a new patient or client about their experience of the service you work in, particularly in relation to first appointment or visit. What did they think about the environment, the language that was used to describe the care they may receive and the approach of the care team?

It may be useful to discuss the outcomes of this discussion with your peers and consider any actions that may need to be taken.

From this activity you may have gained some understanding of how alienating the health service can be on some occasions and for some people. It is, therefore, important to try and remember the following issues at all stages throughout your career:

- To view the organisation and your role in it through the eyes of people visiting it and using it for the first time.
- To hold on to how it must feel to be dependent on others who provide care for their well-being and good health.
- To understand how vulnerable and fearful we all feel when we are unwell and/or very sick.
- To understand that we live in a society where people are used to having 24 hour access to other services – banking, shopping, entertainment for instance, so are not prepared to wait for days, sometimes weeks, for a consultation or treatment.
- To appreciate the impact on working lives for people who may not be able to have time off from work during the day. People who are self-employed, or on piece work risk losing money, or even work, if they can only get an appointment during the normal working day. Imagine the frustration if they plan for an appointment and reschedule their day, and then have to wait a long time, because the clinic is running late?
- To understand the family arrangements that may need to be made for people to keep appointments, for example, those who might have older relatives, children in school, children that are still at home.

Clinical governance is the umbrella term for everything that helps to maintain and improve high standards of patient care and provides a framework to draw these together in a more coordinated way. It is fundamentally about developing a learning culture that is open and shares information. One that is based upon effective multi-professional team working and is about putting the patient first and basing decisions on clinical judgement and what is best for the patient, not just on financial cost. It therefore means that the patient (and/or their carer) is part of the decision-making team.

It is clear from the above, that the individual seeking treatment is balancing lots of different priorities and pressures. Therefore, when that is coupled with anxiety about the diagnosis and the treatment that may be prescribed, it is little wonder that patients and health professionals may describe the consultation in very different ways.

COMMUNICATION AND CULTURE CHANGE

The basis for a lot of the misunderstandings, or lack of comprehension has rightly been put down to communication skills and the provision of good-quality information. All the literature emphasises communication skills (both oral and written) and their importance. Not enough emphasis is put on the ability to listen. Health and social care professionals give lots of reasons for this, chief amongst these being the lack of time. There is, however, reason to believe that time spent early on in the process listening to patients is time well spent. It is at this point that understanding of what patients really want can occur. Understanding the assumptions, expectations, fears and concerns that patients bring to the process will be important in agreeing outcomes and realistic expectations of both treatment and care.

Listening to people and acting on the information they provide is crucial. However, one of the situations patients/clients find hard to understand is that many professionals state that they are short of time for tasks perceived as fundamentally important by those receiving the service, whilst several professionals may have taken the same personal details from them. In this context the question for healthcare professionals is 'what can be done to rationalise the information gathering process in order to be able to release time for issues that patients see as important?'

> **Activity 4.4**
>
> Talk to people who use your service and ask them about their experience of the ways in which professionals gather information and the type of information they collect. Discuss this with a range of professionals with whom you work. Discuss with the team manager whether anything needs to happen about this situation.

PARTNERSHIP WITH PATIENTS AND CLIENTS

The vision for a new, more patient/client-centred NHS is based on the hard evidence that the predominant disease pattern in this country is of chronic rather than acute disease. Increasingly, therefore, it makes good management sense to build on the knowledge and expertise of the person who has the condition. They are the experts on how their disease affects their lives, and the health professional is the expert in the clinical treatment of the disease in general. Bringing the two areas of expertise together in a mutually beneficial and respectful relationship is at the core of creating genuine partnerships between professionals and the client/patient. The aim of working together using the principles that underpin effective partnerships is to seek best solutions for those who use the service. The most important of these principles is creating a relationship where people receiving a service can share their knowledge and insights, can explain their needs and how the disease affects their quality of life, and, where relevant, making information available so that they can live with their condition, and manage it effectively in their everyday lives to gain maximum benefit from the clinical interventions and treatments.

The majority of the voluntary health organisations are for people with a chronic or long-term disease such as arthritis, eczema, diabetes mellitus, mental illness, asthma, stroke and, increasingly, cancers and genetic disorders. People have problems specific to their individual illness but there is also a core of common needs underlying these illnesses. This led some years ago to the creation of the Long-Term Medical Conditions Alliance.

This alliance recognised that the knowledge and experience of patients and their carers was not being used to best effect, either in the development of policy or in the individual management of treatment and care. These core needs include:

- how to deal with acute attacks
- making the most effective use of medicines and treatments
- accessing social and other services
- dealing with fatigue
- managing work
- developing strategies to deal with the psychological consequences of the illness.

Traditionally, these problems have not been comprehensively dealt with by the health service or by other welfare services. However, the nursing profession has long recognised the need for some specialist services and there have been a whole range of appointments made of nurses with a specialist knowledge in one disease area or another in order to attempt to address some of these issues.

Most user groups recognise the benefit of partnerships and good working relationships with health professionals, and work hard to develop and maintain them through training and education programmes, support literature, and often by employing directly, or funding nursing and other staff.

Sharing expertise and building partnership enables the following contributions to be made (Box 4.1):

Box 4.1	
Patient/client	**Clinician**
Experience of illness	Diagnosis
Social circumstances	Disease aetiology
Attitude to risk	Prognosis
Values	Treatment options
Preferences	Outcome probabilities
	(Coulter 2001a)

Where practice is at its best patients/clients are given information and their questions are answered in a reassuring and respectful way. There are a growing number of examples where the person's expert knowledge of her/his condition is developed to the point where they can manage their condition with maximum quality of life, and minimal interruption to their working, social and family life.

Some common experiences of clients/patients are:

- not enough involvement in decisions
- no one to talk to about anxieties and concerns
- tests and/or treatments not clearly explained
- insufficient information for family/friends
- insufficient information about recovery. (Coulter 2001b)

This is despite the observation frequently made by doctors that 'my patient understands her disease better than I do'. In fact, people with chronic long-term disease are experts in their own right for they have had to acquire life skills to cope with the condition and most have the potential to be confident partners with professionals in their care. There is increasing evidence that certain systematic approaches whereby patients/clients – with proper support – take a lead in managing their chronic condition can help to improve health and quality of life and reduce incapacity.

The experience of people with chronic diseases in using health services is very variable. The doctor or nurse may discuss with the person the nature of the treatment and care that he or she needs, and agree a plan for managing the disease. In other situations most attention may be given to the technical aspects of care with inadequate attention paid to the social or emotional consequences of the disease. Too often people with chronic diseases are left to cope with the illness on their own; 'you'll just have to learn to live with it', sometimes feeling – as well as becoming – quite isolated.

The above illustrates how important it is for health- and social-care professionals to use their skills and expertise to help individuals develop knowledge about their disease or condition and at the same time recognising the service users' and carers' insights into the impact of living with the disease day in day out for the whole of their lives. In addition, once the person has developed that knowledge then it makes good sense to continue to enable clients to use that knowledge in order to ensure a person-centred approach to care delivery and, as a result, meet the clinical governance agenda.

Some of the issues which may not be recognised by health and social professionals, but which are critical to patients/clients and their carers are:

- knowing how to recognise and act upon symptoms
- dealing with acute attacks or exacerbations of the disease
- making most effective use of medicines and treatments
- understanding the implications of professional advice
- establishing a stable pattern of sleep and rest, and dealing with fatigue
- accessing social and other services
- managing work
- understanding services available within employment services

- accessing chosen leisure activities
- developing strategies to deal with the psychological consequences of the illness
- learning to cope with other people's response to their chronic illness
- managing the impact of the disease on personal, intimate and family relationships.

One of the difficulties with self-management is that often professionals may use it as an excuse to abdicate responsibility of care to the individual client/patient. This may mean that the person who has a chronic disease is left unsupported and, therefore, disempowered. As such, neither patients nor professionals should see self-management as a replacement for clinical care.

PARTNERSHIP WITH USER ORGANISATIONS

The huge growth of voluntary health organisations has been in part to try to provide some of the above information, as well as offering self help to people who often feel they are the only ones struggling to live with a chronic condition. The impact of these shortcomings is considerable. For the individuals there is the pain and discomfort of the condition, and the limitations which it places on their activity. There are also the more profound consequences for their quality of life and their ability to function fully in society.

In addition, there is also a social cost. These include:

- days lost from work which may result in reduced income for the individual and a loss to both the organisation within which they work and to society
- increased personal expenditure on special treatments, diets, household goods and other aids needed to improve well-being
- the socio-pyschological costs of isolation and social exclusion.

Such costs may be the most damaging to a person who has a chronic condition or disease, and potentially are the least understood of all.

The core component of clinical governance – putting the person first and involving them as part of the decision-making team – is being implemented in the management of chronic disease for all the reasons I have already outlined. Not least of these reasons is that the impetus to change the culture has come from pressure and advocacy over 20 years or more from patient and voluntary health organisations. These organisations and groups have built up an enormous amount of qualitative data on the experience and expectations of the users of services and their carers. These data and information, if used as a base to develop practice, offer healthcare professionals working in the areas of chronic long-term disease unique opportunities to push the boundaries of clinical practice and to challenge old assumptions and ways of doing things.

Activity 4.5

How might you gain information from individuals that you are working with about their wants and expectations in relation to their health care?

Where else might you gain useful and valid information and data about the patient experience in order to inform your practice?

How does this information fit with research-based information?

For healthcare professionals wishing to put patients first and seeking to understand their views there are many ways in which this can be achieved. Many of these strategies already exist and can be found within the following structures and systems:

- through the developing structures within initiatives led by lay people

- engaging with local branches of national voluntary health organisations

- via the self-management movement.

Additional expertise and knowledge to begin the process of changing both culture and behaviour lies within the voluntary health organisations and in the self-management movement. This movement has been strong both here in Britain and also in The Chronic Disease Self-Management Program (CDSMP) developed at Stanford University Patient Education Research Center through a collaborative research project between Stanford and the Northern California Kaiser Permanente Medical Care Program (Lorig et al. 1999). This programme has been developed as a result of 20 years' work with people who have arthritis. The strength of this programme is that it uses professionally trained instructors who have a chronic disease to educate and train volunteer tutors who also have a chronic disease to provide information, support and expertise in areas such as arthritis, diabetes, HIV, stroke and heart disease.

There are five core self-management skills in the CDSMP:

- problem solving

- decision making

- resource utilisation

- formation of a patient/professional partnership

- taking action.

The evidence shows that none of these are in themselves the key to effective self-management. The key is to change the individual's confidence and to generate the belief that they can indeed take control over their life despite their disease. These five skills comprise the toolkit for the individual to deploy as required. A review of the evidence on self-management as a whole, conducted for 'The Expert Patient Task Force' has shown that the benefits of self-management include:

- reduced severity of symptoms
- significant decrease in pain
- improved life control and activity
- improved resourcefulness and life satisfaction.

Within Britain these ideas have been taken forward by a number of voluntary health organisations. For example:

- Self Management Training Programme for Manic Depression begun by the Manic Depression Fellowship in 1998. It is entirely user-developed and user-led. The programme has been designed to enable individuals with a diagnosis of manic depression to gain confidence in their own capacities and to take control of their lives. It is currently the subject of a RCT with good outcomes to date, including improvements in mood sustained 3–6 months after completion of the course.
- Challenging Arthritis (CA) is the name given by Arthritis Care to the arthritis self-management course originally developed at Stanford in 1979. This was launched in 1994. It is also a user-led programme in which all senior staff, self-management trainers and volunteer course leaders are people with arthritis. Over 100 peer-reviewed articles on ASMC have been published since 1980.
- The Multiple Sclerosis Society has begun to train tutors to deliver structured self-management courses based on the Lorig model. The tutors have MS.

A major catalyst in the development of the user-led self-management programmes available to people with chronic long-term conditions was initiated by the Long-Term Medical Conditions Alliance. A 3-year project called Living with Long-Term Illness (Lill) began in September 1998. Lill is reported as having brought about positive benefits for participants, tutors and for participating organisations. In addition, it has provided the basis for research into the CDSMC in the UK and has laid the foundation for the development of generic user-led programmes. During this time there has also been an increase in the number of organisations delivering similar programmes from the two that were in existence in 1998 to thirteen in 2001.

CONCLUSION

This chapter has discussed the role of patients/clients in achieving the aims of the clinical governance agenda. It has focussed upon how patients/clients have knowledge and expertise about their health and well-being that can be used in partnership with expert professional knowledge to provide effective quality care. In particular, it explored the care and support required to meet the needs, wants and expectations of people who use the service in all areas of their life. The issue with regard to clinical governance, therefore, is not whether to involve lay people, patients and carers, or not, but how to do it. In particular, what structures and processes are needed to facilitate professionals and patients to work together in meaningful partnerships in order to achieve a positive outcome for that patient?

REFERENCES

Coulter A 1999 Paternalism or partnership? BMJ 319: 719–720.
Coulter A 2001a The Autonomous Patient – ending paternalism in medical care. The Nuffield Trust.

Coulter A 2001b The Autonomous Patient: ending paternalism in medical care. Class Number: 174.2. Oxford University Press.

Department of Health 2000a The NHS Plan: a plan for investment, a plan for reform. HMSO.

Department of Health 2000b An Organisation with a Memory: Report of an expert group on learning from adverse events in the NHS. HMSO. http://www.doh/gov.uk/orgmemreport/

Holman H, Lorig K 2000 Patients as partners in managing chronic disease. BMJ 320: 526–527.

Jenkins V, Fallowfield L, Saul J 2001 Information needs of patients with cancer: results from a large study in UK cancer centres. British Journal of Cancer 84(1): 48–51.

Lorig KR, Sobel DS, Stewart AL, Brown BW Jr, et al 1999 Evidence suggesting that a chronic disease self-management program can improve health status while reducing hospitalization: a randomized trial. Medical Care 37(1): 5–14.

Meredith C, et al 1996 Information needs of cancer patients in the west of Scotland: cross-sectional survey of patients' views. BMJ 313: 724–726.

UKCC Working Group 2001 Report of the working group. A higher level of practice. Nursing and Midwifery Council. www.nmc-uk.org

---

USEFUL RESOURCES

Arthritis Care
18 Stephenson Way, London NW1 2HD.
Tel: + 44(0)20 7916 1502; Fax: + 44(0)20 7380 6503;
Web: arthritiscare.org.uk

CancerBACUP
3 Bath Place, Rivington Street, London EC21A 3JR.
Tel: + 44(0)20 7920 7233; Fax: +44(0)20 7696 9002;
Web: cancerbacup.org.uk. Provides information, advice and support to people affected by cancer and their carers and health professionals.

Contact a Family (CaF)
209-211 City Road, London EC1V 1JN.
Tel: + 44(0)20 7608 8700; Fax: + 44(0)20 7608 8701;
Email: info@cafamily.org.uk; Web: www.cafamily.org.uk.
Provides help and advice for families who care for children with disabilities, including acute and rare health conditions.

Department of Health Report, The Expert Patient: A New Approach to Chronic Disease Management for the 21st Century. Report and supporting resources for the Expert Patient Programme at http://www.doh.gov.uk/cmo/progress/expertpatient/epp6.htm

Genetic Interest Group (GIG)
4d Leroy House, 436 Essex Road, London N1 3QP.
Tel: + 44(0)20 7704 3141; Fax: + 44(0)20 7359 1147;
Email: mail@gig.org.uk; Web: www.gig.org.uk.
Implications of research in genetics for human health from the perspective of the patient/family.

Long-Term Medical Conditions Alliance (LMCA)
Unit 212, 16 Baldwins Gardens, London EC1N 7RJ.

Tel: + 44(0)20 7813 3637; Fax: + 44(0)20 7813 3640;
Email: rahana@lmca.demon.co.uk;
Web: www.lmca.demon.co.uk. An alliance of over 100 organisations representing people with long-term conditions. Key areas include: influencing policy, membership and self-management.

Manic Depression Fellowship
Castle Works, 21 St Georges Road, London SE1 6ES.
Tel: + 44(0)20 7793 2600; Fax: + 44(0)20 7793 2639;
Email: mdf@mdf.org.uk; Web: mdf.org.uk

Multiple Sclerosis Society
MS National Centre, 372 Edgware Road, London NW2 6ND.
Tel: + 44(0)20 8438 0826; Fax: + 44(0)20 8438 0878;
Web: mssociety.org.uk

Neurological Alliance
PO Box 31287, London NW2 6NL. Tel: + 44(0)20 8438 0902;
Fax: + 44(0)20 8438 0903; Email: info@mssociety.org.uk and nikki@quarryhouse.co.uk. Information provision to member organisations; raising the profile of neurological disorders with government, the NHS and the media.

Picker Institute www.pickereurope.org

Skin Care Campaign
Hill House, Highgate Hill, London N19 5NA.
Tel: + 44(0)20 7281 3553; Fax: + 44(0)20 7281 6395;
Email: plapsley@eczema.org;
Web: www.skincarecampaign.org. Campaigning for improvement in dermatology services, raising the profile of dermatology, running skin information days for health professionals and the public.

Developing and implementing best practice

This section considers a number of the different elements that are essential to the delivery of high quality care and support in order to meet the government's agenda for modernising welfare services. This includes a chapter from Rob McSherry and Shirley Taylor which provides us with an overview of the processes that underpin the development and implementation of best practice. This is further supported by a range of chapters which consider specific aspects of the process such as problem identification, searching for evidence and the role of audit in ensuring that practice has improved and meets the needs of people using the services.

The chapters in this section have been written by people who are very clearly involved in the delivery of evidenced based practice within an NHS context. As such, many of the examples and much of the literature that support these chapters reflects this. However, careful consideration of the concepts included within these chapters should allow the reader to transfer knowledge and techniques to other areas within welfare services.

5

Developing best practice

Rob McSherry
Shirley Taylor

KEY ISSUES

- ◆ The need for evidence-based practice

- ◆ Evidence-based practice: its place within clinical governance

- ◆ Explaining and defining evidence-based practice

- ◆ What constitutes evidence?

- ◆ The various types of evidence

- ◆ Understanding why the methodological approaches were used and the value of utilising more than one type of evidence

- ◆ What is research?

- ◆ Types of research

- ◆ Why do we need it?

- ◆ What is the research process?

- ◆ Skills of critical appraisal

- ◆ The barriers to evidence-based practice within the context of the modernisation agenda.

INTRODUCTION

The purpose of this chapter is to provide a practical guide to the use of evidence-based practice enabling the reader to apply the key principles that underpin evidence-based practice within the context of clinical governance and best value. This will be achieved by providing a general overview of the key attributes akin to evidence-based practice. Furthermore, activities and a case study will be employed throughout the chapter to highlight the interface of evidence within the clinical governance and best value framework. The chapter will open by offering a brief review of the arguments that surround the calls for evidence-based practice within the government's modernisation agenda. Reference will be made to the utilisation of research to inform clinical decision making, which has historically been poorly received across the disciplines. In addition, decision making has also been affected by the lack of evidence from patient/client-centred clinical trials and qualitative studies. As such, an eclectic approach to evidence is called for and to this end a case study will be employed to assist readers in gaining an insight into the key processes that could be employed to integrate evidence into practice. The case study is followed by a section which considers the barriers that have contributed to the apparent lack of enthusiasm for the use of empirical evidence in practice. In addition, this chapter will outline the various and diverse types of evidence that can usefully enhance and advance practice. The approach will implicitly be one that engages practitioners with the realities of maximising the various and diverse sources of evidence available within contemporary healthcare settings. It will encourage practitioners to critically engage with such evidence to enhance decision making at a micro and macro level.

THE NEED FOR EVIDENCE-BASED PRACTICE

The rationale for the development of evidence-based practice is attributed to the perceived decline in the standards and quality of care provision (Scally & Donaldson 1998). The recent raft of measures that have emerged from the government's calls for continuous quality improvement outlined in recent white papers (Department of Health 1997, 1998, 2000) can be seen to have their origins in the following set of factors:

- rising patient/client and carers' expectations
- increased dependency of those who use the services
- technological advances
- demographic changes in society
- changes in care delivery systems
- lack of public confidence in the NHS
- threat of litigation
- demand for greater access to information (McSherry & Pearce 2001).

More importantly, there has also been a growing awareness of the fragility of the knowledge base of the professions. This fragility has led to the development of evidence-based practice being positioned at the centre of clinical governance and best value in the overarching quest for quality enhancement. These factors reflect key changes in society in which lay people have been increasingly exposed to a series of high-profile clinical errors. These have created a loss of faith in what has traditionally been a trusted national institution, that is, the NHS. A recent government quote, 'a series of well publicised lapses in quality have prompted doubts in the minds of patients about the overall standard of care they may receive' (Department of Health 1997, p. 5) reinforces this issue.

Certainly, such issues have resulted in massive costs to the government and increasing scrutiny from external agents. The government's response to this has been the implementation of the concept of modernisation, which has led to the development of a complex set of systems and processes designed to provide a framework for best quality.

Indeed, the system for monitoring the efficiency and effectiveness of these components is currently under the auspice of the Commission for Health Improvements (CHI) and the Commission for Health Inspection and Audit (CHIA) in health, and Social Care Institute for Excellence (SCIE) in social care organisations. A key role of these organisations is to monitor and evaluate the implementation of best evidence as directed by the National Institute for Clinical Excellence (NICE), National Service Frameworks (NSFs) and National Care Standards Commission (NCSC). It is, therefore, imperative that health- and social-care organisations and the professional groups within them are able to internalise and practice from an evidence base. The latter can only be achieved if practitioners have an understanding of the concept of evidence-based practice, how this concept translates in to daily practice and where it relates to clinical governance and best value.

EVIDENCE-BASED PRACTICE: ITS PLACE WITHIN THE MODERNISATION AGENDA

The government's intention is to ensure clear, national standards for services, supported by consistent evidence-based guidance to raise quality standards matching consistency in quality throughout the welfare services with sensitivity to the needs of individual patients and clients, as well as local communities (Department of Health 1999).

From this, it can be seen that support for, and application of, evidenced-based practice is a key feature within the clinical governance and best value agenda. Within this, the needs of individual users of the service are accepted as an important aspect of raising the quality of provision. It is clear from the developments that surround modernisation that the use of research evidence as a basis for service delivery has been formally operationalised within welfare services. It could be argued that this is a significant change in

direction when compared to the focus of the last 15 years during which the concern was ensuring 'financial governance', i.e. financial equilibrium or balancing the books. This focus led to other important organisational issues integral to client care, such as clinical risk, quality, setting standards and measuring client-centred outcomes, receiving little attention. The systems in place within the clinical governance framework are intended to guide the development of an evidence-based approach to care delivery from a macro and micro structure. At a macro level there exists a set of strategies and bodies charged with realising the government's intentions, which include:

- a strategic and managed programme of research to generate the required evidence (NHS Research and Development (R&D) Strategy)
- the systematic appraisal of health technologies (HTA)
- the making available of evidence in the form of expert reviews (National Centre for Reviews and Dissemination)
- the development of research capacity (NHS R&D workforce capacity development)
- the construction of frameworks and standards for specific services (National Service Frameworks and Care Standards)
- a body to decide what treatments should and should not be offered (NICE)
- inspection systems to monitor implementation such as CHIA (Department of Health 1999), SCIE and Registration and Inspections.

At a micro level, practitioners need to be able to situate their role and understand how it fits with the aims of evidence-based practice. Furthermore, they need to be able to utilise effectively the machinery of clinical governance at the patient/client interface. According to Long and Harrison (1996),

Sackett et al. (1997), Cullum et al. (1998) and McSherry and Haddock (1999), to achieve evidence-based practice, an individual needs to have:

- the research awareness skills, knowledge and competence to interpret research material to inform decision making
- a managerial and organisational culture that aids the implementation of research.

Guyatt et al. (2000) add a dimension to this suggesting that such demands are difficult to achieve:

The skills needed to provide an evidence based solution to a clinical dilemma include defining the problem; constructing and conducting an efficient search to locate the best evidence; critically appraising the evidence; and considering that evidence, and its implications, in the context of patients' circumstances and values. Attaining these skills requires intensive study and frequent, time consuming, application (p. 1).

Evidence-based practice is more than just the practicalities of an individual having to read, interpret and utilise research material into practice. To be truly effective, the professional needs to be able to operationalise and integrate several complex components (Box 5.1) into their daily practice. It is evident from Box 5.1, that for a practitioner to provide care, treatment or interventions using an evidence-based approach, they need

---

Box 5.1 Key components required to be operationalised to practice using an evidence base

- Define and explain what evidence-based practice is
- Outline what constitutes evidence
- Describe the various types of evidence
- Understand why the methodological approaches were used
- Value utilising more than one type of evidence
- Resolve the barriers to employing an evidence-based approach to practice.

---

to be informed of and understand the various processes associated with evidence-based practice (McSherry et al. 2001). It is unrealistic to expect a professional to practice using an evidence base if they have not had the underpinning theoretical knowledge or the clinical experience/ exposure, supervisory practice or management/ organisational support to do so. Put simply, you would not expect a car mechanic to change or mend faulty brakes on a car if they did not have the underpinning knowledge and practical experience? Similarly, is it fair to suggest and expect all professionals to practice using an evidence base when they may not have had the underpinning knowledge and practical experience associated with research awareness? Indeed, the complex body of knowledge needed to engage in the repertoire of skills demanded to be an evidence-based practitioner is so vast that pre-appraised evidence is increasingly appealing to busy clinicians.

To ensure that an individual, team or organisation utilises evidence-based practice within the context of clinical governance, it is imperative that organisations support practitioners to be able to develop the knowledge, understanding and skills to practice using an evidence base.

For practitioners to use evidence-based practice within the context of clinical governance and best value, a great deal of demand and pressure is placed upon the individual to work collaboratively and in partnership with other professionals or organisations. This is important in order to acquire the necessary body of knowledge and skills. These factors need to be increasingly debated and acknowledged by those charged with managing and commissioning continuing professional development programmes in an attempt to overcome the diverse backgrounds of the various members of the health- and social-care team. Such diversity has been considered by some commentators (Dingwall et al. 1988, Davies 1996) to create conflict rather than collaboration.

EXPLAINING AND DEFINING EVIDENCE-BASED PRACTICE

The term evidence-based practice has evolved from the desire within the medical profession to ensure the best outcomes for a given treatment or intervention; this is often referred to as effectiveness. The first reference to effectiveness of care was alluded to by Cochrane when making reference to the establishment of the NHS. At this point he suggested that 'all effective treatment must be free'. This concept was expanded upon in the 1970s in the monograph 'Effectiveness and Efficiency' (Cochrane 1972). Despite this history, it is only in the last 5 years or so that the evidence-based agenda has taken centre stage in welfare services. This sudden shift in attitudes and culture could be attributed to changes in the social and economic circumstances imposed on the country by cumulative health- and social-care policy reforms and the impact these have had on services (Walshe & Ham 1997). Health- and social-care management and policy over the past 3 decades have evolved from focusing on efficiency and 'doing things cheaply' to quality and 'doing things better' (Taylor 1997).

EVIDENCE-BASED PRACTICE: A DEFINITION

McMaster University medical school in the 1980s viewed evidence-based medicine as a process that facilitated problem-based clinical teaching and learning that involved students and clinicians in searching for and evaluating the evidence for practice (Taylor 1997). This perception of evidence-based medicine was similar to Cochrane's early works on efficiency and effectiveness, as it focused on the outcome of a given action or intervention. The uniqueness of McMaster's work was the introduction of the 'process' or 'sequential' attributes associated with the concept, yet the processes were not made explicit. A process is defined as 'a series of changes by which something

develops ... a method of doing something in which there are a number of steps' (Collins 1987, p. 671). Relating Collin's definition to McMaster's work, the key stages to practicing using an evidence base begins to emerge:

- a problem is given to the students in the form of a case study
- the students are required to search the evidence associated with the case study
- the evidence is applied to the case study
- evaluation of the effectiveness of their intervention is undertaken associated with the outcome of the case study.

The above confirms that evidence-based practice involves the execution of a series of steps when providing care, treatment or an intervention and in evaluating the effectiveness of that action. Evidence-based practice can, therefore, be viewed as 'the conscientious, explicit and judicious use of current best evidence in making decisions about the care of individual patients' (Sackett et al. 1997, p. 71). Evidence-based practice involves 'the process of systematically finding, appraising and using contemporaneous research findings as the basis for clinical decisions' (Long & Harrison 1996, p.1).

A critical review of Sackett et al. (1997) and Long and Harrison's (1996) definitions confirms that evidence-based practice occurs through the integration of clinical or practice expertise with the best available evidence (Sackett et al. 1996). Essentially, what Sackett et al., and Long and Harrison have outlined is a framework for promoting excellence which fits eloquently within the context of modernisation by encouraging professionals to focus on the problem, the intervention and the outcome.

Essentially, evidence-based practice provides professionals with the confidence that their interventions, practice based, educational or managerial are informed by a current and appropriate knowledge base, where practices and guidelines can be audited and measured against agreed standards (local or national).

The concern for many healthcare professionals is that evidence-based practice may lead to 'cookbook' or prescriptive practices where only one and often the cheapest way is recommended for providing care, a given treatment or intervention. Sackett et al. (1997), Muir Gray (1997) and McSherry et al. (2001) disagree with this notion by suggesting that evidence-based practice is the integration of scientific and experiential knowledge into practice.

Evidence-based practice is not a cookbook approach to care delivery. Evidence-based practice is about professionals using their expertise, practice experience, research awareness and the skills of critical appraisal to decide, on the basis of the best available evidence, the best intervention, treatment or care for the user of the service. Indeed, it replaces 'cookbook' practice, where care was based on authority or tradition because the professional has to provide a sound and rational basis for their decisions. This action alone requires knowledgeable 'doers', professionals who have the skills and expertise to implement evidence and, on occasions, to supervise others involved in providing care and support. To practice evidence-based care, the professional needs to be able to differentiate what constitutes evidence and the various types of evidence.

WHAT CONSTITUTES EVIDENCE?

Muir Gray (1997) addresses the issue of what constitutes evidence and identifies the various types by providing us with a classification that ranks the evidence into a hierarchy of type, and the strength upon which practice can be based (Table 5.1). The strength of evidence is rated I–V, with the best evidence being produced by experimental research in which sources of bias and confounding variables (factors which may influence the results) are controlled.

Muir Gray's work addresses some of the external factors inhibiting the uptake of evidence-based practice by detailing where, how, and the value of certain evidence to informing best practice. The weakness of the information for some practitioners is once the evidence is found it can be difficult to establish its value to practice, again reinforcing the need for health- and social-care professionals to become research aware. A criticism, if any, of Muir Gray's work is the strong emphasis on evidence from a quantitative or scientific research base to support practice as opposed to the value of softer more qualitative approaches.

Quantitative research tests theory (Depoy & Gitlin 1994) in order to provide knowledge on

Table 5.1 Muir Gray (1997) Hierarchy of research evidence

Type	Strength of evidence
I	Strong evidence from at least one systematic review of multiple well designed randomised controlled trials
II	Strong evidence from at least one properly designed randomised controlled trial of appropriate size
III	Evidence from well designed trials without randomisation, single group pre-post, cohort, time series or matched case control studies
IV	Evidence from well designed non-experimental studies from more than one centre or research group
V	Opinions of respected authorities, based on clinical evidence, descriptive studies or reports of expert committees

which to base practice. Concerns have been expressed that if, as DiCenso and Cullum (1998) suggest, the best evidence is developed from randomised controlled trials (RCTs), then some professions such as nursing will be disadvantaged as the methodology may not motivate nurses. In addition, the criteria for such research trials is difficult to adhere to (Reagan 1998, Abbott 2001). Furthermore, Freak (1995) and Abbott (2001) highlight that concern has been expressed about the 'statistical standard' of many published RCTs.

Qualitative research is used to develop theory, insight and understanding (Depoy & Gitlin 1994) and, therefore, plays an essential role in developing the knowledge on which practices can be based. Lloyd-Smith (1996) points out that qualitative research can provide knowledge that quantitative research cannot. Perhaps the most appropriate stance is to value each type of research for what it has to offer, rather than adopt a polarised view of which is the best. The challenge for many professionals is not just about establishing what is quantitative or qualitative research, but about knowing what and how the various types of evidence are relevant to practice. Sackett et al. (1996) regard the best external evidence as research that is not only clinically relevant and frequently from the basic medical sciences, but also related to the accuracy and precision of diagnostic tools and the efficacy and safety of rehabilitative, therapeutic, and preventative interventions.

THE VARIOUS TYPES OF EVIDENCE

Muir Gray (1997) makes good progress in identifying what constitutes best evidence but it does have its limitations. What seems to go unnoticed or unmentioned is the fact that this hierarchy is predominately concerned with completed research outputs and, as such, seems to ignore the basis upon which individuals make decisions relating to the appropriateness of evidence and care delivery. Haynes et al. (1996) and Cullum et al.

(1998) provide an excellent framework outlining the fundamental components of an individual's decision-making processes; these components are referred to as the individual's internal armoury of evidence.

> **Activity 5.2**
>
> Note down what evidence you use to make decisions about client care.
>
> Having undertaken this activity read on and compare your findings with that of the following section in the chapter.

Essentially, the decision-making model outlined by Haynes et al. (1996) and Cullum et al. (1998) uses four internal components or sources of evidence that professionals could enhance and utilise in their pursuit of evidence-based practice. These include: practice expertise, knowledge of research evidence, patient and client preferences, and adequate resources.

Practice expertise

Professionals are accountable for the effectiveness of the care they provide, an approach confirmed by professional regulating bodies such as the Nursing and Midwifery Council (NMC), The General Social Care Council (GSCC) and The General Medical Council (GMC). This perspective essentially makes all professionals:

- personally accountable and responsible for their decisions and actions
- have a duty to monitor and improve their knowledge and competence
- act within their limitations and report any undue concerns.

Taking the above into account practice expertise within the context of evidence-based care, and clinical governance and best value is concerned with providing effective care and support, as well as being able to justify the interventions used by reference to authoritative evidence.

Knowledge of research evidence

It is essential that all professionals are able to access and inform themselves of the latest and highest quality evidence in order to ensure the delivery of the highest quality of care and support (McSherry et al. 2001). To achieve this aim, it is essential that the practitioners are research aware, i.e. have the knowledge, understanding, skills and competence to critically appraise research for its appropriateness to their practice. It is important to note here that while research evidence is at the centre of evidence-based practice, it does not require all professionals to be researchers. This, however, is not to dismiss the complex body of knowledge that needs to be learned for practitioners to competently appraise evidence.

Patient/client preferences

In today's welfare services people are no longer passive recipients of care and support, but expect to be involved and informed in decisions regarding them and their family (McSherry et al. 2001). In order to practice using an evidence base, it is increasingly important to remember that the needs, wants and aspirations of patients/clients and carers must not only be acknowledged, but also integrated into all stages of the care process. Historically, professionals who have been labelled 'disabling' (Pierson 1991, Illich 1976) have played a dominant role in decision making, particularly treating people as passive recipients of their expert knowledge.

The continued emphasis on the risk associated with health- and social-care interventions and informed consent is illustrated through the developments in consumerism and the apparent shift in the relationship between users and welfare services. This shift places individuals at the centre of care delivery with a clear acknowledgement of the person's citizenship and their consumer rights.

Dealing with what are often complex health- and social-care decisions can be daunting for users of the service and the practitioners who work with them. Given the range, and both the perceived and actual risks of many interventions, it is vital that service users are both informed and involved in the discussions surrounding their care, treatment and support. Involving patients and clients in this way, however, requires careful consideration as to the communication of what is often complex information. The professional needs to assess the person's knowledge and understanding of their condition, and involve them in the decision-making processes regarding their care, support, treatments or interventions. To achieve this successfully, the professional needs to be able to access and critically appraise the evidence in relation to the needs of each individual and communicate this information in a style most suited for that person. Inclusion of the service user and their families in the decision-making processes that surround all aspects of their interventions, can result in a better and more qualitative approach to developing and implementing evidence-based practice, which will more effectively meet the modernisation agenda.

Activity 5.3

What approaches could you use to involve service users in developing and implementing evidence-based practice?

In completing this activity you may have considered the use of consumer/patient satisfaction surveys, patient/client stories, complaints, thank you letters, quality of life, and quality of care audits and focus groups.

Resources

Within the clinical governance and best value framework the notion of staff support and resourcing is a fundamental concern in the provision of continuous quality improvements. To assure this for service users it is essential that the organisation reviews and monitors its efficiency and effectiveness. To achieve the goal of an evidence-based organisation research needs to be accessible to professionals. In addition, the professionals must understand the need to base their practice on research, have the critical appraisal skills to evaluate it, time to access it and the skills to implement it (McSherry et al. 2001). The role of the organisation is to ensure that they provide the support, training and education to meet the needs of their workforce. The issue perhaps for some practitioners is not in relating these factors to themselves, but establishing where to find the evidence.

Activity 5.4

Note down what sources of evidence are available to you within and external to your organisation.

Having undertaken this activity read on and compare your findings with the following section in the chapter.

It is evident from Box 5.2 that the resources available to support professionals in accessing the best evidence to develop their practice are vast, varied and sometimes complex to use. For example, searching the various electronic databases for essential evidence can be time-consuming and frustrating. To make this process easier the accessing of evidence could be viewed at two levels: internal to and external to your organisation. To obtain information in the first instance it may prove fruitful to collaborate with other colleagues, departments or local organisations to see if they can help you find the evidence.

Box 5.2	Sources of help and ways of gathering evidence
Internal	External
• Practice development centres	• Local universities
• Audit departments	• King's Fund
• Research departments	• Data search CINAHL, ASSIA
• Organisationally-based libraries	• Internet
• Experts	• Professional bodies
	• Other organisations

Please note that this is not an exhaustive list of resources and sources of help.

For example, contacting your library to see if they provide training and help to enable you to search the electronic databases. If this is unsuccessful then extend your search to external resources and sources such as professional bodies, other welfare services, experts or voluntary organisations. As already stated, the issue for many professionals is not in finding the evidence but in appraising it.

THE IMPACT OF AN ORGANISATIONAL CULTURE ON THE IMPLEMENTATION OF EVIDENCE-BASED PRACTICE

To ensure that evidence-based practice occurs, professionals need to equip themselves with the critical appraisal skills required to rationalise the risks and benefits of care and, indeed, to critique research evidence. To do this effectively requires organisational leadership and service support, sufficient resources and a change in the culture that will enable staff to work in this way. For evidence-based practice to function within the context of clinical governance and best value, and to truly exist and operate effectively, the key components and structures illustrated in Figure 5.1 are required.

According to Figure 5.1 it is essential that efficient and effective channels of communication be established to promote an organisational culture

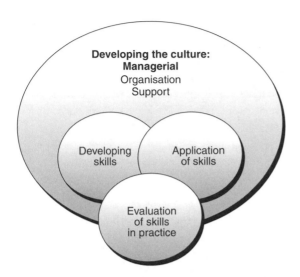

Figure 5.1 Organisation support and evidence-based practice (reproduced from McSherry R, Haddock J 1999 Evidence-based healthcare: its place within clinical governance. British Journal of Nursing 8(2): 114–117, with kind permission).

that proactively develops an infrastructure that nurtures professional and practice development in the pursuit of excellence in practice. This can only be achieved by ensuring that the services provided are staffed with appropriately skilled, knowledgeable and competent practitioners who are then actively supported to further develop, apply and evaluate the skills provided with the aim of improving the quality and standards of care and treatment delivered to patients/clients.

As already suggested, in order to practice using an evidence base within the context of clinical governance and best value it is imperative that organisations provide the necessary resources and support to their staff. As alluded to earlier, in order to practice from an evidence base professionals require regular 'practice exposure and experience'. This is essential for practitioners to become familiar and competent in balancing the risks and benefits of particular treatments, interventions or care and support, that deal with the person's unique set of circumstances. This should be supported by opportunities for the practitioner

to develop skills and competence in relation to new ways of working.

Following the creation of an appropriate environment and culture which supports the development of evidence-based care, the following are needed in order to practice evidence-based care:

- what is research?
- types or approaches to research
- the research process
- skills of critical appraisal (McSherry & Haddock 1999).

What is research?

Ultimately the aim of research is to improve the standard and quality of the service users' life/experience by enhancing the treatments, interventions or care provided. As such, research attempts to 'increase the sum of what is known, usually referred to as a body of knowledge, by the discovery of new facts or relationships through the process of systematic scientific enquiry' (Macleod-Clarke & Hockey 1989). Within clinical governance this is about developing new practices and testing out current practice to ensure the best outcomes for the patient/client/carer and professional.

Types of research

There are two key research approaches; 'quantitative' or 'qualitative' (Seers 1994, Cormack 1996, Burns & Grove 1997). Within these two broad approaches there are a number of different methodologies that can be employed to guide research projects.

Quantitative research is seen as a more systematic, formal or objective approach associated with using numerical and statistical data in the pursuit of answering questions. The research usually attempts to answer questions associated with frequency or occurrences to make reliable and valid measures of a concept in order to produce results that can be generalised. Based upon this quantitative research is seen to test theories (a deductive approach), and uses these as its start point. Examples of research designs include experimental, attitudinal or survey designs (McSherry 2000).

Qualitative research, however, is seen as a more subjective approach that uses life experiences, personal accounts, diaries or observation of a given phenomena or event in order to understand the meanings behind the occurrence. Typically, this is achieved through the use of focus groups, semi-structured interviews or participant and non-participant observation. Unlike quantitative research, qualitative research encourages the development of theories (inductive approach) from the observations of individual or group practices. Qualitative research has much utility in the welfare arena, especially given the increasing emphasis on the user perspective, as it can reveal the experiences and perceptions of the individual.

When considering the value of any research, it is important to consider whether the chosen methodologies are appropriate in the context of the area or issue being explored. Within this, it may be useful to explore the added value that may be given by the use of multi-method approaches.

What is the research process?

The 'research process':

- is a framework made up of a sequence of logical steps within which research is carried out
- provides a chronological list of the tasks to be performed in order to complete successfully a research project
- can be used as headings in writing up your research report (Parahoo & Reid 1988).

The research process (framework) as offered by Hawthorn 1983, Cormack 1996, and Crombie 1997, provides a foundation upon which to build critical appraisal skills essential for developing or examining any research (McSherry 2000).

Skills of critical appraisal

The importance of critical appraisal and its application to practice is well documented (Crombie 1996, Parahoo & Reid 1988, McSherry & Haddock 1999). However, a fundamental issue facing many professionals is the acquisition of the knowledge, skills and experience to critique effectively.

Rosenberg and Donaldson (1995), Crombie (1996) and Sackett et al. (1997) suggests that critical appraisal is about considering the relevance of a research question, evaluating the evidence collected in order to answer the question as well as assessing the effectiveness of the conclusion and recommendations. In a simple way it is about systematically reviewing and questioning the stages of the research process, e.g. literature review, methodology, results, discussion and recommendations (McSherry & Haddock 1999). Crombie (1996) offers the following framework to aid this process:

- Is it of interest?
- Why was it done?
- How was it done?
- What has it found?
- What are the implications?
- What else is of interest? (Crombie 1996, p. 3)

Whilst many professionals are now equipping themselves with the skills of critical appraisal, many are now attempting to identify the interface between this and the implementation of both evidence-based practice and clinical governance. The section that follows explores this in more detail by providing a ten step guide (Fig. 5.2) to improving the standards of record keeping.

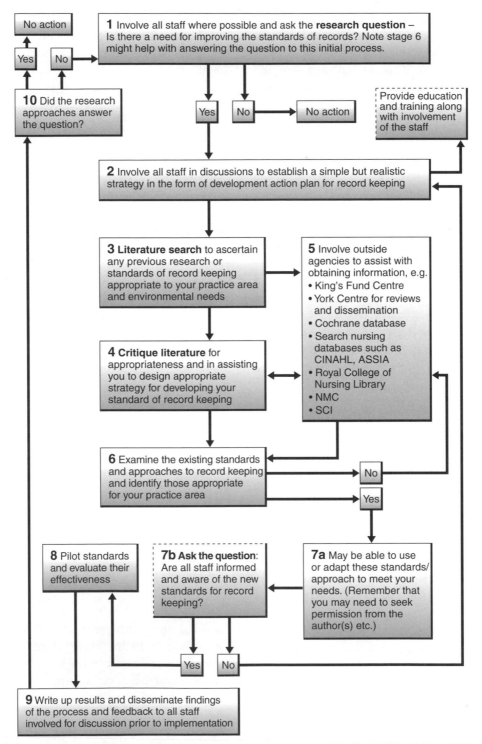

Figure 5.2 Evidence-based practice in action: improving the standards of record keeping (adapted from McSherry 1999, with permission from Nursing Times).

Activity 5.5

As a professional you have become aware that your organisation is concerned about the standard of record keeping. It is their intention to use an evidence-based approach to developing quality standards and you have been co-opted onto the working group.

Write down the processes that you would go through to explore this area of your practice and then compare your notes to the remainder of this section of the chapter.

The following steps are reproduced and adapted with kind permission from Emap Healthcare Ltd. The works of: McSherry R 2000 Researching clinical supervision. In: Bassett C (ed) Clinical supervision: a guide for implementation. Nursing Times Books, London; McSherry R, McSherry W 2001 Putting research into practice. Nursing Times 97(3): 36–37 are acknowledged accordingly.

Figure 5.2 outlines the ten steps to integrating critical appraisal within the evidence-based practice, clinical governance and best value framework. Steps 1–6 support the implementation processes using record keeping as an example and steps 7–10 focus on the evaluation process.

As outlined in chapter 1 the modernisation agenda is about creating an environment in which clinical excellence will flourish. This can only occur where staff are encouraged to participate within the development of new and the evaluation of existing standards and practices. The framework outlined in Figure 5.2 supports this notion by encouraging staff involvement, ownership and collaboration with outside agencies. In addition, it supports the integration of an evidence-based approach, i.e. accessing and critiquing the best evidence. The key points to supporting practitioners to use an evidence-based

approach to clinical governance and best value can best be summarised as follows:

Step 1 – Relevance

Establish whether there is a need to review the current standards in practice.

This can only be done by informing and involving staff, which includes communicating why the concern has come to light, e.g. information from analysing risk management data. Time well spent at this stage in the process can lead to the more effective use of time later in the process.

Step 2 – Staff Ownership

Encouraging participation as this can enable the development of a simple but reliable action plan that is shared, owned and most importantly agreed by all.

If the team are in favour and have a feeling of shared ownership for the project, then the allocation of key roles and responsibilities within the process can be effectively shared.

Step 3 – Literature Searching

Ensure you access all relevant literature, rather than rely on what is easily accessible.

This will ensure that you are appraising the most appropriate data to inform your proposed change.

Step 4 – Involve Outside Agencies

It is important to utilise internal and external sources of help when developing new or evaluating existing standards and practices.

The sources to aid this are enormous and easy to access given the advances in information technology.

Step 5 – Critiquing the Literature

It is important to utilise an established approach to this part of the process. Information should be critiqued for its usefulness and effectiveness in meeting your unique set of practice needs.

Step 6 – Examining the Existing Standards

Examine the existing standards offered in the literature and associated evidence to establish which standards best meet your unit, ward, department, team or individual needs.

Step 7 – Putting the Standards into Practice

Having examined the available standards you may be able to incorporate them into your practice without any changes or with slight modification. You must ensure that approval is obtained from author(s) or you do not breach copyright legislation.

Following the examination of the information some practical considerations and questions need to be asked. In order to demonstrate the essence of this part of the process the example of record keeping will be utilised:

- Why keep records? – records form the basis for planning care and treatment and in obtaining feedback on their progress and in suggesting action for future work.

- Are records legal documents? – this is an essential issue and involves answering questions associated with what constitutes a legal document. Who should sign or write in the records and what should you do if you make a mistake in writing.

- Types of records? – it is essential to establish what constitutes a nursing record for example, and what will be evaluated. Records seem to be unlimited and varied making almost anything pertinent to the patients' care.

- How do you establish a standard of record that could be audited? – there are several written standards/guidelines available outlining ways of evaluating the standards of record keeping such as

the UKCC (1998) and National Health Service Executive (1993).

Having established your newly devised standards, in this example for record keeping, it is essential that they are implemented and evaluated after an agreed period of time (pilot study).

Step 8 – Pilot Study

Test the effectiveness in practice by using a pilot study.

The pilot study will ensure that the standards are achievable and that the new initiative/innovation is practically suitable to your individual, team, ward or department. This is where the quantitative and qualitative approach to research will help. The evaluation of set standards requires the devising of an auditing strategy and template so that the standards can be systematically audited.

Numbers or figures along with the feedback from staff and extracts taken from the audited records can be used to demonstrate achievement of the set standards.

Step 9 – Dissemination of Information

Communicating the information about best practice in order to ensure success.

Once audited the findings can then be reported. After discussions with the team, organisation or other professional colleagues recommendations can be made with regard to the results.

Step 10 – Evaluation

Evaluation of the new way of working will identify how successful implementing the evidence into practice has been. Using the example of record keeping an evaluation strategy could be based on the following:

- Every 2 months two members of staff from different teams evaluate a set of ten randomly selected records and assess the level of compliance against set standards.

- The data are recorded separately for each set of notes resulting in a yearly sample selection of 60 sets of records.

- The findings are established where a summary report comprising of all ten sets of evaluated records is presented to the team or teams, outlining any necessary action to be taken. The yearly results are collated and a report presented on the overall progress in the standards of record keeping.

In conclusion, the case study illustrates how evidence-based practice can be utilised within the context of clinical governance and best value frameworks. In this instance the research process provides a flexible and systematic framework directed towards improving the standards of care. The ten step guide encourages an evidence-based approach by engaging professionals in the processes and, consequently, developing their skills in the gathering of information, literature searching and critiquing the evidence. Furthermore, the guide to promoting evidence-based practice facilitates an evaluative culture by exploring the efficiency and effectiveness of interventions by using audit or bench marking where set standards are measured against recognised guidelines.

The next section explores some of the issues hindering advances in practice and the application of evidence-based care and, as such, highlights the problems that practitioners face when attempting to apply a clinical governance and best value framework.

THE BARRIERS TO EVIDENCE-BASED PRACTICE AND THE MODERNISATION AGENDA

This section of the chapter is reproduced and adapted from the works of McSherry and Pearce (2001) with kind permission from Blackwell Science Publication.

For some organisations, teams and individual practitioners, evidence-based practice and, indeed, clinical governance, is yet another 'thing' imposed on them by the government as a response to high-profile cases that have highlighted inadequate standards and practices. These cases have affected the public's confidence in the welfare services, a confidence that now requires rebuilding. As such, clinical governance 'is much more than a set of bureaucratic systems' (Harvey 1998, p. 8) it is a framework that is designed to improve standards and quality of care. To achieve the aims of clinical governance, i.e. reduce clinical risks, promoting continuous quality improvement and provide best practice based upon the best evidence, a shift in attitudes and culture is needed. Cullen et al. (2000) states that we need to change the culture of organisations; to do this 'we need to unlearn some old habits and develop some new habits'. This view is supported by Davies et al 2000 who states that we need to 'change the way things are done around here'. The barriers implicit within such a culture are outlined in Box 5.3.

Box 5.4 shows that the barriers to implementing evidence-based practice originate from internal and external sources which can affect the organisation, teams and individuals directly or indirectly.

Box 5.3 Examples of perceived barriers to implementing evidence-based practice within the clinical governance and best value frameworks

- Lack of understanding
- Fear
- No clear vision
- It's nothing new, it's a passing fad
- Lack of time
- Lack of resources
- Tool of the management
- Lack of support
- Poor information/no information
- Poor leadership
- Ineffective communication.

Box 5.4 Internal and external factors influencing the implementation of evidence-based practice within clinical governance and best value frameworks

Internal	External
Individual	*Individual*
Lack of knowledge	Lack of support, i.e.
Lack of understanding	peer, management or
Lack of confidence	organisational
Lack of ownership	Lack of resources, i.e.
Fear of what's about or	personnel
being left behind.	Lack of time
Resistance to change	Ineffective
Ineffective communication	communication
Information	Information
Organisation	*Organisation*
Culture: openness, trust	Political pressure
Leadership styles	Increased demand on
Lack of ownership	already overstretched
Management styles	services
Proactive/reactive approach	Increased performance
to change management	targets
Ineffective communication	Public expectations
Information	Increased litigation
	Lack of resourcing, i.e.
	financial backing

Box 5.4 clearly identifies the internal and external barriers affecting the implementation of evidence-based practice within clinical governance and best value and demonstrates the inter-relationship between the organisation, the individual and internal and external drivers. The areas noted clearly fall into a number of themes. These include: culture, management, leadership, communication, education, and training and knowledge.

Activity 5.6

Focusing upon your own organisation, department, ward, unit or team, what are the barriers you face when trying to implement evidence-based care? You may find the above headings useful to organise your thinking.

Culture

Culture is defined as 'the skills and arts, etc. of a given people in a given period; civilization… improvements of the mind, manners etc. …development by special training or care' (Collins 1987, p. 214). The focus upon culture has become prominent within the NHS and other statutory services as a result of the many failures of the systems and processes. This is further reinforced by the high profile professional misconduct cases across all sectors. The use of the word 'culture' or phrases like 'open or closed culture' have emerged following the publication of inquiries into clinical errors in care delivery, as highlighted by organisations such as the CHIA and the National Care Standards Commission. These challenges have resulted in the need for professionals to question the culture they work within and its impact upon evidence-based care, clinical governance and best value.

Activity 5.7

Why is it important to create the right culture in welfare services in order to promote evidence-based practice?

How would you create the right culture for an organisation, team or individuals to provide practices based on best evidence?

As outlined earlier in the chapter, to achieve evidence-based practice within all aspects and provisions of welfare services, professionals should be encouraged and empowered to develop, apply and evaluate their practices at an individual and organisational level. An organisation that nurtures a culture and an environment that is proactive, and recognises the value of sharing and learning is the most effective (Department of Trade and Industry 1997). To engage in and apply the processes associated with evidence-based practice within the clinical governance and best value frameworks the whole notion of having a sharing culture, shared learning, shared effort and shared information are key attributes to high productivity and quality. For evidence-based practice and, indeed, clinical governance and best value to become a reality for any organisation the cultural barriers associated with a lack of openness, mistrust between employees and employers, closed cultures, stifling innovation, undervaluing and not rewarding staff need to be resolved in an open and transparent way. Organisations that are innovative, involving staff from all levels of the organisation and clients/patients/carers are an ideal platform for the implementation of modernisation and the practising of evidence-based care. Haslock (1999) suggests that 'for clinical governance to raise standards in a genuine and lasting fashion it must be developed in a supportive, blame minimizing, educational atmosphere'. The same is true of best value.

The challenge for some organisations, teams and individuals is how to develop such a culture within their work place. In order to achieve this it is necessary to identify the type of culture within your present organisation or team. Hawkins and Shohet (1989) identify five types of culture: blame, bureaucratic, mistrust, reactive and proactive. For evidence-based practice to become the norm within the context of modernising services, a proactive culture of learning from mistakes and each other is the most appropriate. This is because an environment or culture that seeks to apportion blame only leads to secrecy, mistrust and a failure to report mistakes where a knee jerk reaction to resolving the incident is taken.

For example: a practitioner administers the wrong medication to a service user. This results in no harm to the person. The immediate response of the management was to discipline the member of staff who received a written warning on their personnel file. A classical case of reactive knee jerk culture that actively seeks to apportion blame because of failure to rigidly adhere to policy and procedure.

This example demonstrates an example of a culture that is bureaucratic, reactionary, closed and apportions blame. In an organisation that is identified as having a learning or proactive culture, the response may well focus more upon the processes and policies relating to this issue rather than taking any action against the individual. This approach treats the whole incident as a learning opportunity for the individual and the organisation and, where appropriate, offers support to all concerned. As a result, lessons learned from this incident would be disseminated throughout the organisation in a way that avoids naming, blaming and shaming of individuals. Such a culture is more likely to support the implementation of evidence-based practice. This type of culture will be more successful if it is supported by effective management and leadership.

Management, management styles and leadership

The management style of an organisation has a significant impact on how evidence-based practice is perceived and implemented. Management and leadership are often perceived as the same thing, however. Marquis and Hutson (2000) suggest that management is about guiding and directing staff and resources, as well as being concerned with having the power and legitimate authority. Essentially, management is primarily concerned with outcomes and the manipulation of resources to achieve the desired outcome(s).

Conversely, Fagin (1990) defines leadership as the ability to bring about change, whilst Tappen (1995) describes leadership as being about the skills, process and ability to influence others. Slim (1996) articulates the difference as follows:

There is a difference between leadership and management. Leadership is of the spirit, compounded of personality and vision; its practice is an art. Management is of the mind, a matter of accurate calculation ... its practice is a science. Managers are necessary; leaders are essential.

Mullins (1996) identifies leadership behaviours as: mutual confidence and trust, an ability to understand work problems, demonstrating a real interest in the problems and issues of staff, helping with their development, sharing information on all levels, actively seeking opinions about work problems, being approachable, and, finally, giving credit and recognition when due.

Previously in welfare services effective management was valued more than good leadership. Stewart (1996) suggests that in 'difficult times, people need leadership as well as management' (p. 3). As such, this is an approach that has resonance in today's welfare services where leadership is increasingly valued. The impact that an approach in which management and leadership

are integrated can only have advantages in relation to the implementation of evidence-based practice and clinical governance. In this instance, management iscrucial in both highlighting key leaders to take on the roles and responsibilities for advancing care delivery and in empowering staff to do this effectively.

The impact of different approaches to management on promoting evidence-based practice

Marquis and Hudson (2000) identify several theories that have influenced the management of the NHS; these can be categorised under three broad headings, outlined in Table 5.2.

It is evident from Table 5.2 that for evidence-based practice to be implemented successfully within the context of clinical governance the three

Table 5.2 Management styles and their applicability to developing evidence-based practice within the context of the modernisation agenda

Theory	Description	Applicability
Scientific management	Based on scientific principles Efficient and effective use of resources Having the appropriate staff and qualifications Retaining and developing the staff Valuing and rewarding staff Cooperative relationships between managers and personnel	This management style is suited to the development of evidence-based practice because it links nicely to the notion of performance management. Performance management has been associated with the continuous development and rewarding of staff and the monitoring of outcomes based upon best practices or guidelines.
Management functions	Planning Commanding Controlling Coordinating Organising Staffing Directing Reporting	This type of management style is essentially related to the core aspects of the evidence-based practice and the clinical governance framework because it fits with almost all of the key components. For example, command and control are associated with 'accountability'. Staffing and reporting are associated with performance management and clinical risk. The planning and coordinating are related to quality improvement. All of which if managed efficiently and effectively will aid with the development and application of evidence-based culture.
Human relationships management	Involving staff Valuing staff Staff participation Involved and shared decision making	This management style pertains to the humanistic element of clinical governance and best value and the notion of working in teams, sharing and learning from each other when things go well or not so well along with the involvement of the patients who are viewed as an essential asset when developing evidence-based practice.

Adapted from McSherry & Pearce (2001) with kind permission of Blackwell Science Publications.

main management styles need to be applied at the organisation and team levels.

Activity 5.8

What is the management style or combination of styles that exist within your area of work?

How can you manage the situation in order to increase the likelihood of success when implementing evidence-based practice?

Leadership

As mentioned in the previous section managers are essential for the efficiency and effectiveness of an organisation and team. However, this is not to say that all good managers possess the attributes that make them successful leaders. For evidence-based practice to work within the systems and processes aligned to modernisation, we need leaders who can 'make others feel that what they are doing matters and hence makes them feel good about their work' (Stewart 1996, p. 4). This notion of empowering, involving and valuing staff is fundamental in developing the culture in which evidence-based practice will operate effectively. The following are identified as the essential attributes of an effective leader in promoting evidence-based care within clinical governance:

- visionary
- communicator
- facilitator
- advocator
- critical thinker
- doer
- evaluator
- respectable
- knowledgeable
- tactful.

These are demonstrated in Table 5.3 within the context of key leadership styles.

Table 5.3 Leadership style and applicability to promoting evidence-based practice within clinical governance and best value

Theory	Description	Applicability
Authoritarian	Strong control Gives commands Communicates downwards only Does not involve others in decision making Apportions blame	This type of leadership is destructive and inappropriate for the implementation of evidence-based practice within clinical governance. The whole style is at variance with the openness and sharing of the evidence-based philosophy.
Democratic	Less control Directs by guidance Two way process of communication up and down Shared decision making Uses constructive criticism	This is the preferred leadership style for implementing evidence-based practice within modernisation. It offers a strong vehicle for breaking down the barriers by the development of a collaborative, empowering and trusting culture based upon a bedrock of communication and partnership. This is an ideal medium for the sharing and learning from mistakes and good practices
Laissez-faire	Little control Limited direction Communicates well Devolves decision making Group orientated Does not criticise	This style, whilst containing some elements central to the development of an evidence-based culture, is not without its limitations. Constructive criticism is necessary within the context of using evidence-based practice.

Adapted from McSherry & Pearce (2001) with kind permission of Blackwell Science Publications.

Table 5.3 describes how having a democratic leadership style is potentially the most suited for implementing an evidence-based approach. However, the implementation of evidence-based care within the context of clinical governance and best value will not become a reality without efficient and effective channels of communication, training/education and knowledge.

Communication, education/training and knowledge

Communication

Effective communication is an integral ingredient for the successful implementation of evidence-based care and clinical governance. It is through the application of an evidence-based approach to care that effective communications between and within the various systems and processes associated with clinical governance and best value occur. For example, the providing of information to a client by a professional in support of their actions or in explaining a treatment or intervention requires the application of several evidence-based processes. These include: accessing, reading, and critiquing information or data for its or their appropriateness to support the intervention.

A failure in communication between or within organisations, teams or individuals may result in complaints about care delivered. Complaints in the main are linked to a failure in communications associated with 'staff attitudes, poor inter-team communication or lack of information for patients'/clients' (O'Neill 2000, p. 817). For evidence-based practice to become an integral part of the systems and processes akin to clinical governance and best value, open channels of communication between and within all levels of the organisation, teams and individuals are vital. Efficient and effective channels of communication are essential in advancing and enhancing practices and in achieving evidence-based practice. Evidence-based practice is about sharing and

learning from each other where teamwork, partnerships and mutual collaboration are essential ingredients in creating a culture in which excellence becomes the norm. Clinical governance and best value is about creating the right culture. These frameworks are not designed to work in a uni-disciplinary manner; it needs teams and the individuals within the teams to collaborate together. Similarly, evidence-based practice requires individuals to share, learn and network in developing and evaluating new or existing standards of practice. Indeed, for evidence-based practice and clinical governance to become effective, a team-based organisation or system(s) which rely upon the 'direct or indirect support and influences of others, either from their own or other professions or work groups' is essential (Northcott 1999).

One could assume that if we find it difficult to communicate effectively with each other and with clients, what can one expect to find when it comes to reviewing standards and when faced with the challenge of implementing evidence-based practice at an organisational, team or individual level? For evidence-based practice to occur within the context of modernisation, communications should be based on having an appreciation and understanding of your individual roles and responsibilities and having an open channel of communication between and within the organisation, teams and individuals with whom you work.

To practice evidence-based health care you need the ability to:

- actively listen
- express concerns
- trust
- work in teams
- develop partnerships
- collaborate
- respond
- take action.

Education and training

The education and training needs of those who work within welfare services should be considered on an organisation-wide and care-theme basis. To achieve this aim, the education and training of all staff should be based on the premise that knowledge and skills are determined by the individual's role and responsibilities. To ensure that this happens, the employee and employer have a mutual responsibility to ensure that education and training are provided at a local level. The employee should make known through their individual personal development plans that they have a development need associated with evidence-based practice, for example, having the ability to read, interpret, critique research or search the evidence. To address such education and training needs, employers should seek to establish the educational needs of their employees, perhaps through the development and implementation of a staff 'research awareness questionnaire' (McSherry 1997). Likewise local universities providing courses need to develop evidence-based practice modules to educate both their pre- and post-qualifying students about evidence-based practice and its place within the clinical governance and best value frameworks.

The development of any educational programme for teams or individuals should be linked to demands of the local organisation or educational requirement. Any devised education programmes should be evidence based and encompass the following:

- multi-professional approach
- collaborative in nature
- practically focused
- utilise variety of teaching and learning methods
- competency based
- evaluated regularly.

An example of an education programme could be based on the following:

- Aim – to provide an introduction to evidence-based practice within modernisation
- Learning outcomes:
  - to describe what is meant by evidence-based practice within clinical governance and best value
  - to describe the key processes and components of evidence-based practice
  - to describe what evidence-based practice means in relation to individual practice
  - to apply the concept of evidence-based practice to clinical case studies identified from practice
  - how to locate evidence and sources of information
  - to evaluate the effectiveness of the course on the individual's understanding of evidence-based practice in relation to their practice.

All evidence-based practice education programmes should be about learning from the practical experience gained in the workplace. This approach to shared and problem-based learning is more likely to be successful, an approach advocated by the following statements:

Learning in teams, developing multidisciplinary education and training across different agencies, is the way forward for creating learning environments. It will help healthcare professionals to work in partnerships in sharing ideas and solving problems that focus on what is important for patients (Squire 2000, p. 1015).

New approaches to undergraduate medical education, such as the introduction of problem based learning, joint education with other professional disciplines, should in time improve teamworking skills; the importance of team working has been emphasized by the General

Medical Council (Scally & Donaldson 1998, p. 65.)

To foster this approach to shared learning and problem solving relating to the development, implementation and monitoring of evidence-based practice within clinical governance and best value requires financial and resourcing support in enabling staff to have the time and resources to develop their knowledge, skills and understandings of the evidence-based processes and how these relate to the modernisation agenda. The latter cannot be achieved in isolation but in true partnerships formed between employers and employees.

CONCLUSION

Evidence-based practice can be difficult to achieve within current work contexts unless professionals are evidence informed, that is, have the knowledge, skills and understanding of research that is appropriate to their roles and responsibilities. To achieve this within the clinical governance framework in health or social care, an evidence-based culture is needed where managers and leaders support and invest in their professionals to achieve the best standards of practice and outcomes from their staff and service(s). The latter will only become the norm where honest and open channels of communications are developed within the various systems and processes aligned to clinical governance: risk management, practice development, research and audit. Without efficient and effective communication, information gathering and sharing could be hindered resulting in a 'not so good' performance. To ensure that standards are of the best quality, evidence-based practice needs to be supported and encouraged by employers. This involves the development of education and training programmes that facilitate and enable staff to enhance their knowledge, understanding and confidence. This will also help to improve their competence to read, critique, interpret and transfer information to the client/patient/carer or other professionals in support of their actions or interventions using the best evidence or information. Clinical governance and best value provides a framework for professionals to practice using an evidence base because of its close associations with the various systems and processes linked to providing resources and support for staff in developing the skills of research awareness. The challenge for practitioners is in actively seeking to develop their research awareness skills and in gaining the organisation's support.

REFERENCES

Abbott P 2001 Implementing evidence-informed nursing research awareness. In: McSherry R, Simmons M, Abbott P (eds) Evidence-informed nursing: a guide for clinical nurses. Routledge Publishers, London.

Buckingham EJ, McGrath G 1983 The social reality of nursing. Health Service Press, Bristol.

Burns N, Grove KS 1997 The practice of nursing research, 3rd edn. WB Saunders Company, London.

Cochrane A 1972 Effectiveness and efficiency random reflections on the health service. Nuffield Provisional Hospitals Trust, Leeds.

Collins W 1987 Collins Universal English Dictionary. Readers Union Ltd., Glasgow.

Cormack FSD 1996 The research process in nursing, 3rd edn. Blackwell Science Publication, London.

Crombie I 1996 The pocket guide to critical appraisal. British Medical Journal, London.

Cullen R, Nichols S, Halligan A 2000 NHS support team. Reviewing a service – discovering the unwritten rules. British Journal of Clinical Governance 5(4): 233–239.

Cullum N, DiCenso A, Ciliska D 1998 Implementing evidence-based nursing: some misconceptions. Evidence Based Medicine 1(2): 38–40.

Davies C 1996 Cloaked in a tattered illusion. Nursing Times 92(45): 44–46.

Davies HTO, Nutley SM, Mannion R 2000 Organizational culture and quality of health care. Quality in Health Care 9: 111–119.

Deane D, Campbell J 1985 Developing professional effectiveness in nursing. Rector Publishing Company, Virginia.

Department of Health 1997 The new NHS: modern and dependable. HMSO, London.

Department of Health 1998 Quality in the new NHS. HMSO, London.

Department of Health 1999 Making a difference: strengthening nursing, midwifery and health visiting contribution to health and healthcare. HMSO, London.

Department of Health 2000 The national plan. HMSO, London.

Department of Trade and Industry 1997 Partnership with people. Department of Trade, London.

Depoy E, Gitlin LN 1994 Introduction to research multiple strategies for health and human services. Mosby, St Louis.

DiCenso A, Cullum N 1998 Implementing evidence-based nursing: some misconceptions. Evidence-based Nursing 1(2): 38–40.

Dingwall R, Rafferty AM, Webster C 1988 An introduction to the social history of nursing. Routledge, London.

Edwards J, Packham R 1999 A model for the practical implementation of clinical governance. Journal of Clinical Excellence 1(1): 13–18.

Fagin CM 1990 Nursing leadership global strategies. National League for Nursing, New York.

Freak L 1995 Evaluating clinical trials. Journal of Wound Care 4(3): 114–116.

Guyatt GH, Meade MO, Jaeschke R, Cook DJ, Haynes RB 2000 Practitioners of evidence based care: not all clinicians need to apprise evidence from scratch but all need some skills. British Medical Journal 320(7240): 954–955.

Harvey G 1998 Improving patient care. RCN Magazine Autumn: 8–9.

Haslock I 1999 Introducing clinical governance in an acute trust. Hospital Medicine 60(10): 745–747.

Hawthorne P 1983 Principles of research: a checklist. Nursing Times 79(23): 41–42.

Hawkins S, Shohet R 1989 Supervision in the helping professions. Open University Press, Milton Keynes.

Haynes RB, Sackett DL, Muir Gray JA, Cook DJ, Guyatt GH 1996 Transferring evidence from research into practice: 1 The role of clinical care research evidence in clinical decisions. Evidence Based Medicine 125: A–14.

Illich I 1976 Limits to medicine, medical nemesis: the exploration of health. Marion Boyars, London.

Lloyd Smith W 1996 Where's the evidence. British Journal of Therapy and Rehabilitation 3(12): 659–661.

Long A, Harrison S 1996 Evidence-based decision making. Health Service Journal 106: 1–11.

Macleod-Clarke M, Hockey J 1989 Further research in nursing. Scutari Press, London.

Marquis BL, Hutson CJ 2000 Leadership roles and management function in nursing: theory and application, 3rd edn. Lippincott, Philadelphia.

McSherry R 1997 What do registered nurses and midwives feel and know about research. Journal of Advanced Nursing 25(6): 985–998.

McSherry R 1999 Supporting the patient and their family. In: Bassett C, Makin L (eds) Caring for the seriously ill patient. Arnold, London.

McSherry R, Haddock J 1999 Evidence-based healthcare: its place within clinical governance. British Journal of Nursing 8(2): 114–117.

McSherry R 2000 Researching clinical supervision. In: Bassett C (ed.) Clinical supervision: a guide for implementation. Nursing Times Books, London.

McSherry R, McSherry W 2001 Putting research into practice. Nursing Times 97(3): 36–37.

McSherry R, Pearce P 2001 Clinical governance: a guide to implementation for healthcare professionals. Blackwell Science Ltd, Oxford.

McSherry R, Simmons M, Abbott P 2001 Evidence-informed nursing a guide for clinical nurses. Routledge Publishers, London.

Muir Gray JA 1997 Evidence-based healthcare: how to make health policy and management decisions. Churchill Livingstone, London.

Mullins LJ 1996 Management and organizational behaviors, 4th edn. Pitman, London.

National Health Service Executive 1993 Just for the record: a guide to record keeping for health care professionals. Department of Health, London.

Northcott N 1999 Organizational effectiveness. Nursing Times Learning Curve 3(1): 10.

O'Neill S 2000 Clinical governance in action part 4: communication. Professional Nurse 16(1): 816–817.

Parahoo K, Reid MN 1988 The research process. Nursing Times 84(40): 67–70.

Phipps K 2000 Nursing and clinical governance. British Journal of Clinical Governance 5(2): 69–70.

Pierson C 1991 Beyond the welfare state. Policy Press, Cambridge.

Reagan J 1998 Will current clinical effectiveness initiatives encourage and facilitate practitioners to use evidence-based practice for the benefit of their clients. Journal of Clinical Nursing 7(3): 244–250.

Rosenberg W, Donaldson A 1995 Evidence-based medicine: an approach to problem solving. British Medical Journal 310: 1122–1126.

Sackett DL, Rosenberg WM, Muir Gray JA, Haynes R, Richardson W 1996 Evidence-based medicine: what it is what it isn't. British Medical Journal 312: 71–72.

Sackett DL, Rosenburg W, Haynes BR 1997 Evidence-based medicine: how to practice and teach EBM. Churchill Livingstone, London.

Scally G, Donaldson LJ 1998 Clinical governance and the drive for quality improvement in the new NHS in England. British Medical Journal 317: 61–65.

Seers K 1994 Qualitative and quantitative research. Surgical Nurse 7(6): 4–6.

Slim J 1996 cited in Stewart R 1996 Leading in the NHS: a practical guide, 2nd edn. Macmillan Business, London.

Squire S 2000 Clinical governance in action: part 7. Effective learning. Professional Nurse 16(4): 1014–1015.

Stewart R 1996 Leading in the NHS: a practical guide, 2nd edn. Macmillan Business, London.

Tappen RM 1995 Nursing leadership and management: concepts and practice. F.A. Davis, Philadelphia.

Taylor CM 1997 What is evidence-based practice. British Journal of Occupational Therapy, November: 470–474.

United Kingdom Central Council for Nursing, Midwifery and Health Visiting 1992 Code of conduct. UKCC, London.

United Kingdom Central Council for Nursing, Midwifery and Health Visiting 1998 Guidelines for records and record keeping. UKCC, London.

Walshe K, Ham C 1997 Who's acting on the evidence. Health Service Journal 107(5547): 22–25.

6

Problem identification

Kate Gerrish

KEY ISSUES

◆ Reviewing practice through structured
   reflection

◆ Triggers to identifying issues and
   problems from practice

◆ Formulating answerable questions

◆ Types of question: background and
   foreground questions

◆ The components of a question:
   – individual, group or organisational
     issues
   – the setting or context
   – intervention and comparison
     intervention
   – outcomes

◆ Prioritising questions

◆ Linking questions to research evidence.

INTRODUCTION

Achieving best practice through an evidence-based approach requires that practitioners review their professional practice in order to identify areas where their actions may not be the most appropriate and effective for a given situation. In order to set the reader off on the path to achieving practice based on the best available evidence, this chapter begins by exploring the various triggers to identifying issues and problems arising from health- and social-care practice, and it encourages practitioners to actively engage in reflection on practice. Once issues of concern have been identified, it is essential that clearly articulated and focused questions are formulated before embarking on the search for evidence; otherwise precious time may be wasted seeking out evidence that is not of direct relevance to the issue of concern. Techniques for formulating answerable questions are presented and practical guidance given on how to structure such questions in order to guide practitioners towards relevant sources of evidence. Throughout the chapter the term 'practice' is used to encompass clinical, managerial and educational dimensions.

REVIEWING CURRENT PRACTICE

The modernisation agenda (Department of Health 1997, 2000a) of the current Labour government is having considerable impact on the nature of health- and social-care services and, consequently, on the role and function of health- and social-care practitioners. New services are being developed in response to the changing health- and social-care needs of the population, technological advances in health care, the increased expectations of service users and the need to manage the health- and social-care economy more efficiently. Such developments need to be grounded, wherever possible, in research-based evidence concerning the efficacy and efficiency of the initiatives concerned. It is important, therefore, that those involved in commissioning, planning and developing new services are able to identify appropriate evidence to inform the decision-making process. In addition, practitioners are expected to take on new and innovative roles,

adopt more flexible ways of working and engage in multi-professional and multi-agency collaboration. Again, the extension and expansion of professional roles needs to be firmly rooted in the best available evidence.

Activity 6.1

Consider your own area of practice and note down the changes that have already occurred or are being planned as part of the modernisation of health and social care. To what extent have these changes been underpinned by a sound evidence base?

One of the difficulties of trying to underpin new service development with evidence is that the initiative may be so innovative that there is no published evidence to inform the development. In such situations it is particularly important to look for other sources of evidence. These may include:

- evidence from practitioners in other parts of the country who are working on similar initiatives
- networks to share ideas and experiences
- NHS beacon sites, as these were set up specifically with the intention of sharing innovative practice
- databases of practice development and best value initiatives that can be accessed via the internet
- electronic discussion groups also provide the opportunity to post a request for practitioners engaged in similar activities to make contact.

However, it is also important to evaluate the implementation of any new initiatives from the outset and to use the evaluative data to inform the subsequent refinement of the initiative.

Activity 6.2

Think about the changes you listed earlier – how many of these are being formally evaluated?

At the same time as the drive for new service development is taking place, the clinical governance agenda is emphasising the importance of health and social care being firmly embedded in an ethos of quality improvement (Department of Health 1998). Outmoded practices that are based on tradition and a weak empirical base need to be superseded by those supported by a firmer evidence base. Practitioners have a responsibility, therefore, to review their existing practice and be open to considering new ways of providing care. They need to be prepared to continually question their practice and accept that what they do may not always be the most appropriate action in the light of new research findings. The current emphasis on developing learning organisations and instilling an ethos of lifelong learning among health- and social-care practitioners (Department of Health 2000a, b) is in response to a recognition that knowledge gained through initial professional preparation soon becomes outdated and no longer provides an adequate base for practice in a rapidly changing health- and social-care environment.

For many practitioners the day-to-day responsibilities of service delivery can seem overwhelming, and there barely seems time to provide for the essentials, let alone pause to question practice. Often, because things have become over familiar, practitioners no longer pay attention to them and there is a risk that such familiarity can lead to complacency (Johns 2000). Furthermore, when areas of concern are identified it is often difficult to find the time to examine these issues with the degree of detail required. What is important, therefore, is that practitioners develop the skills to identify questions arising from their everyday practice, sift through these questions to determine the relative priority and importance of each question, and then make effective use of their time by systematically seeking out evidence to answer the questions. In some instances the search for evidence will be made easier through accessing published systematic reviews of research on a particular topic. Additionally, summaries of research evidence may be available in an easy-to-use format in journals or as short standalone publications such as the effective healthcare bulletins produced by the NHS Centre for Reviews and Dissemination (2001) at the University of York. In other situations, as Chapter 7 explains, it will be the case of undertaking a detailed search of the literature using electronic databases and the internet to seek out appropriate evidence. In order to maximise these strategies, however, it is important that the professional is aware of what they do and do not know.

REFLECTION *ON* AND *IN* ACTION

Engaging in reflective practice provides a means of identifying areas where practice is perhaps not as it should be or that there are gaps in practitioners' knowledge. Indeed, without engaging in reflection, practitioners may not even be aware of a knowledge deficit. They may have utilised a particular approach over a period of time without recognising that it may have become outdated or have been superseded by other more appropriate techniques. Reflective practitioners are, therefore, curious about their practice and regularly ask such questions as 'why are things as they are?', 'could things be done in a better way?' (Johns 2000).

Reflection entails the process of reviewing an episode of practice in order to describe, analyse and evaluate the experience, and so inform the learning process. Schon (1991) differentiates between two approaches to reflection: reflection *on* action and reflection *in* action. Reflection *on* action entails the retrospective analysis and interpretation of a

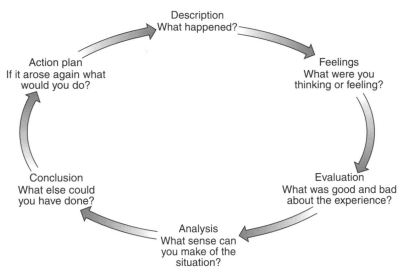

Figure 6.1 The reflective cycle (adapted from Gibbs 1998 and Johns 2000 Becoming a reflective practitioner. Blackwell Science, Oxford, with permission from Blackwell Science and Oxford Brookes University).

particular situation in order to identify the nature of the knowledge used in that situation. The practitioner may speculate how the situation might have been handled differently and what other knowledge would have been helpful (Burns & Bulman 2000).

The reflective learning cycle (Gibbs 1988) provides a useful framework for reflecting on action (Fig. 6.1). By contrast, reflection *in* action is the process whereby the practitioner recognises a novel situation or a new problem and thinks about it while still acting in that situation (Schon 1991). Resolution of the problem can occur if the problem is reframed, i.e. seen differently during the actions, and this may have the effect of modifying the practitioner's behaviour.

Case study: using the reflective learning cycle

Sally Evans is a home-care organiser who has just returned from a re-assessment visit for Elsie Brooks, an 84-year-old lady who has been

receiving home-care services following her discharge from hospital 6 weeks ago. Sally reflects on her visit.

Description

This was my second meeting with Elsie. The purpose of the visit was to assess whether the level of home-care support we were providing was still meeting Elsie's needs. Although Elsie was mentally alert, I was struck by how much frailer she appeared to when I first met her 6 weeks ago. She had great difficulty moving around her ground floor flat and she admitted to having fallen on a couple of occasions recently.

Feelings

I was very worried that Elsie might have another fall and injure herself more seriously. I was frustrated that we had not identified that Elsie was at risk earlier on. I admired Elsie's desire to remain independent and felt that we should endeavour to support her to maintain this.

Evaluation

I was relieved that I had called on Elsie today, as she is at great risk of falling and the sooner we can act the better. It was good that she felt able to confide in me, however, it is worrying that the home-care workers who have been calling three times a week had not identified this problem. I also thought that some simple measures already could have been taken to make the home environment safer for Elsie.

Analysis

The home-care workers appear in this situation to have failed to identify someone at risk and they have not taken the appropriate action in reporting the deterioration in Elsie's general condition. Also, they have not taken simple precautionary measures to make the home environment safer for Elsie. This may be because they lack the skills to monitor an older person's condition and do not have sufficient knowledge of falls prevention.

Conclusion

I should have sought a more detailed verbal report from the home-care workers and actively encouraged them to feedback on Elsie's condition. There is also a need to consider the ongoing training of home-care workers in falls prevention.

Action plan

In addition to addressing the particular issues arising from Elsie's situation, I need to review the training programme for home-care workers on falls prevention. It may be that we could identify a risk assessment tool that would help home-care workers to identify those people who are at increasing risk of falls. There may also be initiatives elsewhere that are targeted specifically on the role of home-care workers in minimising the risk of falls in older people.

Activity 6.3

Identify a recent episode from your practice that lends itself to reflection *on* action. Using the reflective learning cycle make short notes on each of the stages of the reflective process (as in the example above). Develop an action plan that identifies any areas where your knowledge of appropriate evidence may be lacking.

Identifying those aspects of practice that are unsubstantiated by adequate evidence is an important skill to learn. However, engaging in the reflective process can instil feelings of unease and uncertainty about the best course of action to take in a particular situation. It is not always easy to deal with such feelings, as often clients, their carers and more junior colleagues may look on experienced practitioners as experts and expect them to know the answers. However, increasingly, health- and social-care professionals are redefining their relationships with people who access their services to achieve a greater sense of partnership. Schon (1991) describes this as a shift from the position of 'expert' who is presumed to know and must appear to do so, irrespective of feelings of uncertainty, towards that of a reflective practitioner who is prepared to learn with and from clients and their carers.

In considering the unease that practitioners experience when they identify a knowledge deficit, Sackett et al. (2000) differentiate between *cognitive resonance* and *cognitive dissonance*. If a situation calls for knowledge that a practitioner already possesses, the practitioner will experience the reinforcing mental and emotional responses known as cognitive resonance. The practitioner is then able to make rapid decisions regarding the actions to take. But if a situation calls for knowledge that the practitioner does not possess, he or she will experience mental and emotional responses known as cognitive dissonance. A maladaptive reaction to cognitive dissonance may then lead the practitioner either to try to hide the knowledge deficit from him/herself, or to over react emotionally with excessive feelings of anxiety. A more positive adaptive response is for practitioners to recognise their information needs and use their experiences of cognitive dissonance to motivate their learning. Gaps in knowledge can then be developed into questions and, subsequently, answers being sought.

To this end, practitioners should learn to acknowledge and accept that they do not know all the answers. They need to be prepared continually to question their practice and accept that what they do may not always be the right thing, particularly in the light of new research findings. There is a need to be alert to looking actively for signs that may suggest a problem, for example:

- There may be evidence such as feedback from patients/clients or audit findings that suggests that the current approach may no longer be the most appropriate.

- Colleagues may have started to use alternative approaches.

- Articles and news reports in professional journals may suggest practice elsewhere is moving on (NHS Executive Anglia and Oxford 1999).

Reflecting on practice need not be an isolated activity undertaken by individual practitioners. There is considerable merit in meeting with a group of peers to review practice and identify shared areas of concern. It may be possible to ring fence a period of time during a regular team meeting to focus on appraising practice or, alternatively, set up a meeting with this specific intention in mind. The following case study provides an example of a collaborative practitioner-led initiative to review practice.

Case study: evidence-based council

The Northern General Hospital in Sheffield, UK, recently established an Evidence-Based Council for nurses and allied health professionals. The purpose of the Council is to provide a forum for practitioners to meet on a monthly basis to explore issues associated with promoting evidence-based practice in the workplace. Council members are drawn from each of the clinical directorates and are undergoing specialist training in developing skills to facilitate evidence-based practice. Health science librarians attend the Council meetings in order to promote access and utilisation of information sources provided by the library. Council members are responsible for supporting the development of journal clubs in the various clinical settings. While some journal clubs focus on critically appraising journal articles of interest to members, others are more concerned with reviewing practice and identifying issues that are of shared concern. Feedback from the journal clubs to the Council provides the opportunity to gauge the extent to which the issues raised by the individual journal clubs are of general concern and then to consider a collaborative approach to addressing the issues across different directorates.

Activity 6.4

Thinking about the goals of this Council, that is to support the introduction of evidence-based care, how could you set up an approach in your place of work that will achieve similar goals?

IDENTIFYING PROBLEMS AND HIGHLIGHTING ISSUES OF CONCERN

Issues of concern that can subsequently be formulated into questions are most likely to arise from the health- or social-care context in which practitioners work and focus on the services they provide. Often it is the practitioner's interaction with an individual client that is the trigger. For example, there may be uncertainty as to the best way to proceed with an individual's care, or concern over the appropriateness of a particular treatment in a given situation. Sackett et al. (2000, p. 19) identify various aspects of clinical work where questions may arise. These include:

- Clinical findings: how to gather and interpret the information gleaned from completing the patient's/client's history and physical examination.

- Aetiology: how to identify the various causes of a disease.

- Clinical manifestations of disease: knowing when a disease may lead to its clinical manifestations and how to use this knowledge to classify illnesses.

- Diagnostic tests: how to select appropriate diagnostic tests and interpret the findings in order to confirm or exclude a particular diagnosis, whilst at the same time taking into consideration the accuracy, acceptability, expense, safety etc. of the tests.

- Prognosis: how to judge the likely progress a person will make over time and anticipate the complications of the disease that may occur.

- Therapy: how to select the most appropriate and cost-effective interventions.

- Prevention: how to reduce the likelihood of disease occurring by identifying and modifying risk factors and detecting diseases by screening methods.

- Experience and meaning: how to empathise with patients/clients in order to appreciate the meaning they attribute to their experiences and understand how this may influence their health and well-being.

Although this framework provides a useful means of identifying those areas of practice where

issues of concern may be highlighted, it is important to recognise that the questions practitioners identify may not necessarily be those that are of most concern to service users (Sackett et al. 2000). Practitioners need to engage in dialogue with their clients in order to identify those questions that are of relevance. Seeking clients' perceptions of what they see the main problem(s) to be, what treatment options they are aware of, and what their preferences would be, is more likely to lead to patient/client-focused questions that can enhance the quality of care provided (Sackett et al. 2000).

Whilst practitioners' interactions with clients are frequently a key means of identifying issues of concern, other triggers may include:

- Trends or patterns that are observed with a particular client group which had previously been undetected.

- Audit or risk assessment activities that highlight issues of concern and identify variations in practice and/or outcomes.

- A topical issue that has been taken up by the media may cause anxiety amongst clients and raise questions as to the most appropriate advice a practitioner should give.

- An organisational need to provide appropriate clinical and cost-effective services may raise issues regarding workforce planning, resource management and risk assessment etc.

- National policy drivers to develop health- and social-care services may provide the impetus to consider new forms of service delivery, innovative role development or interagency working.

- Service developments may raise educational concerns about ensuring that the workforce is equipped with the appropriate competencies to deliver care.

- Clients and/or carers may raise issues of concern through formal mechanisms such as satisfaction surveys, Patient Advice and Liaison

Service (PALS), or informally through individual interactions with practitioners.

- There may be differences of opinion amongst practitioners as to what constitutes 'best practice' in a given situation.

Box 6.1 provides some examples of the different triggers identified above.

Activity 6.5

Using the triggers identified above make brief notes identifying issues arising from your own practice. It may be that some of the triggers relate to the same or similar issues. You can then use these ideas later on in this chapter to formulate specific questions.

The following case study provides an example of how a group of cardiology nurses observed a trend amongst a particular patient group that stimulated them to undertake an audit. The audit helped to identify important issues that warranted further consideration.

Case study: communication needs of South Asian patients

Nurses in a cardiology unit became concerned that the cardiac rehabilitation needs of patients from South Asian backgrounds were not being met, as few patients were observed to take up the cardiac rehabilitation programme provided by the hospital. It was recognised that new approaches would be needed if the requirements of the National Service Framework for Coronary Heart Disease were to be met and the inequalities in access to services overcome. In order to inform these developments, an audit was conducted to explore the cardiac rehabilitation experiences of cardiac patients of South Asian origin and to identify ways of providing more culturally sensitive and accessible services. The audit confirmed that the low uptake of the cardiac rehabilitation programme was linked to poor communication

---

Box 6.1 Triggers to identifying problems

Trigger	Example
Interactions with individual clients	A GP is unsure whether a young woman who presents with intermittent back pain could be helped by referral to a chiropractor
Trends or patterns within a client group	A school nurse becomes aware of an increase in the number of teenage pregnancies amongst a school's population
Variations in practice identified through audit	An audit of falls occurring in a ward setting reveals a higher than expected incidence
Topical issues identified by media	The risk of deep vein thrombosis associated with long-haul flights
Organisational need to provide clinical and cost effective services	The need to review staffing establishments, workload and skill mix to enable health visitors to extend their public health role
National drivers to develop health and social care	The introduction of intermediate care services for older people raises issues concerning the need for effective interagency collaboration
Educational concern for competent workforce	The need to develop the skills in nurses to undertake intravenous cannulation
Concerns raised by clients and/or carers	A satisfaction survey raises concerns regarding community-based rehabilitation for people who have experienced a stroke
Debates about best practice	Anaesthetists differ in opinion as to whether it is beneficial to give anti-emetics prior to administering a general anaesthetic

between healthcare workers and South Asian patients who did not speak English. Many patients were unaware of the existence of the programme. Moreover, the audit revealed that South Asian patients who were not fluent in English were not always provided with the opportunity to access trained interpreting services in hospital. Poor access to interpreting services put some South Asian patients at a disadvantage in terms of knowledge and awareness of their condition and the support available post discharge. The audit raised important questions regarding how communication between healthcare workers and South Asian patients might be improved.

FORMULATING ANSWERABLE QUESTIONS

Once an issue has been identified that warrants further investigation and current practice has been reviewed, it is necessary to formulate a clear and precise question in order to guide the search for appropriate evidence. It can be tempting if one is pressurised for time to delve straight in from the initial idea to searching for evidence instead of working through the various stages in a systematic way. Yet formulating an answerable question is arguably the most important part of the process (Richardson et al. 1995). A well-formulated question clarifies the particular issue of concern, serves to identify search strategies and helps to focus the limited time available on seeking out evidence that is of direct relevance to answering the question (Sackett et al. 2000).

Types of questions

Sackett et al. (2000) differentiate between two types of question that can be formulated to address an issue of healthcare concern: background questions and foreground questions.

Background questions

These are broad in focus and are concerned with seeking general knowledge about a particular issue. They have two essential components:

- a question root (who, what, where, when, how, why) with a verb
- a particular issue, for example a clinical disorder.

Examples of background questions are:

- What kind of support do carers of an older person with cognitive impairment require?
- How can the incidence of smoking in teenagers be reduced?

Although background questions can be useful for formulating initial ideas about a particular issue, they are too broad to provide the necessary guidance for searching out the evidence. For example, in respect of the support for carers of older people with cognitive impairment it is not clear what kinds of support might be required; it might be that provided by healthcare professionals, social-care agencies or the voluntary sector.

Foreground questions

Foreground questions are more focused and identify the specific knowledge that is required about the particular issue or problem of concern. Such questions generally have five components, although they may not all be evident in every question (Richardson et al. 1995, Flemming 1998, Sackett et al. 2000):

- the individual, group or organisational issue
- the setting or context
- the intervention
- the comparison intervention
- the outcomes.

Whereas this framework lends itself to the identification of clinical questions, it can also be used to formulate questions that are concerned with managerial or educational issues.

Individual, group or organisational issue

This first part of the framework aims to help the practitioner identify where the focus of the question lies. In the case of a clinical problem it may be with an individual client, for example how best to treat a person who has a venous leg ulcer, with a particular client group such as a cohort of people who have hypertension or with a proportion of the population with similar demographic characteristics, for example people over 75 years of age. The characteristics of the individual or group need to be considered, for example in respect of age, gender or ethnicity, as these characteristics will guide the search for the most relevant evidence. An organisational issue might relate to an aspect of healthcare delivery, for example, a breast-screening programme, or the ability to meet targets set for community nurse appointment times. Additional organisational topics could include questions about activity, workload and skill mix or management issues, such as resource management. With regard to an organisational issue, it is important to consider whether the issue is concerned with the organisation as a whole or a particular aspect of the organisation, such as a specific department or staff group.

It is essential at this stage in the process to describe the problem clearly. In the case study concerning the utilisation of cardiac rehabilitation services by South Asian patients outlined earlier, it may be that articulating the problem in a particular way places the 'problem' clearly with South Asian patients' reluctance to access cardiac rehabilitation services. A more thorough exploration of the particular situation identified the problem as communication difficulties between healthcare workers and South Asian patients, arising from the inadequacy of interpreting services provided for South Asian patients. The search for evidence to inform this area of practice would be very different in each of these scenarios.

Setting or context

Having identified whether the issue is related to an individual client, client or staff group or the organisation, it is important to consider the context in which care is delivered. Identifying the setting helps to clarify the particular focus of the question and leads to a more targeted search for evidence. It may be appropriate to focus specifically on primary-, secondary- or community-care settings, or consider rural or urban locations (Chambers & Boath 2001). For example, health education strategies to reduce the incidence of falls among older people are likely to be different in an institutional setting such as a medical ward in an acute hospital than in the person's home environment.

Intervention

The next stage is to consider the intervention of interest. The idea of an intervention is perhaps easiest to conceptualise in relation to a problem relating to a client or client group. Here questions are often concerned with a form of therapy, a particular treatment or a preventative or educative strategy. For example, a midwife may be interested in the benefits of providing specific antenatal classes (the intervention) for pregnant teenagers.

However, the notion of an intervention is not restricted to client-related issues. It can apply equally to organisational concerns. For example, a primary care trust manager may be interested in the benefits of introducing a system of clinical supervision for practice nurses. The intervention is clearly clinical supervision, although at this stage the form that the clinical supervision might take, for example individual or group supervision, has not been specified. Alternatively, questions may be concerned with considering the structures and processes necessary to support new service delivery, such as shared record keeping between health- and social-care workers involved in providing intermediate care services. Whatever the focus, it is important to be clear and specific when stating the intervention, as this will guide the subsequent search for evidence.

Comparison intervention

The comparison intervention refers to an alternative intervention to the one the question is concerned with. The comparison intervention may relate to current practice or to an entirely different intervention that could be introduced. For example, if a district nurse is curious about the benefits of using a new hydrocolloid dressing on a sacral pressure sore, it could be compared with the current dressing in use. Alternatively, the comparison intervention may actually be the 'no treatment' option. If the question is concerned with identifying the benefits of wearing compression hosiery (the intervention) during a long-haul flight to prevent the occurrence of deep vein thrombosis, the comparison intervention would be the hosiery normally worn by the passengers. As with the intervention, the comparison intervention needs to be specified clearly.

Outcomes

Identifying the outcome(s) associated with the question helps to focus the search for evidence. What is needed is a clear indication of how the effects of the intervention can be judged. For example, in the case of using a hydrocolloid dressing to treat a pressure sore it is not sufficient to ask whether the wound heals. What is needed is a clear definition of specific outcome measures, for example, the length of time the wound takes to heal, the frequency with which dressings need to be changed, the cost of an episode of care etc.

Various groups of people may well be interested in different outcome measures. Baker (1998) identifies how the meaning and purpose of outcomes may vary for different stakeholders:

- *Service users* are often concerned with issues of access, information, the opportunity to participate in decision making about their care and satisfaction with their functional abilities and their quality of life.
- *Practitioners* are frequently interested in the effects of specific interventions and the achievement of optimal levels of functioning, particularly in respect of mental and physical health.
- *Service managers* are primarily concerned with the delivery of an effective and efficient service through maximising the utilisation of available resources.
- *Commissioners* are interested in ensuring the highest improvement possible with respect to the health status of the local population. This has to be achieved within resources available and can result in a concern not only with morbidity and mortality associated with particular conditions, but also more specific issues such as the incidence of teenage pregnancy in a particular locality, or the incidence of pressure sores in hospital and community settings.

When formulating a question it is not feasible to consider the different interests of the various stakeholders identified above. Nevertheless, one needs to be clear about whose interests are being served by the particular question.

Once the separate components of the question have been identified, the next step is to consider its structure. The question root selected will depend on what sort of answer is being sought. Questions which ask 'what', 'when', 'where', 'who', 'how' and 'how many' are used to describe or quantify, whereas questions that ask 'why' provide an explanation, and questions beginning with 'is' or 'do' are used to confirm or qualify.

Formulating questions: an example

Consider the following scenario:

A primary healthcare team has decided to review the health education work on smoking that various team members undertake. The team is particularly interested in the impact of different interventions in order to make some decisions about which ones are worth continuing. How might a question be framed to address the concerns of the primary healthcare team?

Patient, group or organisational issue

It is important to consider what the question is actually about. From the information given it is not clear whether the primary healthcare team is interested in the whole or a section of the population they serve, which staff are involved in health education interventions, or what is meant by health education, smoking etc. More attention needs to be given to identifying the specific issue of concern.

Setting or context

The precise focus of interest of the team's activities needs to be clarified. It might be the general practice, a community setting or a particular type of clinic in the practice.

Intervention and comparison interventions

The intervention(s) of interest needs to be clearly identified. There is insufficient information given in the outline of the different health education interventions that the team are interested in, and whether there is an alternative model to which health education might be compared.

Outcomes

The primary healthcare team appears interested in the impact of different interventions; however, it is not clear what is meant by the term 'impact'. For example, it may relate to a change in knowledge or attitudes amongst smokers, the quantity of cigarettes smoked or the numbers of smokers and non-smokers.

From the information provided in the scenario it is only feasible to construct a background question such as 'what is the impact of the range of health education interventions undertaken in primary care on smoking?' However, this does not provided sufficient guidance for focusing a search for evidence. It is necessary to narrow the question down to the specific issue relating to health education about smoking that the primary care team is interested in. For example, if the team was interested in whether they should continue with a nurse-led smoking cessation clinic for mothers of young children, besides looking at attendance figures, patient preferences and opportunity costs, they might want to know 'what is the evidence for the effectiveness of providing individual as opposed to group education about the risks of cigarette smoking for mothers of young children?' This question is sufficiently focused for it to be broken down into its component parts (Box 6.2).

The following case study gives an example of how to formulate a question.

Case study: question formulation

Jane Evans is a 35-year-old school teacher who has presented to her GP with recurrent back pain. On examination there is no evidence of nerve injury and it is recommended that she mobilises. She is concerned about the frequency with which her back pain reoccurs and the effect it is having on her job. She asks whether a course of chiropractic treatment might be more effective in preventing a reoccurrence than the routine back exercises she has been carrying out. From the information provided it is possible to identify the component parts of a potential question (Box 6.3).

Box 6.2

Patient/client, group or organisational issue	Situation – context	Intervention	Comparison intervention	Outcomes
Women with young children	Nurse-led clinic in primary care	One-to-one health education on risks of smoking	Group health education on risks of smoking	For example: Attendance figures Women's preference Knowledge and attitudes to smoking Number of cigarettes smoked

Box 6.3

Patient/client, group or organisational issue	Situation – context	Intervention	Comparison intervention	Outcomes
A 35-year-old woman with recurrent back pain, employed in a non-manual job	Primary care	Chiropractic treatment for repetitive back injury	Routine self-administered back exercises	For example: Frequency of reoccurrence of back pain Severity of back pain Number of days lost from employment

The question itself can then be formulated: 'Is chiropractic treatment more effective than self-administered back exercises in reducing the frequency and severity of recurrent back pain in a woman with a non-manual occupation?'

Activity 6.6

This exercise requires you to formulate a specific question that can then guide the search for appropriate evidence. Look back at the issues you identified in Activity 6.1 (p. 90) and select the one that you find most interesting. Using the framework that has just been presented, make notes under each of the headings. Then go back and review what you have written in order to draft the precise question. Think carefully about the root of the question and what it is you want to find out. Refine and limit the question to what would seem to be relevant to your area of practice, for example, primary or secondary care.

Your question should be shaped by thinking through:

- What is the question really about? Is it concerned with an individual patient, a group of people, a particular population, a practice dilemma, a management problem etc?

- What is the setting or context of the issue of concern? How precisely does it need to be defined?

- What is the intervention and with what is it being compared?

- What are the outcomes of the intervention that you are particularly interested in?

Box 6.4				
Patient/client, group or organisational issue	Situation – context	Intervention	Comparison intervention	Outcomes

Question:

Key words:

- In identifying the root of the question do you want to describe, quantify, explain, confirm or qualify?
- What is the specific question you will ask?

You may find it useful when developing the question to use the grid in Box 6.4.

Having formulated your question, identify up to six key words that best represent the important components of the question. These key words will form the basis of your search for evidence (see Chapter 7).

Finally, when formulating a question it is important to ensure that it is specific enough to provide a clear focus. Specifying fine detail can help ensure that the question is relevant to the particular issues of concern and is likely to lead to appropriate evidence. It can also help ensure that the amount of information retrieved is manageable. However, achieving the fine balance between brevity and detail is not always easy and it may be necessary to refine the question once the search for evidence has been started. It is also important that the question is capable of being answered, is about a topic where change will be possible and important enough to warrant the time devoted to finding an answer (Chambers & Boath 2001). Additionally, if answering the question identifies a need to implement change, such change will be easier to achieve if before embarking on the search to find an answer, the question is agreed and owned by those who will be involved in the change process. For example, if a ward manager was interested in introducing a flexible shift system it would be important to discuss the question with both the senior manager who would need to sanction the change and the staff who would be affected if changes were introduced. The question could then be formulated to address the outcomes that the senior manager, the ward staff and the ward manager deem to be important. It may also be useful to include a provisional timescale as this can help to structure the search for evidence by providing deadlines to work towards. Often it will be necessary to limit the size of the project so that it is manageable within the time available.

QUESTIONS ABOUT CLINICAL AND COST EFFECTIVENESS

Practitioners often want to identify the most clinically and cost effective interventions in order to ensure that limited health- and social-care resources lead to the best possible outcomes (Gerrish & Clayton 1998). However, clinical and cost effectiveness are complex concepts. Although it is beyond the scope of this chapter to consider these concepts in any detail, it may be useful to clarify the terms insofar as it may help to identify issues of concern and formulate specific questions.

The NHS Executive (1996) has defined clinical effectiveness as 'the extent to which specific clinical interventions when deployed in the field for a particular patient or population do what they are intended to do, i.e. maintain and improve health and secure the greatest possible health gain from the available resources'. Questions about clinical effectiveness will, therefore, be concerned with whether a particular intervention achieves beneficial outcomes. For example, a district nurse may be concerned about how effective a new dressing is in promoting wound healing.

Cost effectiveness is a term that is used by health- and social-care practitioners and managers in everyday language to refer to the financial and wider resource implications of delivering a specific outcome or treatment (Benton 1999). It introduces an economic perspective in order to evaluate different treatments, alternative ways of providing services as well as changes in health- and social-care organisation or policy (Chambers & Boath 2001). Such a perspective can provide information that can be used to inform judgements about the value of a particular intervention. Essentially, economic evaluations are concerned with a comparative analysis of alternative courses of action in terms of both costs and consequences (Drummond et al. 1987). They may take one of four forms depending on the precise information that is being sought: cost minimisation, cost effectiveness, cost utility and cost benefit. Øvretveit (1998) clarifies the differences between the various kinds of economic evaluation:

- Cost-minimisation evaluations compare the costs of alternative interventions that have identical health outcomes. Questions concerned with cost minimisation will ask 'how much does it cost and which is the least expensive?'
- Cost-effectiveness studies use one measure of effectiveness, such as the number of lives saved, and compare the cost and effectiveness of interventions with the same treatment objectives.

Questions concerned with cost effectiveness will ask 'if we compare the effects of each intervention on a single simple measure, which intervention gives better value for money?'

- Cost-utility evaluations assess the utility or value of health states produced by different interventions for the same cost. They allow comparison of different interventions used in different health services. Alternative interventions are often measured against a combination of life expectancy and quality of life (a common outcome measure being 'quality-adjusted life-years' [QALYs] Questions concerned with cost utility will ask 'how much well-being do different interventions produce in relation to their cost?'
- Cost-benefit studies value both the resources consumed and the consequences of an intervention in money terms, thus allowing value for money judgements to be made. Cost-benefit analysis compares the incremental costs and benefits of the intervention. Questions concerned with cost benefit will ask 'is the benefit of the intervention more or less than its cost when both are measured in monetary terms?'

What, then, is the relationship between clinical and cost effectiveness in respect of evidence-based practice? An intervention must first be considered clinically effective to warrant investigation into its potential to be cost effective. One needs, therefore, to ask questions of clinical effectiveness before going on to ask about cost effectiveness (Chambers & Boath 2001).

PRIORITISING QUESTIONS

It is often the case that when practitioners start to review their practice and discuss their observations with colleagues, they identify a number of issues or problems that warrant investigation. As there will be limited time and resources available to devote to answering all of these questions, it is necessary to consider how questions can be prioritised. There are a number of factors that need to be borne in mind when deciding which questions need to be answered first. These include:

- the importance to the client or carer of finding an answer to the question
- the importance of the question to the client's well-being
- the likely impact of the answer on service organisation
- the likelihood of the question reoccurring in practice
- the feasibility of answering the question within the time available
- the extent of personal interest in the question.

It may also be helpful to rate questions according to their relative urgency and importance. Urgent questions often relate to the needs of a particular individual and need to be dealt with promptly, whereas important questions generally concern a larger group or the organisation as a whole and the answers are likely to have more widespread impact. It may be helpful to assign each question to a grid depending on whether they are judged to be of high or low urgency and importance (NHS Executive Anglia and Oxford 1999) (Fig. 6.2).

The questions that are deemed to be both urgent and important are clearly the main priorities and those that are neither urgent nor important can be assigned to the bottom of the list. Decisions then need to be made about how best to tackle the urgent questions in order to have time to address the important ones.

LINKING QUESTIONS TO RESEARCH EVIDENCE

Once the question has been clearly formulated consideration can be given to the different sources of evidence that may be appropriate to answering the question. As discussed in Chapter 7, evidence may be drawn from various sources: research studies, organisational information, professional judgement and patient/client preference. With regard to research evidence, the particular focus of the question is likely to lead to different kinds of research (NHS Executive Anglia and Oxford 1999). For example:

- A question about the prevalence of a particular disease in a specific population is likely to lead to epidemiological research.
- A question concerning the effectiveness of a particular intervention may lead to a randomised controlled trial.
- A question exploring patients' experiences of a particular illness may lead to a qualitative study.
- A question about the nature of communication and information giving between patients and practitioners could lead to an observational study.
- A question exploring people's beliefs and attitudes is likely to lead to survey research.

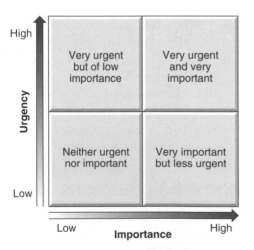

Figure 6.2 Grid for use in prioritising questions (reproduced with kind permission of the Institute of Health Sciences. Asking the question: finding the evidence. Evidence-based health care: an open learning resource for health care practitioners. CASP and HCLU, Luton).

- A question about implementing a change in practice may lead to an action research study.

Although randomised controlled trials are generally regarded as the 'gold star' for establishing evidence-based practice, they are not able to answer all research questions. For example, having undertaken a systematic review of the effectiveness of domiciliary visits undertaken by health visitors, Elkan et al. (2000) conclude that traditional models of economic evaluation based on randomised controlled trials do not necessarily lend themselves to evaluating some health visiting interventions. Just because traditional research methodologies are not able to demonstrate the effectiveness of an intervention, it does not necessarily mean that the intervention itself is inappropriate.

CONCLUSION

Ensuring that practice is based on the best available evidence is an essential requirement of clinical governance. This applies as much to new service development as it does to existing practice. As the pace of change in health and social care is such that existing practices quickly become out-dated, it is all the more important for practitioners regularly to review their practice in order to identify areas where the evidence base may be lacking. Through engaging in reflection *on* practice and being alert to the different triggers to identifying problems and issues arising from everyday practice, practitioners can begin to appraise whether or not they are 'doing the right thing right'.

Having once identified issues of concern, it is important to be systematic in seeking out evidence. Launching straight into a literature search without having clearly articulated the problem is a false economy, as time can easily be wasted pursuing avenues that are peripheral to the central issues of concern. As this chapter has pointed out, formulating clear, unambiguous, focused questions is an essential step in achieving evidence-based practice and paves the way for selecting and finding appropriate evidence.

ANNOTATED READING

NHS Executive Anglia and Oxford (1999) This manual is part of a set of open learning materials which can be used individually or in groups to develop skills in evidence-based health care. It looks in detail about how to formulate answerable questions.

Sackett et al. (2000) One of the classic texts on evidence-based health care. Although the book is written with mainly doctors in mind, an accompanying CD ROM provides

examples relevant to a range of the healthcare professionals. Chapter 2 is concerned with formulating questions.

Chambers and Boath (2001) This is a very readable text that is designed to introduce those working in primary care to the principles of clinical governance and evidence-based practice. The interactive style encourages readers to apply the principles to their day-to-day practice. The first chapter is concerned with asking the right question.

USEFUL RESOURCES

NHS Centre for Reviews and Dissemination (NHS CRD) University of York, York YO10 5DD. york.ac.uk/inst/crd

Centre for Evidence Based Medicine University of Oxford, Nuffield Department of Clinical Medicine, Level 5, The Oxford Radcliffe NHS Trust, Headley Way, Headington, Oxford OX3 9DV. cebm.jr2.oc.ac.uk

Centre for Evidence Based Nursing University of York, Information Service, Heslington, York YO1 5DD. york.ac.uk/deps/hstd/centres/evidence/ev-intro.htm

Netting the Evidence sheffield.ac.uk/~scharr/ir/netting

REFERENCES

Baker J 1998 Measuring the outcomes of care. In: Pickering S, Thompson J (eds) Promoting positive practice: nursing older people. Baillière Tindall, London.

Benton D 1999 Clinical effectiveness. In: Hamer S, Collinson G (eds) Achieving evidence-based practice: a handbook for practitioners. Baillière Tindall, Edinburgh.

Burns S, Bulman C 2000 Reflective practice in nursing: The growth of the professional practitioner, 2nd edn. Blackwell, Oxford.

Chambers R, Boath E 2001 Clinical effectiveness and clinical governance made easy, 2nd edn. Radcliffe Medical Press, Abingdon.

Department of Health 1997 The new NHS: Modern, dependable. The Stationery Office, London.

Department of Health 1998 A first class service: quality in the new NHS. Department of Health, London.

Department of Health 2000a The NHS plan: a plan for investment, a plan for reform. Department of Health, London.

Department of Health 2000b A Health Service of all the talents: Developing the NHS workforce. Department of Health, London.

Drummond M, Stoddard G, Torrence G 1987 Methods for the economic evaluation of health care programmes. Oxford Medical Publications, Oxford.

Elkan R, Robinson J, Blair M et al. 2000 The effectiveness of health services: the case of health visiting. Health and Social Care in the Community 8(1): 70–78.

Flemming K 1998 Asking answerable questions. Evidence-Based Nursing 1(2): 36–37.

Gerrish K, Clayton J 1998 Improving clinical effectiveness through an evidence-based approach: meeting the challenge for nursing in the United Kingdom. Nursing Administration Quarterly 22(4): 55–64.

Gibbs G 1988 Learning by doing: a guide to teaching and learning. Further Education Unit, Oxford Polytechnic, Oxford.

Johns C 2000 Becoming a reflective practitioner. Blackwell Science, Oxford.

NHS Centre for Reviews and Dissemination 2001 Accessing the evidence on clinical effectiveness. Effectiveness Matters 5: 1.

NHS Executive 1996 Promoting clinical effectiveness: a framework for action in and through the NHS. NHS Executive, London.

NHS Executive Anglia and Oxford 1999 Unit 2: Asking the question: Finding the evidence. Evidence-based Health Care: An open learning resource for health care practitioners. Critical Skills Appraisal Programme (CASP) and Health Care Libraries Unit (HCLU), Luton.

Øvretveit J 1998 Evaluating health interventions. Open University Press, Buckingham.

Richardson WS, Wilson MC, Nishikawa J et al. 1995 The well-built clinical question: a key to evidence-based decisions. ACP Journal Club 123(3): A12–13.

Sackett DL, Straus SE, Richardson WS et al. 2000 Evidence-based medicine: how to practice and teach EBM, 2nd edn. Churchill Livingstone, Edinburgh.

Schon D 1991 The Reflective Practitioner, 3rd edn. Josey Bass, San Francisco.

GLOSSARY

Background questions: Questions that are broad in focus and are concerned with seeking general knowledge about a particular issue. They comprise a question root (who, what, where, when, how, why) with a verb and identify a particular issue, for example a clinical disorder.

Foreground questions: Focused questions that identify the specific knowledge that is required about the particular issue or problem of concern. Such questions generally have five components: the individual, group or organisational issue; the setting or context; the intervention; the comparison intervention; and the outcome.

Outcome: The impact of an intervention on, for example, a patient's previous health state. Outcome measures assess the end result of the intervention.

PALS: Patient Advocacy and Liaison Service to be established in every NHS Trust as part of the NHS Plan.

Reflection: The process of reviewing an episode of practice in order to describe, analyse and evaluate the experience and so inform the learning process.

Reflection on action: The retrospective analysis and interpretation of a particular situation in order to identify the nature of the knowledge used in that situation.

7

Finding, appraising and using research evidence in practice

Carl Thompson

KEY ISSUES

◆ Experience *alone* is not sufficient basis for practice

◆ Reducing the uncertainties in practice calls for a systematic approach to searching, appraising and using research evidence

◆ Tried and tested search strategies, technologies and filters exist which can improve the efficiency and effectiveness of searching

◆ Critical appraisal need not be onerous and design-specific checklists make the task simpler, quicker and more accurate

◆ Implementing the outcomes from research is complex and relies on a good diagnosis of the barriers to change in your area, the deployment of good-quality theoretical models of change, and the adoption of evidence-based multifaceted intervention strategies.

INTRODUCTION

This chapter begins with a simple statement: nothing in health and social care is certain. The accuracy of the diagnosis you receive from a practitioner, the effects of the intervention they prescribe, the prognosis of the disease or condition that they offer, and even the way *they* think *you* might be experiencing the care they deliver are all surrounded by uncertainty. Such uncertainty generates information needs on the part of the clinician, policy maker or service planner. The same can be true of social care settings. It is meeting and handling these information needs that are the focus of this chapter. Specifically, the chapter will show how a range of approaches can provide a fighting chance of recasting uncertainty into a format for evidence-based practice, successfully retrieving evidence that is fit for the purpose of reducing this ambiguity, establishing a bottom line for your patients/clients or the service and getting the evidence into practice in a sustainable way.

To those readers who have experience of trying and failing in the arenas of practice development and the introduction of evidence into practice this last paragraph might sound a little optimistic (to say the least). Of course, like most claims of this nature, there are a few caveats. This chapter is intended to act as a starting point from where the reader can begin an informed foray into the wealth of text based and on-line resources offering far more guidance than a single chapter in a book can offer. I would strongly encourage the reader to seek out the further reading at the end of the chapter and to follow up the on-line links appearing in the body of the text and in the resources detailed at the end.

Finally, whilst it may seem a bit strange, I would like to present the 'take home' message of this chapter right at the beginning so that it is remembered. Specifically, finding and using evidence is a bit like a large maze: it can be complex, and the best way of handling this complexity is to adopt a systematic approach. If a systematic approach is your guiding principle then it *is* possible to emerge relatively unscathed.

WHY BOTHER BEING SYSTEMATIC?

The success of the welfare system (in terms of delivering good outcomes for patients and clients) is dependent on the quality of the decisions taken within it (Muir Gray 1997). These decisions take many forms (Box 7.1 for example details some of the decisions faced by nurses) and have almost infinite foci, but they have one thing in common: sometimes you may not always know the outcomes of the choices that you are faced with.

Box 7.1 Decision types and associated clinical questions

Decision type	Exemplar decision	Exemplar question
Intervention/effectiveness: these kinds of decisions involve choosing between interventions.	Choosing a mattress for a frail elderly man who has been admitted with an acute bowel obstruction.	In elderly and inactive patients, who may require surgical intervention, which is the most suitable pressure relieving mattress to prevent pressure sores?
Targeting: this is, strictly speaking, a subcategory of intervention/effectiveness decisions outlined above. These decisions are of the form, 'choosing which patient will most benefit from the intervention'.	Deciding which patients should get anti-embolic stockings.	Is there a risk assessment tool available that will accurately predict which group of patients will benefit most from anti-embolic stockings?
Timing: again, a subcategory of intervention/effectiveness decisions. These commonly take the form of choosing the best time to deploy the intervention.	Choosing a time to commence asthma education on newly diagnosed clients.	When to commence asthma education on newly diagnosed clients?
Communication: these kinds of decisions commonly focus on choices relating to ways of delivering and receiving information to and from patients, families or colleagues. Sometimes these decisions are specifically related to the communication of risks and benefits of different interventions or prognostic categories.	Choosing how to approach cardiac rehabilitation with an elderly patient following acute myocardial infarction who lives alone with family nearby.	Would I be better talking and explaining rehab with the patient's family present so that a clear understanding is obtained prior to the patient's discharge?
Service organisation, delivery and management: these kinds of decisions concern the configuration or processes of service delivery.	Choosing how to organise handover so that communication is most effective.	How should I organise handover so that the most effective form of communicating information results?
Experiential, understanding or hermeneutic: these relate to the interpretation of cues in the process of care.	Choosing how to reassure a patient who is worrying about cardiac arrest after witnessing another patient arresting.	How best do you reassure a patient who has witnessed someone having a cardiac arrest?

Activity 7.1

Consider the types of decisions you make on a day-to-day basis. Using the information in the box above identify the category they fall into. What does this mean about your understanding of the way in which you make decisions?

The problem of anticipating the outcome is a significant one; research into decision making reveals that rapid, regular choices have to be made, and that these choices generate information needs. In medicine, Covell et al. (1985) found primary care physicians generated two information seeking questions for every three patients they saw. Thompson et al. (2001) found that nurses make even more decisions – although of course not all will be associated with the need for research information. For example, one staff nurse observed on an acute medical ward made a total of 18 decisions in a 3 hour period of observation, a total of one every 10 minutes.

As already stated, these decisions generate the need for information. Sometimes these information needs can be met by drawing on one's own practice or, more generally, life experience. However, practice-based decisions usually require *validated information*. For example, it is unlikely that the accuracy of a diagnostic test (the degree to which it avoids false negatives and false positives – its specificity and sensitivity) can be accurately determined with reference to one's own practice experience alone. Similarly, it is unlikely that a single practitioner will ever amass enough practice experience of similar patients/clients to rival a large randomised controlled trial with upwards of 1000 participants, all of whom have an equivalent control, and from whom a reliable estimate of the effect of an intervention can be determined. In essence, this is what research knowledge does: it offers insights that cannot be gained anywhere else. This research insight, when combined with one's own practice expertise, the resources you have available to help you and the preferences of the client are the raw ingredients of an evidence-based decision. The due weight you attach to research knowledge determines your claims to be an evidence-based practitioner.

The dangers of relying on experience

Because practice (and life in general) is a complex phenomenon, human beings employ a series of workaday 'shortcuts' to help them process the masses of information which they are confronted with in daily life. These shortcuts – or heuristics – are incredibly useful in daily life, indeed, if we did not use them life would grind to a halt, but they can cause problems when they dominate practice decisions. Specifically, heuristics are associated with the introduction of systematic bias into decision making – they distort the reality of a situation.

There are many sources of bias that can arise because of these heuristic shortcuts, but five of the most common are: overconfidence, hindsight, base rate neglect, availability and anchoring.

Overconfidence

Individuals are often overconfident when assessing the correctness of their knowledge. Ironically, this often occurs in situations when we have least knowledge. In the laboratory there are a number of classic studies showing this. They include two-choice general knowledge questions (Lichenstein & Fischoff 1977, Gigerenzer 1991): impossible tasks involving perception, such as assigning the continents of authors by their handwriting, or predicting the rise of stocks based on limited knowledge of previous performance (Lichenstein & Fischoff 1977, Fischoff 1975); and guessing the true value of a quantity (Lichenstein & Fischoff 1977).

Hindsight

Most practitioners will be aware of exhortations to be more 'reflective'. Our experiences amount to rich repositories of information that can be used in our decision-making processes. Using experience in this way can be a necessary and positive force in decision making. However, experience alone is not a sufficient prerequisite for good practice-based decisions. Hindsight artificially increases the estimate of the outcomes of events that happened in the past, increases the estimated chances of medical diagnoses and produces favourable distortions of memory.

Base rate neglect

Professionals have a tendency to neglect the underlying base rates of disease or the associated symptoms when diagnosing, assessing, and meeting the health- and social-care needs of individuals (Dowie & Elstein 1988). The classic example is illustrated by Kahneman and Tversky (1973) who examined biases of people when presented with stereotypical descriptions of individuals. In their experiment they presented people with the knowledge that there was a 30:70 ratio of engineers to lawyers in a sample. Decisions that the person was likely to be one of the smaller group of 30 engineers (when there was a higher chance of being a lawyer: 2.3 to 1) appear to have been based upon information such as marital status, political allegiance and hobbies. Therefore, it seems that people made their choices based on subjective information rather than on a rational decision-making process.

Practice encourages attention to base rates (how often do you think about the eight out of 10 patients/clients who seem to recover from a myocardial infarction or other condition?); this however is not a sufficient knowledge base for such decisions. Amassing enough experience with similar clients/patients is problematic, and the role of hindsight and other forms of bias mean that experience-derived base rates alone are likely to be distorted by knowledge of the person in front of you.

Availability

People tend to use information that is closest to hand when making decisions. The problem with this approach is that what is closest to hand (cognitively speaking) is not necessarily the same for each individual, and so variation in decisions can result. People tend to recall either very recently presented information (the recency effect) or information from further back in time (the primacy effect). If you are more prone to the recency effect you are more likely to recall recent similar instances of a decision problem to that in front of you, which may not necessarily be the most appropriate match for this particular problem.

Anchoring

When people make decisions they draw on *anchors* to help them do so. Anchors are cognitive

reference points from which people work outwards. Cioffi (1997) uses the example of the midwife who describes the colour of a baby following an assessment for jaundice, 'every baby has a colour of his own … hopefully every baby is pink, or if they're a couple of days old, they may be a little yellow.' For this nurse, the initial anchors are her colour values of 'pink' and 'yellow', from which she can work in order to describe the jaundice. Cioffi (1997) implies this kind of heuristic is valuable, even desirable, in professional practice. Certainly there is little doubt that some approaches to professional expertise – the Dreyfus' (1986) and Benner (1984) models being good examples – imply that these anchors are legitimate and useful. Experts are commonly classified as experts because they are skilled in deploying these anchors. This skill is often seen to be as a result of considerable practice experience. The problem with such anchors, as we have seen, is that other kinds of heuristic and error types can distort their construction, and it is difficult to amass enough experiences of a similar nature to construct them for every situation.

The dangers of unsystematically gathered evidence

At this point the reader might be thinking, 'OK so I know that experience alone is not enough for good practice-based decision making, so what is wrong with the literature review that you find by accident (or if you are an optimist – serendipity) in the library in your lunch hour?' In an important piece of work, Mulrow (1987) examined 50 reviews published during June 1985 to June 1986 in four major medical journals. Assessments were based on eight explicit quality criteria adapted from published guidelines for the synthesis of information. Of the 50 articles, just 17 met three of the eight criteria; 32 satisfied four or five criteria; only one satisfied six criteria; and non achieved all eight criteria. Whilst most reviews had clearly specified purposes ($n = 40$) and conclusions ($n = 37$). Only one had clearly specified methods of identifying, selecting and validating the information included. Results were synthesised mainly using qualitative techniques ($n = 43$); quantitative synthesis was rarely used ($n = 3$). Unsystematic reviews do not routinely use scientific methods to identify, assess, and synthesise information. Because of the influence of subjectivity (and all the biases and heuristics associated with it), unsystematically reviewed information can be as biased as relying on experience alone.

Complexity requires imaginative and well-constructed solutions

Getting evidence into practice is a complex business. As well as the strength of the evidence, you need to balance the views of likely stakeholders and juggle the opportunity and the marginal costs involved in development. In addition, you may have to fundamentally alter the ways in which you work, and I am sure the reader can think of

---

Box 7.2 Clinical decision making, uncertainty, bias and the need for systematic approaches: a summary so far

- clinical practice involves making clinical decisions
- decisions can have an almost infinite clinical focus but many revolve around a limited number of categories such as diagnosis, treatment and the presentation of information (such as prognostic information)
- these decision types represent (and generate) information needs in clinicians
- relying on clinical experience alone is insufficient basis for practice
- research offers access to the experience of hundreds and thousands of patients and/or clinicians and can be of enormous benefit
- research evidence varies in its quality
- information-based solutions can be complex and a systematic approach is required to manage this complexity
- the evidence-based healthcare approach is one such systematic way of achieving this.

---

any number of the myriad of other challenges that await the practitioner or manager trying to change behaviour. Managing this complexity means having an array of tools to draw on to help you. Later, the chapter will show that the ingredients of change management: diagnosing challenges to change, engaging with theories of change, evaluating progress, is a science in itself requiring a systematic approach to deployment. However, the beauty of an evidence-based approach to practice is that, despite the complexity of the end result, the process and techniques involved are quite simple. The starting point for this process is converting uncertainty into a format you can work with. The device for this transformation is the focused practice question.

FORMULATING A CLINICAL QUESTION
Why formulate questions?

With the growth of access to information and communication technology it is often tempting to simply tap a couple of key words into an on-line database such as PUBMED (a free version of MEDLINE available at http://www.ncbi.nlm.nih.gov/entrez/query.fcgi) and see what comes up. This is a really inefficient way of doing it (we will see why later in the chapter when examining searching). Before dashing to a computer terminal, a much more reasonable starting point is to think about what bits of a practice situation are prone to uncertainty: the population or situation, the intervention or the outcome.

What's in a practice-based question?

There are three components to a well-structured question:

The situation or population

This is the individual, group or problem that is likely to be affected by the decision being made – or the results of the research being applied. Examples include: individual patients/clients, groups of patients or clients with similar problems (for example, insulin dependent diabetes) or services (for example, district nurses).

The intervention

This is the course of action, care, treatment that the population is to be exposed to. For example, suppose you are interested in the effectiveness of audio tape diabetic self-care educational packages in improving the control of blood sugar levels. The intervention in this case would be the self-care educational package. Sometimes questions may relate to a choice between two distinct treatment options – for example, between audio tape and computer-based self-care packages in fostering better blood sugar management. In questions like this, there is clearly an added dimension: the counter intervention (in this case the computer-based packages).

The outcome

Whilst identifying who and what you are looking at, it is sometimes easy to forget why you are looking in the first place. Usually there are things that we like to encourage (such as wound healing), and things that we like to try and prevent (such as premature mortality). Of course, we often want to promote or avoid multiple outcomes. For example, when trying to decide which is the most appropriate urinary catheter for your patient/client you may want to prevent re-catheterisation and simultaneously avoid infection.

Activity 7.2

Using the components identified in Box. 7.3 formulate a question that will help you to address a problem you wish to consider in your area of practice.

Box 7.3 PICO focused clinical questions

Focused clinical questions have three (and sometimes four) elements:

- The **population** or **problem**
- The **intervention**
- A **counter intervention** (sometimes)
- An **outcome**

An example: in patients aged 16–60 years with insulin-controlled diabetes which is more effective in improving the control of blood sugar levels: audio tape diabetic self-care educational packages or computer-based self-care educational packages?

Under PICO headings:

- **Problem or population** – patients aged 16–60 years with insulin controlled diabetes
- **Intervention** – audio tape diabetic self-care educational packages
- **Counter intervention** – computer-based self-care educational packages
- **Outcome** – control of blood sugar levels

DIFFERENT SOURCES OF EVIDENCE FOR DIFFERENT QUESTIONS

For each of the different types of questions you develop there are particular types of research design which are appropriate to use. This 'best fit' occurs because it is the design that minimises the biases that can lead to misleading results in studies. So, for a practice question that deals with the effectiveness of different decision options (such as selecting wound care treatments), the design which is least likely to lead to a misleading answer (i.e. an over- or underestimation of the true effect of a treatment) is a systematic review of randomised controlled trials. This idea of appropriate research designs for particular questions is what is referred to when the 'hierarchy of evidence' is discussed. A hierarchy of evidence for questions relating to clinical effectiveness is outlined in Figure 7.1 and the most appropriate types of research design for particular questions outlined in Box 7.4.

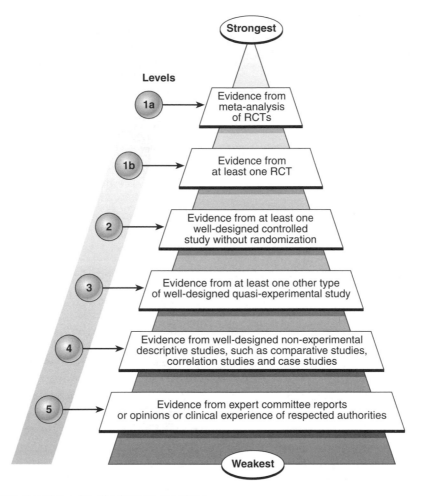

Figure 7.1 Hierarchy of evidence for effectiveness questions.

Box 7.4	Types of practice question and the most appropriate research design to look for	
Type of question	**Example**	**Best design**
Effectiveness of treatment/ prevention, adverse effects of treatments	Does compression bandaging increase the healing of venous leg ulcers compared with no compression?	Systematic reviews of randomised controlled trials
Causation	Are people who have had a deep vein thrombosis more likely to get a leg ulcer than people who have not?	Cohort study
Feelings, understanding, perceptions	How do people with venous leg ulcers feel about their health and their lifestyle?	Qualitative techniques or survey
Diagnosis	What is the most accurate means of diagnosing venous leg ulcers in clinical practice?	Studies comparing the test to a 'gold standard'

SEARCHING FOR EVIDENCE

Having constructed a focused question you are now ready to start thinking about searching for the best form of evidence to answer your question. The most important point is to think strategically; failure to do so will heighten your chances of becoming distracted by articles and evidence that will not answer your questions, and will lengthen the time you spend away from practice.

How phrasing the question differently can help in your search for evidence

Before delving into the library it is worth writing down all the synonyms (different words for the same phenomenon). This includes American spellings or versions of words (for example pediatrics and paediatrics, learning disability and mental retardation), and lay terms (for example, shingles for herpes zoster). If you do this for each of the components of your question the chances of retrieving relevant information are much higher.

Activity 7.3

Thinking about the area you wish to change and the question you have already formulated write down all the other words that may be relevant to your question. Do not forget to consider the areas mentioned above as a guide.

Thinking about where you will look

Having written down all the alternative words associated with your search, the next stage is to think about where you will look for evidence. The four sources of evidence that are most useful in practice are:

- Evidence-based journals – these journals usually follow a similar format: they take the best quality research published in ordinary scientific peer reviewed journals, summarise it, provide a clinical bottom line, and usually a commentary from an expert in the field. Examples include, *Evidence Based Nursing, Evidence Based Mental Health* and *Evidence Based Medicine.*

- The Cochrane Library (http://www.cochrane.org) and the NHS Centre for Reviews and Dissemination (http://www.york.ac.uk/inst/crd/) – these sources are repositories of high-quality systematic reviews of rigorous research. They also offer valuable links to groups of researchers and practitioners interested in similar problems as well as training, searching and critical appraisal resources.

- On-line computerised databases such as MEDLINE (a computerised version of the Index Medicus) and CINAHL (the Cumulated Index of Nursing and Allied Health Literature). These databases are bibliographic reference sources. What this means is that they do not conventionally offer the full text of a reference, just the citation and the abstract (where available). The exception to this is PUBMED (which is also free) which offers hyperlinks to selected full text resources, such as the BMJ and JAMA. PUBMED is available at http://www.ncbi.nlm.nih.gov/entrez/query.fcgi and offers a full feature gateway to MEDLINE. One valuable feature of PUBMED is its ability to be able to match the references it provides in a search to the question you are asking via its 'clinical queries' section. When using on-line databases it is worth getting to grips with search filters; more on these in a moment.

- The internet (world wide web) – whilst the internet contains much which is of very poor quality, there are sites which are increasingly applying filters to the sorts of information being presented. Moreover, the internet is also a valuable gateway to resources such as the National Electronic Library for Health.

When you get there

If you have chosen your evidence source well, then the tasks required once you arrive there will be minimised. For example, if your question is one of effectiveness, then it is quite feasible that simply typing a key word into the search screen of the Cochrane Library will reveal some useful evidence. However, some sources – particularly the ubiquitous 'on-line bibliographic database' – need more effort if you are to find useful evidence more effectively and efficiently. The most powerful resources (on-line databases) are also the least reliable in the hands of the inexperienced. The three strategic components to bear in mind when using an on-line database are:

- Revisit your synonyms and make use of them when working up your search.

- Seek to perform as broad a search as possible in the first instance using either text words or MESH headings (MESH – medical subject headings – are the labels used by MEDLINE and CINAHL and other databases to categorise citations and abstracts) – this stage will commonly involve using the combining word 'or'.

- Narrow down the broad search by excluding the least relevant studies – use key words, only include studies which are the right kind of design for the question you want, and use the joining phrase 'and'.

Activity 7.4

Using the information identified in Figure 7.2 and Box 7.5 carry out the search for evidence required to answer your question.

Search filters

We have already encountered the idea of 'matching' the right kind of evidence to the right kind of

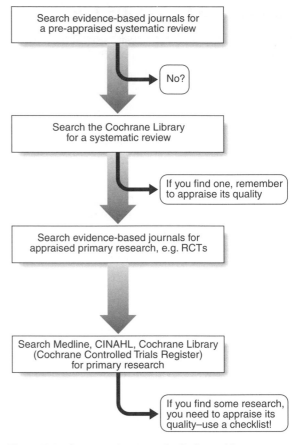

Figure 7.2 Suggested strategy for finding evidence on effectiveness.

Box 7.5 The main stages of a search strategy

- Develop your clinical question
- Write down all the key words and synonyms (alternatives) you can think of (consider American spellings)
- Decide in advance where you are going to look: see Figure 7.2
- Do as broad a search as possible based on the subject area (intervention, population outcome) using the 'or' operator
- Narrow the search down by rejecting the inappropriate and or unhelpful studies (use the AND/NOT operators)
- Review your success and rework the strategy if necessary (i.e. broaden or narrow it further).

question. One way of transferring this idea to your search strategy (above and beyond looking at the right source – see Fig. 7.2) is by the use of specialist search filters. These filters all work by restricting the kinds of evidence retrieved to those which are most likely to answer the question you propose. So if your question is one of the accuracy of diagnostic tests for Down's syndrome, a good search filter will look primarily for systematic reviews of studies which compare tests to a 'gold standard'. Alternatively, if your question is concerned with the most effective means of pressure-sore prevention, a useful filter will extract those references based primarily on systematic reviews of randomised controlled trials. One of these filters is built into PUBMED already in the form of the 'clinical queries' section of the site. This section of the site enables you to specify the type of question you are asking and to restrict the results accordingly.

Getting the search filter into your strategy when you do not use PUBMED

One way of getting the filter into the software you are using is to type in the filter line by line and then save it as a 'history' file (with the extension .his in Silverplatter). This only has to be done once for each of the kinds of filter (effectiveness, diagnosis, prognosis, qualitative) you want to use, as you can then load the filter into subsequent strategies and adapt it for the specifics of that search. In many ways this is preferable to the alternative (downloading an off-the-shelf filter from a site such as the University of Rochester (http://www.urmc.rochester.edu/Miner/Educ/Expertsearch.html)), as you will learn the syntax and correct term construction for your software, thereby helping you develop your generic computer package skills. Box 7.6 gives an example of one filter which looks for references based around qualitative research.

Box 7.6 A search filter for qualitative evidence (adapted from University of Rochester for the Silverplatter search software)

qualitative studies	purpos* adj sampl*
ethnographic research	emic or etic or hermeneutic* or heuristic or semiotics
phenomenological research	data adj saturat*
ethnonursing research	participant adj observ*
grounded theory	heidegger* or colaizzi* or spiegelberg*
explode 'qualitative validity'/all topical subheadings/all age subheadings	van adj manen*
	van adj kaam*
purposive sample	'merleau ponty'
explode 'observational method'/all topical subheadings/all age subheadings	hussel* or giorgi*
	field adj (study or studies or research)
content analysis or thematic analysis	lived experience
constant comparative method	narrative analysis
field studies	discourse* adj analysis
theoretical sample	human science
discourse analysis	life experiences
focus groups	explode 'cluster sample'/all topical subheadings/all age subheadings
phenomenology or ethnography or ethnological research	
#1 or #2 or #3 or #4 or #5 or #6 or #7 or #8 or #9 or #10 or #11 or #12 or #13 or #14 or #15	#16 or #17 or #18 or #19 or #20 or #21 or #22 or #23 or #24 or #25 or #26 or #27 or #28 or #29 or #30 or #31 or #32 or #33 or #34 or #35 or #36
qualitative or ethnon$ or phenomenol$	DT = 'STUDY'
qualitative or ethnon* or phenomenol*	#37 and (DT = 'STUDY')
grounded adj (theor* or study or studies or research)	
constant adj (comparative or comparison)	

Quick and dirty alternatives to bespoke filters

An alternative to the full blown search filter is to use the 'fields', which MEDLINE and CINAHL use to classify references. These fields – for example, author, publication type and language of publication – can be used to good effect when searching. For example, a search on 'childhood asthma' AND 'systematic review in PT' (PT is the field for publication type) on CINAHL will identify only papers which are systematic reviews that relate to childhood asthma.

I cannot stress enough the benefits of utilising the skills of your subject librarian, although in the 21st century the term 'information broker' is probably a more apt description. These individuals serve a number of useful functions for the practitioner:

- They are one gateway to accessing on-line resources such as MEDLINE, CINAHL, ASSIA, EMBASE. More importantly, they offer a guide service enabling mistakes to be corrected and the full texts of articles to be retrieved more readily.

- They are a source of expertise. Obviously librarians have busy jobs just like the rest of us, but their expertise is marshalled most effectively when they are given the best raw materials to be able to deploy it. Having developed the skill of asking focused questions and writing down synonyms, you will have an advantage on your peers who do not possess these skills and the librarians task is made that much easier; increasing the chances of you receiving a fruitful set of search results.

- They are a source of education, training and support.

- They are cost effective disseminators. Some librarians filter, appraise and target information to practice areas as a means of keeping units up to date.

QUESTIONING THE EVIDENCE: CRITICAL APPRAISAL

Why bother appraising research evidence?

The research evidence that is available varies enormously in its quality. Because of this variability it is essential to critically appraise any research evidence we wish to factor into our decision making. There is a strong case for arguing that using inaccurate or unreliable evidence is probably worse than not using evidence at all.

Critical appraisal in practice focuses upon three key areas of the paper you are reading: its validity, what the results actually mean, and how could it be applied to the decision or patient/client you are faced with? Before we look at appraisal questions, and the checklists we can use to ask them quickly and easily, it is worth expanding on these three aims of appraisal generally.

Establishing the validity of the research

The purpose of asking questions regarding the validity of the research is to establish whether it was of sufficient quality in its design and execution that you can trust the results (having of course ascertained what they are). In other words, you scrutinise the research by asking questions designed to identify any systematic errors (bias) or one off flaws in the study. The presence of such negative features in a piece of research determines the extent to which the study will accurately and reliably achieve what it set out to achieve. Almost all appraisal checklists (more on this in a moment) start with a series of questions designed to assess the validity of a piece of work. It is better to ask four or five questions which will help you ascertain whether a piece of research is worth reading. This is better than wasting time working out the clinical significance of the paper only to find that the randomised controlled trial you were examining was neither properly randomised nor blinded, does not provide any details on the statistical tests used or was on too small a sample of people to be of any use in practice.

Establishing what the results mean: statistical significance and its relevance to practice

Having established that the study you are examining is worthy of further scrutiny and that you can trust whatever it has to say, the next stage of any appraisal process is to isolate the actual results of the study. There are two main elements to any such estimation: did the results occur by chance (i.e. are the results *statistically* significant?) and are the results important (i.e. are the results significant to your area of practice?). It is important to recognise the difference between these two concepts (statistical and practice significance). The oft-reported 'p value' (as in $p < 0.05$) simply tells you the probability that the results occurred by chance, so in this example the reported p value is telling us that there is a less than 5% probability that the result being reported occurred by chance. This information is useful but it *does not* give any indication of the importance of the result in a practice context. Any study, if it is large enough, will be able to demonstrate a statistically significant difference or association between the groups or variables being examined. In order to ascertain the significance for practice, we need to look at other characteristics, such as the outcome being measured (mild ear ache or preventable death), and the size of the effect of any intervention or causal relationship. The best way of examining this last point is by understanding the idea of confidence intervals. These will be discussed later in the chapter.

What do the results mean for me: how can I apply them to my decisions or to my work with clients/patients?

An evidence-based decision is one which balances the preferences of patients/clients, the expertise of the practitioner, the available resources and the strength of the research evidence. Having established that the research results are valid and relevant for practice, one needs to grapple with how the results can be applied to one's own practice. There are formal decision support tools (such as decision analytic approaches) to help with this process (Lilford et al. 1998). However, ordinarily it involves asking tricky questions around the similarity of those to whom you are providing a service to those in the study, the feasibility of applying it in your setting, the harms and benefits to the individual patient/client or problem (rather that the population from where the evidence is derived), and whether you have the necessary skills to actually employ the valid and important research results.

Appraisal checklists

As already alluded to, appraisal in practice needs to be efficient and effective if it is to become a part of evidence-based care delivery. The most efficient and effective means of making appraisal a reality is to utilise checklists specifically designed to establish the validity, results and applicability of research evidence. Crucially, these checklists are associated with particular research designs (and by default, the related questions) and are easily mastered. Because there are as many checklists as there are research designs, a full explication lies outside the scope of this chapter and the reader is directed to the text and on-line resources at the end of the chapter for more information. Appraisal checklists have been developed by a number of organisations (CASP – the Critical Skills Appraisal Programme;

CEBM – Centre for Evidence Based Medicine) and are available on-line, in journals, and in text books. Two examples are the Centre for Evidence Based Nursing's NT learning curve series and the excellent JAMA users' guides to the medical literature (see end of the chapter for more information). Whilst different organisationally derived checklists may differ in the detail, they all share the same central concerns with establishing the validity, results and applicability of the research being scrutinised.

Eleven questions to ask of all research evidence

Although checklists should be matched to the research you are faced with there are 11 generic appraisal questions which should be asked of all the research evidence you encounter.

Does the paper clearly state the aims of the research?

Research needs to clearly state the aims that underpin it; failure to do this means it is difficult for the reader to assess whether the aims are achieved. In quantitative research in particular, clear aims are the basis for clear and limited hypotheses, which are stated before data collection and analysis and are a sign of good-quality research. Fewer hypotheses in a study usually means fewer comparisons (statistical tests) between the variables being examined – this is important for many reasons, but the main one is about reducing the effect of chance. If the researcher uses the conventional 5% cut-off point (as in $p = {<}0.05$), then out of a 100 comparisons we could expect five 'significant' results to occur by chance. Expressed alternatively, one result out of every 20 could be spurious. The more comparisons a study has the greater the probability that the results occurred by chance alone.

Does the paper clearly justify the sample size?

Most (quantitative) research designs aim to detect differences or associations between variables. A study needs to be large enough to detect these differences. Conversely, it also needs to be large enough to avoid the mistake of saying that there is a difference between two variables when in reality there isn't. A well designed study will take into account previous research results for the intervention, population and outcome being examined, and the size of effect that is desirable and produce an *a priori* (specified in advance) power calculation (as in establishing the sample size necessary to be powerful enough to detect true differences and prevent spurious claims of difference).

Many kinds of studies looking at interventions that professionals deploy need large sample sizes to accurately detect differences or associations (because the treatment effects or outcomes are not always large). For a quick retrospective check on the adequacy of sample size in a paper, look at the confidence intervals that are reported. Confidence intervals provide the range within which we can be confident (typically reported as either a 95% or 99% confidence interval, indicating that we can be either 95% or 99% confident in the results) that the true effect (i.e. the effect in a population rather than a sample of that population) will occur. Confidence intervals take the form of a lower and an upper figure, with the 'true' average or other measure lying anywhere between these two points. So, for example Buchkremer and colleagues (1995) looked at the impact on people with schizophrenia of having their relatives participate in a therapeutic group. They showed that you could be 95% sure that the odds of committing suicide while your relatives participated in this therapy were between 0.05 and 3.65 (odds of 1 – or evens – would be an equal chance of committing suicide whether in the intervention or control group). This information tells us that a person could be more likely to commit suicide whilst part of this programme or just as plausibly much less likely to commit suicide. Clearly this doesn't help reduce the uncertainties associated with the kinds of decisions likely to arise in this situation – should I refer a family to a group counselling service? Should I establish such a service? The study was too small with only 99 people in it. The larger the study, the smaller the confidence intervals, and the more accurately we can assess the importance of the findings (and the adequacy of the sample size).

Are the measurements used in the paper valid and reliable?

Often research sets out to 'measure' phenomena or concepts. Sometimes these entities are relatively easy to measure, such as mortality, but concepts such as depression or quality of life are more of a challenge. A valid measure is one that accurately captures the phenomenon it seeks to measure. Consider asking an alcoholic how much their daily intake of alcohol is. You may not get an entirely accurate answer. A more valid (but invasive and expensive) measure would be to measure the blood levels of alcohol present on a daily basis. Good quality research pays attention to, justifies and discusses the measures that are used, and identifies the trade offs (pragmatic and academic) that are involved.

Reliability of the measures used is another important consideration in appraisal. Even very reliable measures, such as blood pressure measured via a sphygmomanometer, are subject to systematic and random variation according to the position of the arm, the position of the patient and the technique of the practitioner. Studies will often present statistical information on the reliability of the measures that are used, i.e. the degree to which a measure will produce the same results on subsequent occasions, such as the Kappa coefficient. In addition, statistical information can indicate the degree to which two halves of a questionnaire purporting to measure the same concept, such as depression, produce similar results, for example, the Cronbach's alpha split half reliability coefficient. Quality research will provide an indication of the reliability of the measures used. For example, a measure with a Chronbach's alpha score of more than 0.8 would be a very reliable measure, between 0.6 and 0.8 less so, and less than 0.6 not very reliable.

Does the paper adequately describe the statistics used?

Most well constructed studies will use the most appropriate tests for the data types and questions used. The most appropriate tests are well known and include t-test, ANOVA, simple correlation and regression and chi-square; because they are the most appropriate they are also the most common. Unusual tests should be accompanied by a detailed justification for their use. All statistical tests are based on sets of assumptions about the data they are applied to, for example, the distribution of scores, the type of data, the independence of the measures generating it. Good researchers will always reassure the reader that these assumptions have been met; this usually occurs in the analysis section of a report. If in doubt regarding the suitability of the application of a particular test, then consult someone who has the necessary knowledge, for example, a research and development lead, a clinical governance or best practice lead, or a researcher.

Did any unplanned or untoward events happen during the course of the study?

Well planned studies will take into account (either prospectively or retrospectively) untoward events, such as subjects excessively dropping out of the study or the non-compliance of participatory research sites. Untoward events can usually be forecast reasonably with experience, however, some are truly beyond the control of the research teams involved. For example, imagine a situation in which a public health professional wished to establish the prevalence of depressive symptoms in the UK farming population and half way through the data collection period a foot and mouth outbreak occurs. Of course, such events have significant implications for the research results and should be brought to the attention of the reader.

Does the paper adequately describe the basic data?

Applying the results of good quality research is made very difficult if the reporting of an otherwise excellent study is let down by the presentation of very basic data on the subjects involved. All studies should provide details of the basic numbers of people or subjects involved (often referred to as 'n', as in $n = 55$) and some indication of the degree of variance around a measure of central tendency such as the mean (or average). The most common indication of the variance around a mean or other measure of central tendency (such as the median) is the standard deviation (often referred to as the 'sd', as in the mean age was 55 years, sd = 3.4). The purpose of presenting such information is to give the reader enough detail to be able to understand the composition of the subjects involved in the study. Consequently, reporting demographic and biographical data (age, sex, social class) is a must for a good quality research study.

Do the numbers presented in the text or tables add up?

This is obviously only an issue for quantitative studies. It is common these days for researchers to use computer packages, for example SPSS or MINISTAT, to do the more laborious calculations that are associated with handling large amounts of data. Theoretically then mistakes in calculation should be kept to a minimum. However, mistakes still occur in reporting the results of studies, and occasionally researchers, for a variety of reasons, sometimes fail to use the data from all the subjects in a study (missing data points). In small studies even small discrepancies between groups can result in large differences in the results. As an example, if you half the number of people in a sample, you quarter the standard error associated with the population's variability around the mean (the standard error is the measure of variability used to construct confidence intervals). Consequently, small shifts in sample size, for example by leaving people out of the analysis, can exert a significant effect on the results. Moreover, one should always assume that people left out of an analysis, for whatever reason, suffered negative outcomes, consequently, the results of studies become much more conservative – perhaps needlessly so.

Does the study present results in terms of their statistical significance and, if so, how?

As we have seen the statistical importance of a result (did it occur by chance?) is not the same as the importance and relevance to practice. Nevertheless, something cannot be important in practice if it occurs by chance and, therefore, you have no reliable way of reproducing the results with patients/clients or in the service. For this reason the p value is still an important feature of interpreting any research results and should be presented where the authors are advocating that the outcomes of their research are applicable to a wider context.

How do the authors interpret null (negative) findings?

Many research projects do not isolate statistically significant negative results in relation to the questions asked: it is rare to see 'result X failed to reach statistical significance' reported in research papers. However, whilst these negative findings are frustrating for researchers, they are important for appraisers. Often such results arise because studies are too small (examine the confidence intervals, if they range from positively harmful to positively beneficial then the study is probably too small) or one of a myriad of other potential reasons. The important point for the appraiser is that the researcher should explain why the results have occurred.

Does the paper miss important effects?

Researchers, like all human beings, are occasionally prone to only analysing and presenting selective information. People tend towards seeking evidence that fits rather than challenges their preconceived views and arguments. Of course, this tendency is unhelpful in research as the 'truth' uncovered by a project relies on the picture built up by systematically challenging ideas in the form of seeking to disprove null hypotheses. A useful tip here is to draw one's own conclusions from the results presented and to see if the author also reaches the same ones – if not, why not?

What do the findings of the study actually mean?

Once you have determined that the results did not occur by chance, the next task is to ascertain what the results mean in the practice context. We have already encountered the idea of confidence intervals as one way of making sense of the size of an effect or the practice significance of a set of results. Confidence intervals can be constructed for a whole range of different measures, such as proportions, the difference between two means and likelihood ratios. For more details on these calculations see Altman et al. (2000) and Sackett et al. (2000).

Interpretation of the confidence intervals are not the only way of determining the importance of the results. Use your own experience and knowledge to decide whether the results make biological or theoretical sense. Good quality research will always discuss the results in the context of current knowledge and previous research, and this makes this appraisal task a lot easier. Identifying these links between knowledge, previous research and the study's results is easier for some designs than others: systematic reviews, for example, are generally easier to appraise than a piece of qualitative research. Systematic reviews adhere to a reasonably universal format and have less flexibility in the ways in which they are reported.

> **Activity 7.5**
>
> Having found the evidence you need for your question, appraise each piece of evidence using the 11 questions outlined above. Obviously, if any of your material is qualitative in nature you will need to select the appropriate questions to use.

More on checklists

These 11 generic appraisal questions should be applied to all research that you encounter as a result of formulating a question and applying your search strategy. However, as already mentioned, there are supplementary questions that should be asked of all research designs (Box 7.7 provides the questions that should be asked of reviews, for example). The reader is strongly encouraged to make use of the links to appraisal resources at the end of the chapter for more examples of checklists for particular research designs.

IMPLEMENTING THE EVIDENCE – DEVELOPING AN EVIDENCE-BASED TOOLKIT?

Having searched for and appraised the evidence and decided that it is worthy of application in the

---

> **Box 7.7** Appraisal checklist – review articles
>
> **Are the results valid?**
> *Primary guides*
> Did the review address a focused clinical question?
> Were the criteria used to select articles for inclusion
> appropriate?
>
> *Secondary guides*
> Is it unlikely that important, relevant studies were
> missed?
> Was the validity of the included studies appraised?
> Were the assessments of studies reproducible?
> Were the results similar from study to study?
>
> **What are the results?**
> What are the overall results of the review?
> How precise were the results?
>
> **Will the results help me in caring for my patients?**
> Can the results be applied to my patient care?
> Were all clinically important outcomes considered?
> Are the benefits worth the harms and costs?
>
> **Reference**: JAMA 1994; 272: 1367–1371

workplace, how should one proceed? As a researcher I often hear the plaintive cry that 'there is nothing out there which tells us what works when we want to change practice'. In fact, we know quite a bit about changing behaviour and managing the transition from abstract research knowledge into improved, and research-informed, professional decisions. The Cochrane Collaboration's (http://www.cochrane.co.uk) EPOC group produce systematic reviews on just this topic, the results of which have been summarised in an Effective Health Care Bulletin (NHS CRD, 1999), journal articles and policy reports over the past 6 years (Oxman et al. 1995). More recently, the service delivery and organisation (SDO) arm of the UK NHS R&D strategy has produced a substantive review of the literature on organisational change (Lies & Sutherland 2001).

Start small – developing your own workplace information resource

Professionals have limited time available for accessing written information, many resources

are out of date and few appear explicitly evidence based. As a starting point then (and with the earlier broad strategy of thinking about the best *source* for information), it is probably worth concentrating on compiling only explicitly evidence-based resources. This strategy will mean less fruitless searching and less unnecessary appraisal, leaving more time for practice. Some examples of evidence-based written sources of knowledge are presented in Box 7.8.

In order to keep track of all this information it is important that professionals acquire the skills to handle information effectively. Practitioners need to develop the computer and keyboard skills necessary to use a personal referencing system or on-line database. For those people also engaged in academic development, these skills are transferable to and from that environment.

Diagnosing the challenges and barriers to use of evidence

The importance of diagnosing the likely barriers to changing practice is an essential component to any strategy designed to increase the use of research knowledge in the decisions made in a service. There are a variety of diagnostic methods available to the practitioner ranging from qualitative enquiry with key stakeholders to the diagnostic scales represented by tools such as the BARRIERS scale, developed by Sandra Funk and colleagues (Funk et al. 1995, Retsas 2000). Space precludes a detailed exposition of the techniques involved, but the important point here is that the reader should be aware of the crucial nature of diagnosis. For without a firm diagnosis it is difficult to accurately target messages or initiatives. Again there are a number of models available (such as social marketing and precede-proceed), which can help the strategist organise and focus their activity (NHS CRD 1999).

Having diagnosed what the likely environmental barriers are and considered the approaches to organising the actions required, there are

Box 7.8 Sources of evidence-based healthcare knowledge for a ward/unit library	
Source	Description
Effective Healthcare Bulletins	Based around systematic reviews of effectiveness and cost effectiveness studies. Produced by the NHS CRD at the University of York. Dealing with a range of clinical and management topics.
Effectiveness matters	Complements Effective Healthcare, provides updates on the effectiveness of important health interventions for practitioners and decision makers in the NHS. Covers topics in a shorter more journalistic style, summarising the results of high quality systematic reviews.
CRD reports	Detailed reports of the systematic reviews carried out by CRD (in-depth, detailed and comprehensive)
Evidence based journals	Journals such as Evidence Based Nursing, Evidence Based Medicine, Evidence Based Mental Health, Evidence Based Healthcare Management, ACP Journal Club offer concise summaries and clinical commentaries of the best quality research evidence.
Epidemiologically based needs assessments	Published by the NHSE to support the commissioning process.
Health technology assessments	Some of the NHS HTA program consists of systematic reviews. Available on-line from http://www.hta.nhsweb.nhs.uk/
Clinical Evidence	Clinical Evidence is a six monthly, updated compendium of evidence on the effects of common clinical interventions, published by the BMJ Publishing Group. It provides a concise account of the current state of knowledge, ignorance, and uncertainty about the prevention and treatment of a wide range of clinical conditions based on thorough searches of the literature. It is not a textbook of medicine nor a book of guidelines. It summarises the best available evidence, and where there is no good evidence, it says so. http://www.clinicalevidence.com/
Cochrane Library	The Cochrane Library is actually 4 databases which can be accessed via the internet (and NHS Net) and local CD Rom: • Cochrane Database of Systematic Reviews: a database of systematic reviews and planned reviews carried out for the Cochrane Collaboration • Database of Abstracts of Reviews of Effectiveness (DARE): critically appraised abstracts of systematic reviews. The abstracts are produced by reviewers from the NHS Centre for Reviews and Dissemination at the University of York • Cochrane review methodology update: articles, links, and resources for those considering or undertaking a review • Cochrane Controlled Trials Register: a register of controlled trials identified by reviewers for the Cochrane Collaboration (http://www.cochranelibrary.com)
National clinical guidelines	The Royal College of Nursing is beginning to carry out guidelines (so far in the management of leg ulcers and pain in children). The National Institute for Clinical Excellence is set to produce clinical guidelines based on reviews of good quality research evidence. At present organisations such as the Scottish Intercollegiate Guidelines Network and the North of England Guidelines Group also produce evidence based clinical guidelines.

specific techniques which practitioners should consider in any overall change strategy. These should be informed by the knowledge that planned, multifaceted approaches based on a good diagnosis are likely to yield the best results (Oxman et al. 1995).

Continuing educational approaches

Continuing professional development (study days, CPD courses, conference attendance), are common features of most professionals' working lives. It is not clear, however, that when this is the only component of professional development that they are very effective. Five systematic reviews (Bertram 1977, Lloyd 1979, Beaudry 1989, Waddell 1991, Davis 1995) have examined the impact of educational approaches to changing healthcare professional behaviours. Results are mixed with most reviews reporting at least some effect but hampered by the poor quality of many of the primary research reports. Perhaps significantly, the systematic reviews of the highest calibre (Davis 1995) conclude that continuing educational approaches are a largely ineffective way of changing practice. Conversely, reviews of lesser quality tend towards viewing initiatives such as study days as more effective (Waddell 1991).

Clinical and practice guidelines

Clinical guidelines have proved very influential in health care, the Royal College of Nursing's guidelines on venous leg ulcers (RCN 1998) being a good example. However, as with continuing professional development, guidelines should not be assumed to be a panacea for changing practice. Thomas and colleagues (1999) looked at the role of clinical guidelines as a way of lessening inappropriate variations in practice. They found 18 good quality studies and concluded that guidelines are limited in their ability to change practice. Research has not yet revealed which modes of dissemination and implementation work best in relation to guidelines or whether any apparent effects are sustainable. The only real conclusions are that evidence-based theoretical perspectives (Grol 1992) as well as adaptation of national guidelines to local circumstance can be useful (NHS CRD 1999). Guidelines can also be useful when used in conjunction with supportive educational strategies and specific reminders.

One approach which incorporates many of these elements are integrated care pathways. These are commonly based around local systems and processes, supported by clinical and managerial teams, use a guideline format and have reminders built into the accompanying documentation and monitoring. However, there is only limited evidence of their success (Marrie 2000) and, as yet, they need large scale evaluation.

Some systematic reviews look at broad dissemination and implementation strategies (Oxman 1995, Yano 1995, Wensing 1998): providing research information alone, management approaches, and social influence approaches. Most concur with Oxman's (1995) conclusion that 'no magic bullets' exist for changing professional practice or attitudes. Multifaceted approaches to change, whilst more expensive, seem to have the most impact. This impact, however, is unpredictable and not always reliable.

Specific approaches

In contrast to the broad approaches outlined above there are some specific techniques you might want to consider. One way of classifying these is according to the impact that you can expect from employing them: consistently effective, mixed, or little/no impact (Bero et al. 1998).

Consistently effective

Educational outreach/detailing. Academic or educational detailing – involves trained individuals going out to practice environments to help promote the utilisation of research findings in practice. This approach has been used in the area of compression bandaging for venous leg ulceration as well as in the area of prescribing; the work in the latter area has proved to be particularly successful. Up until now, most of the work has been conducted in North American settings with doctors, but this strategy may be useful in attempting to change practice in this country. The effect of outreach is maximised when conducted alongside a social marketing framework. The National Research Register (http://www.update-software.

com/NRR/) gives contact details of researchers currently examining the value of educational outreach in the UK. Examples include: 'An evaluation of the effectiveness and cost effectiveness of audit and feedback and educational outreach in improving nursing practice and outcomes', and 'Educational outreach in diabetes to encourage practice nurses to respond to guidelines to control hypertension and hyperlipidaemia in primary and shared care (EDEN): a randomised trial using a blocked reciprocal control design'. Generally, 'interactive' approaches to educating groups of professionals may yield positive results (Bero et al. 1998).

Reminders. Whether manual or electronic, reminders have been shown to be effective in improving preventative care (Shea 1996) and general management of patients/clients, their effect in relation to improving diagnostic behaviour is uncertain.

Multifaceted interventions. Combining two or more of audit and feedback, reminders, local consensus processes (see below) and marketing approaches in an overall change strategy offers the highest chance of success (Davis et al. 1995, Wensing 1994).

Mixed effect

Audit and feedback. It is doubtful that audit, on its own, is a sufficient mechanism for sustained change. Those studies looking at whether audit and feedback approaches to change, result in improved behaviours (Buntinx et al. 1993, Balas et al. 1996, Thomson et al. 1999) report at best only moderate effects and see it as less effective than less labour intensive methods such as reminders. Audit and feedback, as part of a wider strategy, have some merit, but as a stand-alone approach to change should not be relied upon.

Local opinion leaders. Thomson et al. (1999) report that local opinion leaders as conduits for change have mixed effects on professional practice. However, we do not always know what local opinion leaders do and descriptions of their characteristics are often lacking. Thomson et al. (1999) suggests that further research is required to determine the identifying characteristics of leaders and the circumstances in which they are likely to influence the practice of their peers. Bero et al. (1998) suggest that colleagues nominated by peers as 'educationally influential' might be a useful characteristic to focus on. Thompson et al. (2001) suggests that 'clinical credibility', in the form of experience, rather than research competence or awareness is influential in getting nurses to engage with imparted information. Local opinion leaders (often those embodying the clinical nurse specialist role) were a powerful force for change.

Local consensus approaches. Mulhall and LeMay (1999, p. 200) recognise that 'ownership of the [change] project is important'. Bero et al. (1998) report that inclusion of stakeholder professionals in discussions to ensure their perception of the change problem as 'important' is essential. However, the results of their scrutiny are mixed and consensus alone should not be relied upon.

Patient/client-mediated interventions. If a patient asked you to justify your choice of wound dressing or urinary catheter would it change your approach? This kind of question lies at the core of mediated interventions. By providing information to patients/clients that they can use in a specific way in interactions with professionals they can, in theory, exert an impact on the behaviour of practitioners. For example, many professionals are increasingly encountering the 'internet informed' person and, anecdotally, GPs have reported that this 'makes them think twice' about the sorts of information and care provided. However, here too results are mixed and patient/client-mediated approaches are not a sufficient stand-alone mechanism for cultural shift.

Little or no effect

Worryingly, those sources of research-based knowledge which many professionals rely on, such as didactic lecture style study days, passively disseminated practice guidelines, lecture notes, educational videos and protocols, seem to exert the least (if any) effect on professional practice. Freemantle et al. (1999) in a review of printed educational materials found no statistically significant improvements in practice. Similarly, Bero and colleagues (1998) report that didactic style educational meetings are not a useful route for inducing change in practice.

A NOTE ON CLINICAL AUDIT

Evaluation of the process of implementing evidence-based practice is vital in order to determine whether or not changes have influenced practice and ultimately patient/client care. One should remember though that audit is a cyclical process. Whilst definitions of audit are multifarious (Crombie et al. 1997), one characteristic which all approaches share is that practitioner effort during clinical audit should focus on fulfilling the key stages of an audit cycle. The basic audit stages of observing current practice, setting standards of care, comparing practice with the standards and implementing a change, should be addressed in a continuous and iterative way. There should be no pre-determined end point for stopping the cycle. Limited space and scope preclude a detailed discussion of clinical audit and its role in clinical governance, and it is covered elsewhere in this book.

CONCLUSION

This has been a chapter which has had to cover a lot of ground in a short space. Consequently, it has only been possible to scratch the surface of the complex field of finding, appraising and using evidence in practice. By now you should be familiar enough with the exhortation to use the further reading and resources after you have finished this chapter. That said, it is possible to draw some conclusions regarding the identification, appraisal and implementation of research evidence, and their link with the clinical governance and best value agenda.

First, be clear about why you need the literature. Fostering this clarity means reviewing the uncertainties you face in practice and which are associated with the choices (practice decisions) you make. Capturing this uncertainty is best promoted via the device of the focused question. Get into the habit of asking these questions – at information exchange meetings, when writing reports, when reflecting on practice and in supervision sessions. The opportunities are limitless and the rewards high.

Second, do not rely on chance or serendipity for success in either searching, appraisal or implementation. Going to the local academic library and casually grazing on a few of your favourite journals is *not* the way to acquire information that is fit for the purposes of reducing your uncertainty, and if it does so it probably does so erroneously. Think about the sort of information you need, match the research design underpinning the information to the questions you want answered, be systematic in development of your search strategy, and choose an appropriate appraisal tool or checklist and work through it sequentially. Do not be afraid to reject evidence on the basis of such systematic appraisal.

When it comes to implementation, it is worth reiterating Oxman's (1995) mantra that there 'are no magic bullets'. However, acquiring a good diagnosis of the likely barriers and promoters in your area, adopting a theoretical framework as a way of organising activity, and basing strategy on multifaceted interventions that will give you more than a fighting chance of success is one good way of starting.

Finally, do not be disheartened in your early efforts. Searching, appraisal and implementation involves knowledge, skills and techniques that improve with practice and experience. Your learning curve will be swift, your results (and hopefully decisions) will improve, and your own portfolio of skills and knowledge will be richer for it. It is through the improving of your decisions and the implementation of research-based evidence that we will move closer to the goals of modernising welfare services.

FURTHER READING AND RESOURCES

The essential site is SCHARR's excellent web resources page: shef.ac.uk/~scharr/links.htm; especially good is the 'netting the evidence' section, providing links to appraisal sheets, search filters and on-line training.

The University of Rochester's evidence-based search filters are useful (and easily adapted to whatever front end software you use, such as Silverplatter or PUBMED): urmc.rochester.edu/Miner/Educ/Expertsearch.html.

Once you progress with appraisal you might like to enhance your estimation of the clinical bottom line for your patient or service with some quantitative estimates of risk, benefit, harm and other measures of effect. The excellent family medicine site has more calculators and spread sheets than you are ever likely to need: fammed.ouhsc.edu/robhamm/cdmcalc.htm.

In terms of teaching (and learning about) evidence-based medicine the original (albeit the 2nd edition) is still the best. The 2nd edition also has sections relating to nursing and PAMs on the accompanying CD ROM: Sackett D, Strauss SE, Richardson WS, Rosenburg W, Haynes RB 2000 Evidence based medicine: how to practice and teach EBM. Churchill Livingstone, London.

For a more detailed treatment of clinical audit have a look at: Crombie IK, Davies HTO, Abraham SCS, Flare CDuV 1997 The audit handbook: improving health care through clinical audit. John Wiley, London.

Periodically JAMA publish commissioned pieces of work entitled the Users Guide to the Medical Literature. These are excellent and represent (in many cases) the state of the art in terms of appraisal and use of research evidence. Similarly, the Evidence Based Medicine/ Evidence Based Nursing notebooks and editorials in the journals of the same name make for a valuable learning resource.

With regard to the impact of organisational culture on the change management process the following text is a useful resource. Thompson C, Learmouth M 2001 Creating an evidence based organisational culture. In: Craig J et al. (eds) Evidence based healthcare handbook. Baillière Tindall, Edinburgh.

REFERENCES

Altman DG, Machin D, Bryant TN, Gardner MJ (eds) 2000 Statistics with confidence. 2nd Edition. BMJ Publishing, London.

Balas EA, Austin SM, Mitchell J et al. 1996 The clinical value of computerized information services: a review of 98 randomized clinical trials. Archives of Family Medicine 5: 271–278.

Beaudry JS 1989 The effectiveness of continuing medical education: a quantitative synthesis. Journal of Continuing Education in the Health Professions 9: 285–307.

Benner P 1984 From novice to expert: excellence and power in clinical nursing practice. Addison-Wesley, Menlo Park CA.

Bero LA, Grilli R, Grimshaw JM et al. 1998 Closing the gap between research and practice: an overview of systematic reviews of interventions to promote the implementation of research findings. British Medical Journal 317: 465–468.

Bertram DA, Brooks-Bertram PA 1977 The evaluation of continuing medical education: a literature review. Health Education Monographs 5: 330–362.

Buchkremer G, Schulze M, Holle R et al. 1995 The impact of therapeutic relatives groups on the course of illness of schizophrenic patients. European Psychiatry 10: 17–27.

Buntinx F, Winkens R, Grol R et al. 1993 Influencing diagnostic and preventative performance in ambulatory care by feedback and reminders. A review. Journal of Family Practice 10: 219–228.

Cioffi J 1997 Heuristics, servants to intuition, in clinical decision-making. Journal of Advanced Nursing, 26: 203–208.

Covell DG, Gwen C, Uman RN, Manning PR 1985 Information needs in office practice: are they being met? Annals of Internal Medicine 103: 596–599.

Crombie IK, Davies HTO, Abraham SCS, Flare CDuV 1997 The audit handbook: improving health care through clinical audit. John Wiley, London.

Davis DA, Thomson MA, Oxman AD et al. 1995 Changing physician performance: a systematic review of the effect of continuing medical education strategies. Journal of the American Medical Association 274: 700–705.

Dowie J, Elstein A 1988 Professional judgement. A reader in clinical decision making. Cambridge University Press, Cambridge.

Dreyfus HL, Dreyfus SE 1986 Mind over machine: The power of human intuition and expertise in the era of the computer. Free Press, New York.

Fischoff B 1975 Hindsight & foresight: the effect of outcome knowledge on judgement under uncertainty. Journal of Experimental Psychology: Human Perception and Performance 1: 288–299.

Freemantle N, Harvey EL, Wolf F, Grimshaw JM, Grilli R, Bero LA 1999 Printed educational materials to improve the behavior of health care professionals and patient outcomes (Cochrane Review). In: The Cochrane Library, Issue 1, Update Software, Oxford.

Funk SG, Tornquist EM, Champagn MT 1995 Barriers and facilitators of research utilization. Nursing Clinics of North America 30(3): 395–407.

Gigerenzer G 1991 How to make cognitive illusions disappear: beyond 'heuristics and biases'. European Review of Social Psychology 2: 83–115.

Grol R 1992 Implementing guidelines in general practice care. Quality in Health Care 1: 184–191.

Kahneman D, Tversky A 1973 On the psychology of prediction. Psychological Review 80: 237–251.

Lichenstein S, Fischoff B 1977 Do those who know more also know more about how much they know? The calibration of probability judgements. Organizational Behaviour and Human Performance 20: 159–183.

Lies V, Sutherland K 2001 Organisational change: A review for healthcare managers, professionals and researchers. NCC SDO R&D, London.

Lilford R, Pauker SG, Braunholtz D, Chard J 1998 Decision analysis and the implementation of research findings. In Haines A, Donald A (eds) Getting research findings into practice. BMJ Publishing, London.

Lloyd JS, Abrahamson S 1979 Effectiveness of continuing medical education: a review of the evidence. Evaluation and the Health Professions 2: 251–280.

Marrie TJ, Lau CY, Wheeler SL, Wong CJ, Vandervoort MK, Feagan BG 2000 A controlled trial of a critical pathway for treatment of community-acquired pneumonia. Journal of the American Medical Association 283(6): 749–755.

Muir Gray JA 1997 Evidence based healthcare: how to make health policy and management decisions. Churchill Livingstone, Edinburgh.

Mulhall A, Le May A 1999 Nursing research: dissemination and implementation. Churchill Livingstone, London.

Mulrow CD 1987 The medical review article: state of the science. Annals of Internal Medicine 106(3): 485–488.

NHS Centre for Reviews and Dissemination 1999 Getting Evidence Into Practice. Effective Health Care Bulletin 5(1). NHS CRD, York.

Oxman AD, Cook DJ, Guyatt GH 1994 Evidence based medicine working group users guide to the medical literature VI: how to use an overview. JAMA 272: 136–171.

Oxman A, Thomson MA, Davis DA, Haynes RB 1995 No magic bullets: A systematic review of 102 trials of interventions to improve professional practice. Canadian Medical Association Journal 153(10): 1423–1431.

Retsas A 2000 Barriers to using research evidence in nursing practice. Journal of Advanced Nursing 31(3): 599–606.

Royal College of Nursing Institute, Centre for Evidence-Based Nursing, University of York and the School of Nursing, Midwifery and Health Visiting, University of Manchester 1998 The management of patients with venous leg ulcers. RCN Publishing, London.

Sackett DL, Strauss SE, Richardson WS, Rosenberg W, Haynes RB 2000 Evidence based medicine: how to practice and teach EBM. Churchill Livingstone, London.

Shea S, DuMouchel W, Bahamonde L 1996 A meta-analysis of 16 randomized controlled trials to evaluate computer-based clinical reminder systems for preventative care in the ambulatory setting. Journal of the American Medical Informatics Association 3: 399–409.

Thomas L, Cullum N, McColl E, Rousseau N, Soutter J, Steen N 1999 Clinical guidelines in nursing, midwifery and other professions allied to medicine (Cochrane Review). In: The Cochrane Library, Issue 1, Update Software, Oxford.

Thompson C, Learmonth M 2002 How can we develop an evidence based culture? In: Craig JV, Smyth RL (eds) The evidence based practice manual for nurses. Churchill Livingstone, Edinburgh, pp. 211–239.

Thompson C, McCaughan D, Cullum N, Sheldon T, Thompson D 2001 Nurses' use of research information in clinical decision making: a descriptive and analytical study. National Coordinating Centre for Service Delivery and Organisation, London.

Thomson MA, Oxman AD, Davis DA, Haynes RB, Freemantle N, Harvey EL 1999 Outreach visits to improve health professional practice and health care outcomes (Cochrane Review). In: The Cochrane Library, Issue 1, Update Software, Oxford.

Waddell DL 1991 The effects of continuing education on nursing practice: a meta-analysis. Journal of Continuing Education in Nursing 22: 113–118.

Wensing M, Van der Weijden TRG 1998 Implementing guidelines and innovations in general practice: which interventions are effective. British Journal of General Practice 48: 991–997.

Yano EM, Fink A, Hirsch SH et al. 1995 Helping practices reach primary care goals. Lessons from the literature. Archives of Internal Medicine 155: 1146–1156.

8

Audit: the beginning and the end of the change cycle

Marc Saunders

KEY ISSUES

◆ Descriptions and definitions

◆ The case for clinical audit

◆ How audit works

◆ Engaging in audit

◆ Audit in the real world

◆ Preparing the team.

INTRODUCTION

In many ways clinical governance and best value are like a machine waiting for the mechanism to be fitted before it can work effectively. There are lots of parts to this machine each with their own contribution to make, and these are discussed in other chapters. Audit is a pivotal component if the modernisation agenda is to make good the promise of better welfare services for those that use the service as well as more predictable outcomes that are more efficiently delivered.

The concept of audit is remarkably uncomplicated. It evolved out of a desire to ensure welfare services were provided in line with good practice and delivered the kind of outcomes that might reasonably be expected. Despite this, some practitioners still lack the confidence to engage in audit, particularly as the dissemination of results throughout the service is not uniform either in terms of its quality or in the level of audit activity.

However, audit continues to be a powerful vehicle for change providing this change is rigorously pursued. Those who look to facilitate the process of audit often use the term 'closing the circle'. The circle is only closed when the audit cycle has been completed, a change in practice has occurred and that practice is embedded in the new order of things. This chapter sets out to consider why we choose to use audit as a method of developing quality and where audit sits within clinical governance and best value. A substantial part of the chapter looks at the practical application of audit in a variety of service settings.

DESCRIPTIONS AND DEFINITIONS

At this early stage it is important to dispel a few myths and mysteries with respect of audit. Firstly, audit is not complex: not unless you want it to be. It can and should be a shared experience, particularly as a multi-disciplinary approach is more likely to be successful. We should not forget that the only reason for engaging in audit is to deliver changes in practice for the benefit of those that use the service. Reviews and evaluations are useful and important; however, audit is concerned with the introduction of necessary change. This chapter acknowledges that audit can be a time-consuming activity, and rightfully so. However, it is our responsibility to ensure that this investment in scarce resources results in real and significant changes for those who use the service.

So, what is audit? There are many definitions that succinctly describe audit and what it is designed to achieve. From a policy perspective, one of the first explicit references to audit within health care can be found in the white paper

Working for Patients:

> ... *a systematic, critical analysis of the quality of medical care, including the procedures used for diagnosis and treatment, the use of resources and the resulting outcome for the patient ... It is a means of ensuring, through peer review of medical practice, that the quality of medical work meets acceptable standards (Department of Health 1989, pp. 39–40).*

Having found enthusiastic support in a national policy document, the concept of audit found mainstream acceptance in many healthcare settings. Subsequently, there were a number of significant publications designed to promote our understanding of audit. Shortly after the publication of *Working for Patients* a further document aimed particularly at nurses was published which defined nursing audit as:

> ... *part of the quality assurance cycle. It incorporates the systematic and critical analyses by nurses, midwives and health visitors, in conjunction with other staff, of the planning, delivery and evaluation of nursing and midwifery care, in terms of their use of resources and the outcome for patients/clients, and introduces appropriate change in response to that analysis (NHSME 1991, p. 4).*

Subsequently it became clear that different professional groups were auditing their own professional practice, and although there was value in this, it ignored one of the critical aspects of care delivery; that is, that it is nearly always a multi-disciplinary activity. As a result audits were likely to either miss significant elements of the care process or result in one profession auditing the work of different professional groups without their explicit support and involvement. This was not conducive to the care team having ownership of the issues raised as a result of the audit and made the process of change more difficult to achieve than might have been anticipated. The great leap forward that followed saw uni-professional audit evolve to become a multi-disciplinary process often referred to as clinical audit. The guidance from the Department of Health reflected this:

Clinical audit is a professionally-led initiative which seeks to improve the quality and outcome of patient care through clinicians examining their practices and results and modifying practice where indicated (NHSE 1996, p. 16).

Following these and other policy developments, in parallel with a substantial drive within services and the professions, the concept of audit became better known and understood. It delivered changes in practice that had real benefits for those who use services. However, it still was not clear whether the outcomes justified the investment in time and resources. A review of audit activity in England was a little more optimistic; however, Buttery et al. (1995) acknowledge that some audit activity did not result in changes to practice. For the most part, audit still seemed to operate on the periphery; showing us interesting things, but not having the impact on practice the effort deserved.

The question then became how to continue to move audit into the mainstream of service provision? Clinical governance and best value may well be the vehicle through which to achieve this, as it places audit in a framework, that organisations have to be accountable for that is designed to improve the process of care as well as the outcomes for people who use services.

THE CASE FOR CLINICAL AUDIT

Whatever our professional background, there is a requirement to keep ourselves up to date and to pursue best practice. This is often made explicit through our respective professional codes of practice. Increasingly, practitioners are being called upon to demonstrate that they abide by their code and practice accordingly. Audit is not the answer to

every issue, nor will audit act as some kind of substitute for good practice. However, it is a useful tool for practitioners and teams as a means of reviewing and evaluating their practice and introducing necessary change.

So why is audit an important development in welfare services? The act of caring for someone is often viewed as a simplistic, manual task. However, care is complex. People are complex. If we are to effectively meet the needs of the people who use services then it is essential we adopt systems that support the effective delivery of care. This has to be contextualised within the constantly changing knowledge base from which we all operate. It is possible to be the most knowledgeable professional in the service; this does not, however, automatically ensure good-quality care delivery. In order to achieve this goal such knowledge has to be used in a systematic and structured way to inform care delivery. Audit is one way this can be achieved.

Codes of practice and an ever-increasing knowledge base is only part of the overall picture. The last 15 years have also witnessed an enormous change in society that has become much more consumer conscious and litigious. We should have high expectations of our services because users themselves will have high expectations. Audit is not purely about litigation avoidance, it is about making sure that services are operating in line with good practice in the first place. The people who use our services want to know that we know what we are doing and why we are doing it. However, it is clear we still cannot be confident about the effectiveness of many interventions. Until such time audit should not be seen as a luxury, but should be viewed as a fundamental requirement of service provision.

HOW AUDIT WORKS

Defining audit and an overview of policy is a helpful starting point. However, it is important to

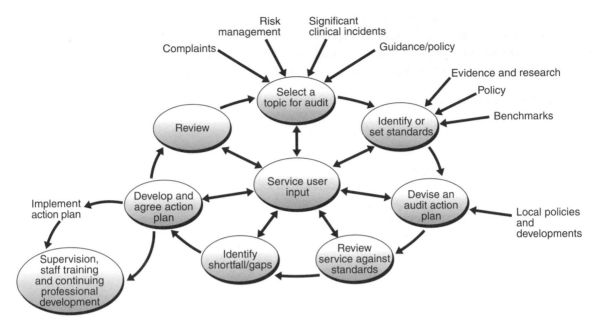

Figure 8.1 The audit process in the context of clinical governance and best value.

have a clear idea about the processes that combine to make audit what it is. There is a simplicity in the concept of audit that has much to commend it. It is logical, the steps which need to be taken naturally follow one another, and the product is a visible and measurable change in practice.

Many texts describe audit as a cyclical process. These texts are clear and informative (Malby 1994, Buttery et al. 1995), but the modernisation agenda now encourages us to look again at the cycle and to consider how the principles which underpin clinical governance and best value can be reflected in the audit cycle (see Figure 8.1).

Figure 8.1 illustrates how the audit cycle interlocks with other related elements of clinical governance and best value. More than ever we should ensure we understand audit and its relationship with the other components of change management. There are other methods of introducing change into welfare services, however, most do not reflect the rigour or the systematic nature of audit as a way of achieving effective services

based on evidence and research. *A First Class Service* states that clinical governance is '... the framework through which NHS organisations are accountable for continuously improving the quality of their services...' (Department of Health 1998, p. 33). In this context audit will have been seen to fail if real improvements in service delivery are not visible. What follows is a brief note on each step of the audit process and how this relates to clinical governance and best value.

Involving the service user

A number of significant policy documents have been published over the last 3 or 4 years: *The New NHS: Modern, Dependable* (Department of Health 1997), *A First Class Service* (Department of Health 1998), *the NHS Plan* (Department of Health 2000), *Valuing People* (Department of Health 2001). Within these, there is a consistent theme that supports a greater role for involving those who use services in the management and development of those services. Despite these recent policy developments it is clear there continues to be limited involvement of people who use services in the process of audit.

Where a decision is made to involve users in the process of audit, then it seems sensible for people to be involved from the outset. Service users could contribute to the selection of the audit project and to many of the other stages of the process. It should be noted that people who are new to audit, or who may have other specific needs, will require preparation, training and support to become involved. The curse of tokenism will be upon us if we do not plan and resource user involvement properly.

What should we audit?

As audit grew in our collective consciousness, the process of selecting what to audit was largely a case of local practitioners arriving at a decision. However, there was a danger that this did not reflect the most pressing issues within the service. This was often to avoid contentious audit programmes or in an attempt to keep the workload at a manageable level. The problem with this approach was that the real priorities for improving services could potentially be missed.

Clinical governance and best value is an opportunity to ensure that audit priorities reflect both the service and the user priorities. A team might wish to consider:

- views of users of the service
- complaints management data
- risk management data (including trends/incident reviews etc.)
- significant incidents (or what are sometimes called 'near misses')
- guidance, policy and advice on best practice (effectiveness notices)

- National Service Frameworks, Health Improvement Programmes (HImPs), Joint Investment Plans (JIPs), Local Delivery Plans (LDPs) and Strategic Health Authority Franchise Plans.

This does not preclude teams arriving at their own decisions; however, it does encourage or even compel practitioners to work in those areas where the real concerns can be identified.

Identifying or setting standards

Standard setting is not a new concept in services. Nurses are very familiar with the 'structure, process, outcome' approach to setting standards (Royal College of Nursing 1990), which gained significant currency in services during the late 1980s and early 1990s. However, whilst this process has its merits, it quickly became recognised as a cumbersome way of ensuring services achieved what they were designed to achieve. Figure 8.1 underlines how clinical governance and best value contributes to the setting of standards.

What both clinical governance and best value provide is a framework through which information can be collated, and which can advise the process of setting standards. These standards do not need to be written in the 'structure, process, outcome' style, so long as the standard is relevant to the issue identified and is written in a way that facilitates measurement. In many cases the standards already exist and it is just a case of identifying them and working with them locally in order to be able to complete the audit process.

In many cases standards arrive via the policy and guidance route. For example, the National Service Frameworks (NSFs) contain standards that could be justifiably placed into an audit programme. Similarly, a number of benchmarking activities mean that information is available from which services can compare their performance with that of other areas. For example, see the publication *Essence of Care* (Department of Health 2001b). A significant source of advice on the setting of standards is through searching the available evidence on the identified issue. This means that the standard, once written, should reflect what could be considered best practice. Some organisations are making meta-analyses available on a range of issues (where all the known research on a particular issue is reviewed) so that evidence in a useable format is increasingly available.

There are also standards to be found in any number of documents; some designed with the intention of directing the reader on the implementation and subsequent audit of standards. There is no shortage in this respect. The cautionary note when considering auditing against set standards concerns trying not to do too many things too quickly. In addition, we should be wary of visiting the welfare standards 'supermarket' and merely selecting a few 'off-the-shelf' ideas.

Reviewing service provision and identifying shortfalls

Once the standards have been identified, designed and agreed, the work of measuring the service against the standards can begin. A structure will need to be in place to achieve this. This may mean utilising approaches from which relevant information can be gained; usually some sort of audit pro-forma. These are most successful if they are:

- simple to complete
- quick to complete
- uncomplicated (if 'yes' go to question x, if 'no' go to question y designs are not always helpful)
- related to a process which happens as part of the routine

- understood by everyone who completes them (training)
- available.

Some audits can be carried out retrospectively by reviewing documents and records that have already been completed. These are just as valuable as newly designed audit tools.

There is clearly a skill in working to identify or design standards that underpin any audit activity. However, there is also a skill in using the information gained to identify shortfalls or gaps. The clinical team will need to spend time on data analysis and the subsequent interpretation of that data. If the standard is well written then most of the analysis will be self-explanatory: this happens 85% of the time, this only happened 23% of the time; 48 people of 60 reported less pain, 12 people reported no difference and so on.

Finally, it is also important to remember that audit is about acknowledging good practice where this is already happening. Often we are too quick to look for the faults in what we do when we should also look for the positive aspects.

Developing and implementing an action plan

Unless audit results in a change in the service and in clinical practice, it will merely take the form of evaluation and monitoring of standards. Whilst there is some value in carrying out evaluation, the real value of audit lies in the implementation of change. There are clear links between the modernisation agenda and the change component of audit. There have been a number of high-profile cases where proper consideration of audit data and action thereafter may have made a difference. Clinical governance and best value are part of the incentive to take seriously the results of our audit work and to act accordingly.

The action plan should be clear to all members of the team so that whatever new practices or methods of working are advocated, they are understood by all those involved. Change is often not as straightforward as we would wish and the plan may need to consider some milestones on the route so that progress can be checked. The process might be interfaced with supervision for staff so that everyone can continue to consider their role in responding to the outcome of the audit data analysis.

The audit may also indicate where continuing professional development might mean a programme of training and development for the team. This does not have to mean training. It might mean looking at other services to see how particular issues are dealt with, it might also mean working on a small piece of research or reviewing further the literature in relation to the service.

Review

If change indicated by audit has been implemented, then the cycle has been completed. However, there is some justification for reviewing the work undertaken. Initially, it is worth considering whether further work is needed on the main issues identified through the audit. For this reason it is not unusual to repeat the audit cycle so that the standards can be re-visited once the changes have been made; this has clear links with the concepts underpinning the modernisation agenda. An additional reason for undertaking a review of the whole process is to give credit where due and to celebrate successes.

ENGAGING IN AUDIT

The gap that exists between theory and practice is often cited as a contributing factor when considering the difference that exists between what is known as best practice and what happens at an operational level. The basis for these differences are many and varied. What is clear is that to a relative of someone adversely affected by

welfare services, a catalogue of reasons about why a service was not following the most up-to-date research or guidance will not be acceptable. The good news is that audit, if properly implemented, can bridge the gap between theory and practice in a way that does not feel artificial to those in direct care roles. The process described in the previous section is logical and sensible and we can see why it should work. This part of the chapter considers how audit can actually be applied in the field and develops a model that can be used directly or adapted by practitioners and others as a way of most effectively implementing audit within their service.

The text in Box 8.1 might be considered a menu from which you can select or identify a number of components when designing and developing an audit project. Audit is part of the fabric of clinical governance and best value, but only if measures are taken to ensure its place within this structure. Based upon Figure 8.1 earlier in the chapter, there are a number of sections, each with a selection of choices and ideas that can be used to shape an audit. The menu is written in the present tense merely out of convenience, and could be used in the process of developing an audit project, or to review one that has been completed or is currently in progress.

AUDIT IN THE REAL WORLD

The NHS Plan (Department of Health 2000) is aimed at breaking down barriers: barriers within as well as between services. Other documents published subsequent to *the NHS Plan* have similar and re-affirming aspirations. The phrase 'seamless service' is often used. To this end, this section considers an example of audit in action which crosses service boundaries. Inevitably what follows can only be an illustration of the process, however, it does reflect the key points for consideration and raises a number of issues along the way.

Box 8.1

1. Selecting a topic for audit

- Service users are involved in identifying an issue that could be the focus of an audit.

- National guidance is consulted or reviewed in the process of considering what to audit.

- If your organisation has a Risk Manager or a Risk Management group, have any priorities been identified?

- Carry out a risk analysis in your own area. Look to where you might find trends or patterns of events that indicate a need to review how care is provided.

- Have there been any near misses in your services? Think about something that nearly went wrong and might indicate the need for a change in practice.

- This work could be described as high volume.

- There is research indicating that a change in practice is needed and the team can identify this.

- There is a significant element of risk associated with this work.

- The team can describe why this particular audit is a priority.

- The team feels that change is necessary insome form.

- This is an area of practice which could be described as high volume or high risk.

- The whole clinical team feel that this is a priority for action (or a majority).

Commentary

The relationship between clinical governance and best value and the selection of an aspect of service delivery for audit is very powerful. You might consider this is clinical goverance and best value in their purist form. In order to ensure that a service is working towards an evidence based framework it first needs to take a look at what it is doing in the light of research and current best practice.

The points raised on the involvement of users can be raised throughout the audit process. There are some complex decisions to be made here. Many services will concern users with whom communication is an issue. This will need to be managed. In primary and secondary care there is the challenge of representation, i.e. how do you find a small number of users who will represent your population? Ensuring that people have a genuine rather than a token role in the process is essential.

When standard setting first became a familiar concept, teams were anxious to describe much of what they did

and tended to focus on the 'non-issues'. Clinical governance and best value is the pursuit of the antithesis of this where efforts are made to concentrate on the important issues. The team should identify that the need for change is more likely rather than less likely. For example, considering where the issue is a high volume activity (e.g. prescribing/ giving medication) or high risk (e.g. certain forms of surgery, ECT) is one way of evaluating the nature of the proposed project.

Risk management data, 'near miss' reports and so on will only be available if your organisation has systems in place to deliver these. This information is an important aid to deciding where to focus your audit, however, teams can illicit some of this information for themselves by, for example, keeping a record of medication errors, equipment failures, unexpected deaths and so on.

Most importantly is to select a focus that is worthy of the time and effort which is about to be spent on it.

2. Identifying and setting standards

- Standards currently published in recent policy initiatives are included? For example, National Service Frameworks (NSFs), *Essence of Care* (DoH 2001b) DoH reference documents etc.

- Where there is existing good practice guidance and internal policies and procedures based on good practice then standards are drawn from these (or do not contradict these).

- Current research is considered and reviewed. Standards of practice are designed with reference to this research.

- Research is reviewed by members of the team with critical appraisal skills or outside advice and support is sought in pursuit of this.

- Users are involved in identifying the standards against which the service will be measured.

- A small (representative if possible) group of practitioners, users and others have agreed those standards upon which the audit will be based.

- Other services have been approached to see if standards have been developed elsewhere which would be relevant to the audit being implemented.

(continued)

Box 8.1   *(continued)*

Commentary
Developing standards is one way of working most directly within a clinical governance and best value framework: a method for getting best practice (practice based on good evidence) into the work carried out by a team.

This can only happen if team members have access and time to gather evidence for consideration. Access to Information Technology (IT) is clearly needed. But this is insufficient. Some members of the team need to have the skill to critically appraise the evidence as it is presented. There is a lot of good research to be found, and a lot of poor quality work or work which is insufficiently rigorous in order to justify changes in practice.

Some organisations do actually publish what are referred to as 'meta-analyses' of research. For example see the Effective Healthcare Bulletins on drug treatment for schizophrenia (NHS Centre for Reviews and Dissemination 1999) and the bulletin on acupuncture (NHS Centre for Reviews and Dissemination/The Royal Society for Medicine Press 2001). Key research on these issues is drawn together and required actions in line with best practice are identified. It is always worth exploring to see if there is a meta-analysis on the subject of the proposed audit.

3. Devising an audit action plan

- Only data required to support the audit are collected.

- The process for collecting data (the audit tool) is clearly described and is understood by the team.

- A system for analysing the data is identified and agreed.

- The data analysis model is straightforward and understood by members of the team.

- Those events/service users who fall outside the scope of the audit project are clearly identified.

- Confidentiality of serivce users is maintained as part of the audit plan.

- If consent is required on behalf of service users then there is a system in place to ensure this.

- If service users wish to see information on the audit this is presented in a format that is usable by them.

- There are clear instructions on the use of the audit tool.

- The audit tool has been tested prior to commencing the audit and adjustments made as appropriate.

Commentary
Collecting data to support an audit project does have some pitfalls. There are questions to be addressed such as who does it, how and when is it carried out, what is outside the scope of the project and so on? One mistake made by many is the attempt to turn the audit into some kind of research project. For the most part the team should not be looking for generalisable results. The project should interest itself in the work being done by the team concerned.

In addition, there is also a tendency to become 'data hungry' and over-complicate the data-collection process. A better picture is nearly always obtained by keeping the data collected to an absolute minimum designed to support the set standards.

Wherever possible it is advisable to use an existing tool which has already been tested. This is not always possible so the design of an audit tool should be made with

reference to the points raised above. Where a locally devised tool is being used, take the opportunity to test it before going on with the audit. This can be done in another area; the data obtained are less critical than the ease of use of the tool itself, especially if it has to be used as part of the daily routine.

The team should carefully consider the issue of confidentiality and consent. This is not research so it is unlikely that many service users will notice that an audit project is underway (this would defeat the object of doing the audit) so ethics committee approval may not be essential, but do not rule this out. However, we are entering an age where the service user is much more central to the process of care and information and involvement should be carefully considered.

4. Review the service against the identified standards (collect the data)

- The data collection method is applied as agreed in the audit project plan.

- Efforts are made to ensure the data collection process is consistently applied by all those involved.

(continued)

Box 8.1   *(continued)*

- Where appropriate, service users are supported to contribute to the review of the service against the audit standards.

  – This can be tested by two or more people completing the audit tool for the same event/care episode etc. and comparing the results obtained to ensure there is no significant discrepancy.

Commentary
The need to test whether two or more people 'agree' on their view of a particular episode/event or so on is based on the concern for consistency. In research terms this is sometimes referred to as inter-rater reliability. In the case of collecting numerical data there is usually small scope for debate, e.g. the number of times an event happens, the time taken to carry out an intervention etc.

However, where some qualitative analysis of a situation is needed then there is scope for discrepancy between participants. Talking about the data-collection process can reduce this; reviewing some scenarios and taking care to acknowledge these differences when considering the data collected will also be necessary.

This is also an opportunity to test the data analysis process.

5. Identify shortfalls and gaps in service provision

- The data analysis is carried out in line with the audit project plan.
- The differences in what happens within the service and what is required by the standards are clearly identified and clearly described.
- All members of the team have the opportunity to review the data collected and the data analysis.

- Service users are supported to contribute in identifying shortfalls and gaps in the service.
- The identified shortfalls/gaps/areas for development are reflected in the data analysis and are not merely a reflection of the interests of the team or individuals within the team.

Commentary
There is room for some disagreement in this part of the process. This is concerned with the analysis of data and the subsequent interpretation in terms of what these data suggest from the point of view of changes to service delivery.

User involvement could be the key to this where

there is some tempering of the practitioner's view of how things should be.

Most importantly, identifying differences between what happens 'on the ground' and what is required by the standards used should be very carefully reflected in those gaps and shortfalls identified.

6. Develop and agree an action plan for change

- The action plan is developed following the analysis of data.
- The action plan for change is clear and is understood by all members of the team/department.
- The action plan is, in its own right, measurable and identifies goals and milestones in order to monitor its implementation.
- The action plan contains rewards and reinforcers for staff designed to help to ensure its successful implementation.
- The plan has a timetable.
- The audit action plan is realistic and deliverable by the team.

- All team members have signed to agree to implement the action plan.
- Training and supervision are provided if these are required as part of the action plan (this includes time to engage in these activities if required).
- Supporting educational and information technology are available to staff if required.
- Where there are clear barriers to implementing the changes required then the action plan includes strategies to overcome these.

(continued)

Box 8.1   *(continued)*

- The plan is dynamic and can be changed to reflect changing circumstances within the service.

- The intergrity of the standards or the purpose of the audit is not compromised by, for example, altering the

Commentary
As with most of the audit process when considered in the light of recent policy developments, for example, *The NHS Plan* (DoH 2000) the issue of user involvement in all aspects of healthcare delivery should not be overlooked.

Critically, this is probably the most important part of the audit process and reflects the drive and direction of clinical governance. The issue of change and change

standards so that the service is meeting the standards identified.

- Service users have contributed to the audit plan.

management is considered elsewhere in the book, however, change is an essential part of the audit process and without it the process is reduced to a version of service review and probably does not deserve the level of time and effort put in. In short, if it does not have an impact upon the care of service users, should we consider this a priority use of time?

7. Implementing and reviewing the plan for change

- All team members contribute to implementing the action plan.

- The action plan is implemented in line with the identified timetable.

Commentary
One way of reviewing the whole process is to re-visit the audit either in full or in a slightly curtailed format. This will be the acid test to see if changes have been

- All resources are provided as necessary.

- The audit has been repeated and no shortfalls/gaps in service provision are identified (or a reduction in the shortfalls/gaps is reported).

consistently implemented and that there has been an impact upon the care given to service users.

Case example

Those who are at risk of serious self-harm, or have a history of self-harm, are the business of a number of agencies and services. In the first instance, let us consider who might have an interest in this:

- The Department of Health and service commissioners have noted suicide rates worthy of consideration in the mental health NSF (Department of Health 1999).

- Care Trusts and Mental Health NHS Trusts who provide services to those people at risk of self harm.

- Primary Care Trusts will provide care to individuals with these needs.

- Social Services will provide a critical aspect of the care package to someone at risk from serious self-harm.

- Secondary and tertiary services will often deal with the consequences of self-harm.

In this setting there are a number of options from which an area of concern can be identified. Options may include:

- How do we identify those at risk from self-harm before the self-harm occurs?

- What treatment and intervention options should be used when working with people who self-harm and are there different intervention types for differing presentations?

- Multi-agency working.

- What outcomes can be expected from services provided to people whom self-harm?

- Systems for communicating with service users.

- Risk assessment and risk management in this area.

As already stated, choosing an audit project is an important part of the audit process. The involvement of service users in this respect is important, but also achievable on the basis that there is probably a defined population of people to consider. People who self-harm also have families and relatives who may also be legitimate contributors to this process (confidentiality and issues of consent notwithstanding).

Quite often, individuals with issues such as these have already formed into support groups of one sort or another, and more often than not are waiting for the opportunity to contribute to services. So, for example, this audit project could include people from an established mental health support group as part of the team.

However, we should not underestimate the difficulties in involving service users in what is, at times, an almost impenetrable world of professional speak, jargon, concepts and protocols. If those who use services are to contribute on an equal footing, then we have to be prepared to sweep some of these barriers aside, even if there is a personal cost or discomfort in doing so.

Clinical governance and best value are, however, more than ensuring the involvement of those who use services. As highlighted earlier, there are a large number of stakeholders, many of whom might wish to consider the ongoing publication of policy and guidance, the high risks associated with working with this group of people, as well as the human cost of ineffective practice. All of these are important factors in deciding where to focus energy and resources. On this basis, and for the purpose of this illustration, let us assume that we might wish to audit the systems we have for identifying and assessing people for whom there may be a risk of self-harm.

The next stage is concerned with the identification and setting of standards. There is a temptation to believe that those who use services cannot be involved in this part of the process. It is our job to consider how we might overcome this. Ensuring that the user is an equal part of the project team can counteract the pursuit of ideological purity over pragmatism.

The project focus has already been identified. The process now moves on to finding or developing standards which will inform the team on how service provision measures against what might be considered best practice. Information and ideas can be gained from a number of sources:

- accessing the internet to draw on research into current practice
- special interest groups and experts
- government policy and guidance
- research databases
- meta-analyses of research in this area
- those that use the service
- service users' families and significant others.

There is a lot of work to be done and it is not always feasible for the whole team to engage in all of this process. It is also worth considering that this is an issue that stretches over health and social care boundaries. A team may include:

- psychiatrist
- social worker
- community mental health nurse
- GP or practice nurse
- mental health unit nurse
- accident and emergency department representative
- voluntary sector
- a person who has self harmed and their family.

Let us assume that the team identify a number of standards which seem reasonable to use in order to audit the services provided. A small number are identified here. Please note, this is an illustrative example set in a particular context. Your work in your own area will define different priorities and different standards.

Standard one

All people admitted to the local accident and emergency department with injuries that could be considered to have been caused by the person themselves are referred to mental health services for review.

Standard two

A risk assessment is carried out on all people who have expressed thoughts of harming themselves or who have previously harmed themselves.

Standard three

New admissions to residential facilities are assessed with regard to the possibility of self-harm within 7 days of their admission.

Standard four

Those people who present to their GP with depression are reviewed with regard to the likelihood of engaging in self-harm and referrals made to a psychiatrist if necessary.

Standard five

New referrals to the community mental health team are screened with regard to self-harm.

Standard six

Social workers identify changes in mental health status and will contact the community mental health team if there is an increased likelihood of self-harm occurring.

The standards described above could have been from a number of sources. The next stage is to identify and implement a system for collecting data. For brevity, the illustration will focus on Standard one and Standard two.

There are a number of ways in which this audit could be approached and like so many issues concerned with the behaviour and welfare of people, there is no one right way. When choosing the methodology, both the context and location will be important influencing factors. The following is an example of how an audit can be undertaken.

In these circumstances the team have decided to carry out as much of the audit as possible through reference to existing records. It is possible to gather good information by pursuing a retrospective audit of records. This also clarifies why it is important to have a working team with a range of backgrounds and from across the agencies involved. Once the decision is made on how best to address the questions raised through the standards identified, it will be necessary to design an audit tool. Any decisions about the tool should, as with all decisions, be based upon sound evidence and a clear rationale.

Part of the audit tool might look something like this. For Standard one, the team decided to:

1. Random sample 1000 records from the A&E department.
2. Review each record and identify:
    a. group 1: there is a cause that can be discounted as self-harm, e.g. heart condition, CVA etc.
    b. group 2: it is unclear whether the cause is self-harm
    c. group 3: the admission is identified as someone who has self-harmed.

3. Those who are identified in the second group – further review is carried out to ascertain whether or not self-harm is the likely cause (e.g. history of depression, previous history of self-harm etc.). These are then filtered appropriately into the first or the third group.

4. Identify record by record, whether the clients in group 3 were referred to mental health services.

For Standard two (see p. 143), the team has agreed to take the following steps:

1. A random sample of 250 records from the mental health service records office should be identified.

2. Each record is screened and assigned to one of the following groups:
   a. group 1: those who have expressed no intention of self-harm and have no history of harming themselves
   b. group 2: those who have expressed thoughts of self-harm
   c. group 3: those who have a history of harming themselves
   d. group 4: those who have expressed no intention of self-harm and have no history of harming themselves, however, the clinical team identify this person as necessary for review.

3. For the records in groups 2 and 3, identify those which contain a risk assessment, those which do not contain a risk assessment and those where the assessment of risk has been started, but is not current or is inadequate for the purposes needed.

There will need to be a time scale agreed by which point the capture of the initial data needs to be completed. In this case, unless people are actually given time within which to complete the audit, then the audit will not be as effective as it needs to be. Analysing records is time-consuming and does have its own specific challenges (poorly recorded care episodes, bad hand-writing, missing records, records which are not located in one place even in the same agency).

A straightforward matrix can be devised to record the data. For illustration purposes the

Table 8.1 Standard one

Group	No. of cases	Referred to the mental health team
Group 3: the admission is identified as someone who has self-harmed	62	37

following data have been identified and summarised for the team.

For Standard one, the first stage of the audit shows that 847 cases fell into group 1, 63 into group 2 and 40 into group 3. The subsequent stage re-assigned 41 cases to group 1 and 22 to group 3. Of the 62 in the self-harm set (group 3), 37 were referred to the mental health team. This is summarized in Table 8.1.

For Standard two, the data in Table 8.2 was collected and summarised.

It is clear from this very basic data that there are gaps between what the service is providing and what is seen as good practice. For Standard one, the referral to mental health services was only happening in 37 out of 62 cases. In part, this was a practice issue, but also an issue of identification.

In Standard two, for those expressing feelings of self-harm, there is a difference in the number of people who should have a risk assessment and those who have an adequate risk assessment. Therefore, there is an issue of both professional practice in terms of knowing when to carry out a risk assessment as well as a quality issue. More positively, for those who had previously self-harmed there is a higher level of adequate risk assessments in evidence (36 out of 53). However, considering these are people who have self-harmed in the past, and that this can be considered an indicator of future intention, there is still a significant gap in terms of the service provided to this group of people.

Once all the data have been analysed, an action plan can be developed to change systems and

Table 8.2 Standard two

Group	No. of cases	Adequate risk assessment	Inadequate risk assessments	With no risk assessments
Group 1: those who have expressed no intention of self-harm and have no history of self-harm	115	n/a	n/a	n/a
Group 2: those who have expressed thoughts of self-harm	65	21	17	27
Group 3: those who have a history of harming themselves	53	36	14	3
Group 4: those who have expressed no intention of self-harm and have no history of harming themselves, however, the team identify this person as necessary for review	17	n/a	n/a	n/a

Table 8.3

Action	Lead person	Review date
Training for all current and new medical and nursing staff at the A&E department on the identification of people who have engaged in self-harm	AW	31.10
Design a standard referral letter template to speed up the contact between A&E and mental health services	PG	24.01
Quarterly review meetings to be held between A&E and mental health service representatives	AW	17.05 and on-going
Set up an on-call arrangement with mental health services to review patients within the A&E department	LS	30.11
Training for staff in mental health services on developing and implementing a risk assessment	AR	31.10
Ensure that forms and guidance on carrying out a risk assessment are readily available in mental health services	JG	15.07
Set in place a review process so that care plans can be checked to ensure risk-assessment recommendations are included	SWS	21.08
The need for skills and experience in carrying out risk assessments to be incorporated into job descriptions	JG	13.05

practice. For the two standards in this illustration a brief action plan may look something like Table 8.3.

The group who led the audit can be the overseeing body for ensuring that the change management part of the process is actually completed. A repeat of the audit is recommended to ensure that changes have been properly implemented and that the desired outcomes are being achieved. It is possible that, even though the changes have been made, other factors are at work to prevent the standards being met and further action is needed.

PREPARING THE TEAM

If audit is to be effectively applied in any service setting it seems appropriate to take action in order to prepare the team to carry out this work. An assumption is made that team members, as far as possible, are able to carry out their role, have kept up to date and have a desire to see services develop. What follows are some ideas for the sorts of things that may help team members contribute more effectively to the audit process with particular reference to clinical governance and best value.

If the audit is to depend upon standards that reflect current best practice, there are a number of areas for staff development:

- critical appraisal skills
- time management
- networking skills
- audit and continuous quality improvement
- library skills
- IT and computer skills (including internet access skills)
- supervision
- accessing databases.

There will also be a demand on resources. Access to appropriate materials and resources will need to be reviewed by the team. Resources such as:

- funding to carry out training as identified above
- subscriptions to appropriate journals
- data analysis software if needed
- subscription to on-line databases
- access to library facilities
- time to carry out the audit without impacting on service user care
- time to network/contact and visit other services etc.

One of the most important resources is a team leader with the foresight to support people to gain ideas and skills which will, in turn, contribute to the development of audit projects and, therefore, to the pursuit of clinical governance and best value within the service.

CONCLUSION

Health- and social-care professionals work in an increasingly challenging environment. The demand to provide efficient and effective care that is free from error and at the forefront of good practice is greater than ever before. Clinical governance reflects these pressures but provides us with an opportunity to live up to the high expectation users have of us and we have of ourselves.

Audit is part of the design of clinical governance. It offers us the chance to rigorously check how services operate against a backdrop of best practice and then to make changes based on what we find. It is a multi-disciplinary process that must enjoy the contribution of service users so that proposals have some legitimacy with those who, in the end, will receive the service. The only remaining barriers are those of attitude and culture. Change is not the product of audit, it is the only reason to pursue audit, and in doing so, the aims of clinical governance will come to be realised.

REFERENCES

Buttery Y, Walshe K, Rumsey M et al. 1995 Provider audit in England: a review of twenty-nine programmes. Caspe Research, London.

Department of Health 1989 Working for patients. Cmnd 555. HMSO, London.

Department of Health 1997 The new NHS: modern, dependable. Cm 3807. The Stationery Office, London.

Department of Health 1998 A first class service: quality in the new NHS. Department of Health, London.

Department of Health 1999 National service framework for mental health: executive summary. Department of Health, London.

Department of Health 2000 The NHS plan: a plan for investment, a plan for reform. Cm 4818-I. The Stationery Office, London.

Department of Health 2001a Valuing people: a new strategy for learning disability for the 21st century. Cm 5086. The Stationery Office, London.

Department of Health 2001b Essence of care: patient-focused benchmarking for health care practitioners. Department of Health, London.

Malby R 1995 The whys and wherefores of audit. In: Malby R (ed) Clinical audit for nurses and therapists. Scutari Press, London.

NHS Centre for Reviews and Dissemination/The Royal Society of Medicine Press 2001 Effective health care vol. 7 no. 2. Acupuncture. University of York, York.

NHS Centre for Reviews and Dissemination, the University of York 1999 Effective health care vol. 5, no. 6. Drug treatment for schizophrenia. University of York, York.

NHSE 1996 Promoting clinical effectiveness: a framework for action. NHSE, London.

NHSME 1991 Framework of audit for nursing services. HMSO, London.

Royal College of Nursing 1990 The dynamic standard setting system. RCN, Harrow.

Accountability and risk

Many areas of welfare services are currently experiencing significant pressure in relation to accountability and risk. The chapters within this section provide numerous examples from both health and social care where this has been case. In this context it is vital that practitioners consider both the risks associated with any proposed developments as well as the accountability issues both personally, professionally and organisationally. As such, these chapters provide the reader with significant information to support them in such activity.

9

Accountability and professional self-regulation

Sue Merrylees

KEY ISSUES

◆ The concept of accountability

◆ Models of accountability

◆ Professional self-regulation

◆ Accountability and the policy context

◆ Accountability and professional self-
  regulation – the clinical governance
  agenda
  – practitioner issues
  – best practice and accountable service
    delivery
  – continuing professional development
  – leadership issues.

INTRODUCTION

This book has explored a range of issues within the clinical governance agenda. This chapter aims to address one of the many key themes within clinical governance and best value, that is, accountable practice. Accountability has become a key concept in the delivery of public services. Both across health- and social-care sectors, the nature and focus of accountability has evolved. The consequence of this is that it has now created a discipline in its own right.

Within this chapter it is intended to discuss a range of both theoretical and practice issues. This will be achieved by exploring the development of the concept of accountability. This will initially be through discussions about the contemporary meaning of accountability within service delivery. In doing so, the scope and range of issues are presented along with a brief overview of models of accountability. This allows the reader to explore the many different aspects of this concept. A brief discussion on the origins of accountability and an exploration of the mechanisms within the health- and social-care professions is presented to provide a background to the current debate on professional self-regulation. The changes to the systems for professional self-regulation are also included in this section.

The chapter subsequently moves on to explore the emerging political drivers concerned with the delivery of accountable practice. From this, an exploration of concepts of quality, partnership and clinical governance emerge. Bringing together each of these elements provides a framework for the development of clinical governance within a framework of accountability. Working within the constraints of each of these concepts is a challenge for all concerned within health and social care. Through the use of examples, brief case studies and activities, the chapter moves on to address some of the problems and issues facing both professionals and lay people. In conclusion, the challenges and opportunities for the future are explored.

ACCOUNTABILITY – THE CONCEPT

Presented simplistically, accountability is being asked to account for one's actions. Within health and social care, however, the complexity of the structures and organisations involved means this ability to account is difficult. Accountability affects every organisation, structure and system involved in the whole range of health- and social-care

activity, including commissioning, strategic planning and training, some of which are not always seen within this context.

The range and variety of activities involved in the actual day-to-day delivery of health and social care is all underpinned by systems that rely on accountability. It is little wonder, therefore, that the systems, structures and methods of accountability are equally complex and varied. In order to consider these issues, an exploration of the definitions associated with accountability is necessary. As there are countless definitions of accountability it is the intention of this chapter to provide only a flavour of what accountability means in practice.

Activity 9.1

Think about what accountability means to you as an individual, in relation to the work you do.

Nurses will be familiar with the United Kingdom Central Council for Nursing, Midwifery and Health Visiting's (UKCC) definition of accountability:

Each registered nurse, midwife, and health visitor shall act, at all times, in such a manner as to safe-guard and promote the interests of individual patients and clients; to serve the interests of society, justify public trust and confidence and uphold and enhance the good standing and reputation of the professions (UKCC 1992).

In medicine, the General Medical Council has a similar approach and offers the following guidance:

Patients must be able to trust doctors with their lives and well being. To justify that trust we as a profession have a duty to maintain a good standard of practice and care and show respect for human life (GMC 1999).

The principles espoused in both of these apply to all forms of professional self-regulation.

A different way of describing accountability is offered by Stacey (1995)

Accountability is based on legal requirements and moral expectation. Whether in the NHS or the private sector, patients consulting and receiving treatment from health care professionals should be able to trust them to be competent at their jobs (p. 35).

So far these definitions have focused on the concept of professional accountability. There are, of course, other spheres of accountability and it is important to consider at least some of the legal aspects. Young (1994) draws the distinction between statutory law and case law. Young describes statutory law as parliament made laws. For health- and social-care practitioners there are numerous examples of the laws that affect practice. Examples include the Health and Safety at Work Act (Home Office 1974), Mental Health Act (Department of Health 1983) and NHS and Community Care Act (Department of Health 1993).

Tingle and Cribb (2002) discuss case law as having a very strong impact on practice. In this instance the principle of the 'Law of Tortuous Liability' applies. They offer a simple explanation of this. For negligence to have occurred:

- A duty of care must be established (the very nature of the professional care role establishes such a duty of care).
- There must have been a breach of this duty (either by act or omission).
- The person making the complaint has suffered as a result of the act or omission.

It is important to note that health- and social-care practitioners are accountable under both of these systems. Within either context an important

consideration is that action of any practitioner is judged in law in the context of the actions of any reasonable competent practitioner faced with similar circumstances. This means that when a professional steps outside of their usual role they will be judged by a different standard. This issue has implications for professional practice for those individuals who accept advanced or extended roles. In nursing there is guidance under the Scope of Professional Practice (UKCC 1992). The Nursing and Midwifery Council (NMC) came into being in April 2002, and in July 2002 they published the updated codes of professional conduct. Other professional bodies offer similar guidance.

A further aspect of accountability that must be considered is that of employment status and, therefore, the accountability of both the employee and employer. As an employee, a health- and social-care professional is accountable for the way in which they undertake their role. This inter-relationship is not always straightforward. For example, Seedhouse (1995) explores the difficulty of being able to 'do the right thing' when resources are scarce. Situations such as this can give rise to conflict between the different spheres of accountability.

In addition, accountability has a moral aspect, particularly as the relationship between the practitioner and service user is built on trust. Being able to account to oneself for one's own action is an important part of the human psyche. The chapter is too brief to explore this issue in depth, but a good source of further reading on this is the ethical work of Tschudin (1992). Walsh (2000, p. 97) likens accountability to gravity: 'It's an invisible yet powerful force exerted in well defined directions towards various bodies'. For me, this summarises some of the dilemmas in accountability.

In the current context of service delivery, clinical governance and best value do appear to offer a collective and structured means for working through some of these very complex issues. The next section explores a framework within which this may occur.

MODELS OF ACCOUNTABILITY

Models of accountability emerge from the many definitions that exist. It is helpful to explore some of these as they can be used as tools to enhance the application of clinical governance to situations in which accountability plays a key role.

Hallett (2002) describes several components of accountability. These include the expectations of society and factors central to the role of the professions. Societal concerns include:

- the cost of care and economic factors
- public expectation and increasing awareness
- the organisational structure and lines of accountability.

This means that those who provide care have to be accountable for these factors. With increasing cost, issues of value for money and prevention of waste are a key component, particularly in relation to fiscal accountability. The idea of a better-educated public has been central to a number of debates and the Audit Commission Report 1999 (Audit Commission 2000) cites public expectation as a key driver in health care in the future. The third of the above points relates to the fact that accountability is seen as an integral part of fiscal management.

Factors internal to the professional are described by Hallett as 'running sideways with concern for other colleagues, being free to weigh up the pros and cons leading to autonomy and job satisfaction' (2002, p. 95).

All of the above factors indicate a move towards increased professionalisation within welfare services. Accountability within a profession can be seen as an indicator of the maturity of that profession. This is reinforced by Moloney (1986) who describes how accountability is an important facet of professional practice.

Dimond (1995) discusses four arenas of accountability. She describes these as being the:

- Public arena – accountability in law.
- Patient arena – accountability through civil means.
- Professional arena – for example accountability to the Nurses and Midwives Council (NMC) for this group of professionals.
- Employment arena – contractual accountability.

In exploring the wider issues of accountability it can be seen that such a model is likely to apply across both health and social care. However, there are key differences in the structures and arrangements that support accountability.

Walsh (2000) highlights a model that explores consistency, quality and responsiveness, all of which are central themes of both accountability and clinical governance. This model has three components:

- Corporate accountability – this is the setting up of clear lines of accountability within the organisation.
- Internal mechanisms – these include personal accountability and professional self-regulation.
- External mechanisms – an example being the Commission for Health Improvement or Social Care Institute for Excellence.

Walsh (2000) again offers a set of key principles that, when applied, could be considered as a model for practice. These include:

- personal
- involving measurable goals
- requires mutual trust and a more equal relationship between managers and the managed.

STRUCTURES AND SYSTEMS

The principles and processes underpinning accountable practice is supported by a range of systems and structures. These have evolved as welfare services have developed. The professional bodies have emerged as the central focus for the self-regulation of professional practice. Each of these bodies has their own structures and processes, which are discussed in more detail in the next section.

In addition, executive structures have emerged within health and social care in support of corporate accountability. These lines of accountability exist both within organisations and in the way they account to external commissioners. It is important that individual practitioners understand these structures and the way in which they apply to the service in which they work. Consequently, good management systems are essential in the delivery of competent services and in support of the individual and their personal accountability. Essentially, therefore, clinical governance, best value and good management can be seen to have an almost symbiotic relationship.

The concept of accountability is further supported by the legal system within the UK and much publicity has been given to the increase in litigation in both health and social care. As a consequence, practitioners are becoming increasingly aware of the legal aspects of their practice. However, in some areas there is a growing feeling that one of the main drivers in service delivery is the growing fear of litigation. For example, in obstetrics and midwifery, litigation is becoming such an issue that their professional organisations now offer advice to their members with regard to accountability.

This section has introduced the fact that accountability has a variety of complex interfaces, including the inter-relationship of individual, corporate and legal accountabilities. It has also introduced the case for using clinical governance and best value as

a means to develop and monitor accountable practice. This section has begun to develop a framework to work through clinical governance and best value issues, but before the chapter moves on, there are two key issues influencing the accountability agenda that must be addressed. These are:

- the concept of professional self-regulation
- the effect of the current government's modernisation agenda.

PROFESSIONAL SELF-REGULATION

Professional self-regulation is the method by which individual practitioners monitor the quality of those people practising within their own profession. When exploring the concept of professionalisation, the process of gate keeping is seen as a key component of professional activity. This means that the profession regulates the number and nature of the individuals who may enter the profession. There is also a role in setting standards for conduct and the regular revalidation of practitioners. All regulatory bodies have a role in removing undesirables from their register and all have a health monitoring process. Whilst professional self-regulation has emerged as a key driver for quality improvement within health care, this is not yet as well developed within the social care sector.

In order to explore the issues relating to self-regulation in sufficient depth, it is necessary to consider each of the professions separately. For the purposes of this chapter a distinction is drawn between medicine and nursing, and the healthcare professions, as this reflects the current approach to self-regulation.

HEALTHCARE PROFESSIONS

The term 'healthcare profession' has been coined as an umbrella term for practitioners involved in the delivery of care that do not fall into either medicine or nursing. There are some distinctive features relating to the professionalisation of practitioners within this group, particularly as each of the professions involved tends to be small and distinctive in its own right. Within this group, most practitioners undertake a period of pre-qualifying preparation involving studying to at least degree level. However, all have struggled for recognition as a legitimate profession. These are some of the factors that make them distinctive from both nursing and medicine.

In terms of professional self-regulation, there have been several different professional groups who formed part of what was 'The Council for Professions Supplementary to Medicine' (CPSM). These included: radiographers, occupational therapists and physiotherapists, amongst others. This collective approach to self-regulation appears to have been of benefit to these groups, as it not only created a critical mass, but also allowed for some external scrutiny. This lack of external scrutiny has been one of the criticisms levelled at other professional bodies, particularly the General Medical Council (GMC). Some healthcare professionals belonged to a different regulatory body; these include: those for opticians and pharmacists, and, more recently, those bodies overseeing groups such as chiropractors and osteopaths (Davies 2000).

Essentially, there were at least six regulatory bodies concerned with professional self-regulation in the healthcare professions. Inevitably, difficulties in this matrix of provision arose and, given the earlier discussions on the wider complexity of accountability issues, a review became necessary. Subsequently, JM Consultancy were asked to consider professional self-regulation in the healthcare professions. Davies (2000) identified that, amongst other things, there was a need to refocus on the purpose and practice of self-regulation. In addition, the report stated that regulatory bodies should not be involved in the process of accrediting courses and that there should be a new overarching body: the Council For Health Professionals (CHP).

MEDICINE

The role of professional self-regulation in medicine has a long history. The first body was set up in 1858. As with all the professional bodies, the role of gate keeping is a key function and the GMC has traditionally dealt with this issue for the medical profession. Stacey (1995) identifies some of the special privileges that have resulted from this. Most notable is that of clinical autonomy. Davies (2000) notes an additional factor and points to the role that gender has played in the development of self-regulation in medicine and the unique flavour that the predominance of males has given it. Despite such criticism, one cannot ignore the fact that the GMC was established in a time before the NHS, when organised health care was chaotic and inadequate. This too has contributed to its current framework. Essentially, the GMC has played an important role in the regulation of the medical profession over the years.

Recently, the debate on the future of professional self-regulation has gained momentum. A Health Service Journal (HSJ) comment (15th November 2001) highlights how complaints against doctors have risen by a dramatic 49% to a record high in the year 2000. Against this backdrop there have been some very high profile cases, such as Harold Shipman, Alder Hey and the Bristol Inquiry. The Bristol Inquiry resulted in the publication of the Kennedy Report (Bristol Royal Infirmary 2001). This has prompted a review of the role and the function of the GMC. Much criticism is levelled at the methods of professional self-regulation and the perpetuation of outmoded forms of inquiry. The issue of public protection has, it is suggested, become buried in the annals of medical privilege.

NURSING

The development of self-regulation in nursing can be traced back to 1919 and the advent of the General Nursing Council (GNC). In 1948 at the inauguration of the National Health Service, the role and function of the council was reviewed and other areas of nursing, such as psychiatry and learning disabilities, came into the fold. In 1971, the Report of the Committee into Nursing described some of the problems facing the nursing profession as being linked to both its size and the many various routes and outcomes of training. Many of these criticisms have been addressed over the years.

As nursing remains the largest professional group within health care today, the regulation of such a workforce has become an enormous task. In 1983 this was acknowledged and there was a division in the body to form:

- the UKCC – responsible for conduct and professional standards
- the National Boards for Nursing, Midwifery and Health Visiting – responsible for standards of practitioner preparation.

This move towards regulation and, therefore, professionalisation has resulted in a mixed response. On the positive side is the recognition of the contribution of the role of the nurse to health care and a recognition of the importance of professional preparation. However, as with medicine, there have been a number of high profile failures. The Allitt case, for instance, resulted in the implementation of the Clothier Report (Clothier 1994); this includes recommendations on vetting applications for training and appointments.

More recently, there has been an increasing sense of dissatisfaction with the way that professional self-regulation has been managed in nursing. There has been a perception that the messages emanating from the UKCC and the National Boards have not been consistent or clear. In 1999 the government commissioned JM Consultancy to undertake a review of the UKCC. The results were far reaching with a suggestion that nursing was more concerned with it own tribalism than with its prime function: the protection of the public. JM Consultancy has recommended a series of changes to the regulatory framework which were implemented from April 2002. This has resulted in the formation of the Nursing and Midwifery Council (NMC).

SOCIAL WORK

Social work presents with a very different history in terms of professional self-regulation. There have been no internal mechanisms within social work for accountability in the form of an overarching professional body. Structures within social services have developed very differently to those in health and the role of the elected body in the form of the local government has meant that systems of accountability are vastly different in the social care sector. There is also a greater difference in the ratio of unqualified workers to professionally qualified workers in the social care arena, compared to many parts of health care. This creates an additional dynamic with respect of self-regulation.

The lack of a traditional professional body appears to have been an anomaly in professional practice. Social work students have undergone professional preparation overseen by a training body, the Central Council for the Education and Training of Social Workers (CCETSW). The modernisation agenda in the health- and social-care sectors has allowed a review of the regulation system in social care. Once again, the feature of high profile cases has been an important factor within this review process. In social work in particular, much blame has been levelled at practitioners involved in the much publicised failures in the child protection system.

Modernising Social Services (Department of Health 1998a) has been instrumental in the changes to the social work profession. There has been the development of the General Social Care Council (GSCC), which came into being in April 2002; their initial focus was the registration of qualified social workers. On completion of this, the GSCC will move to register the non-professionally qualified social care workforce.

THE FUTURE?

All key stakeholders predominantly agree that there is a need for professional self-regulation.

Davies (2000) sees this as following some of the emerging themes from the establishment of the GSCC. She argues that this will become a model for regulation and will act as a watchdog, advocate and source of information.

Taking the proposals of JM Consultancy into account, the refocusing of the professional self-regulation systems into a prime concern with public protection in mind seems essential. In order to do this, the bodies are to concern themselves more with this function and concentrate less on internal professional mechanisms. The result is that bodies are expected to be smaller with an equal representation of lay and professional members. An acknowledgement of the Human Rights legislation is central. Davies discusses this as a new way for the professionals to view the public: she describes them as being 'A grown up Public' (p. 287).

Another key challenge laid down through reform is the speed and efficiency of internal processes, as the bodies are commanded to become more professional themselves. There are changes too in the way that education at a pre-registration/qualifying level is organised and validated. An example comes from nursing, with the dissolution of the UKCC and the National Boards. New systems in place will rely on collaboration between the Quality Assurance Agency in Higher Education (QAA) and the Personal Development and Life Long Learning Unit and the Nursing and Midwifery Council (NMC).

Stacey (1995) refers to the possibility of what she terms the most radical proposal afoot. This is

the creation of a Health Standards Inspectorate. The National Health Service Reform and Health Professions Bill (Department of Health 2001a) makes provision for the establishment of a 'Council for the Regulation of Health Care Professionals'. This body will oversee the activities of the various regulatory bodies of the healthcare professionals. It provides for the council to provide good practice guidelines and other aspects of the regulatory bodies' work, and for it to encourage the regulatory bodies to act in the interests of patients and others. Specifically, the council will oversee the GMC, the General Dental Council, the General Optical Council, the General Osteopathic Council, the General Chiropractic Council, the Royal Pharmaceutical Society of Great Britain, the NMC and the HCP. The Bill provides for the council to 'have the right of appeal in cases determining practitioners' fitness to practice and examining if there has been an instance of professional misconduct where the decision of the regulatory body seems harmful to the protection of the public' (p. 2 & 3).

The development of this new council has far-reaching implications on the future autonomy of the regulatory bodies. Whist not creating an overarching body, the council will monitor and regulate the activities of the regulatory bodies. Additional mechanisms are emerging for the monitoring of service standards. An example of this is seen in the Health Service Journal comment mentioned earlier (15th November 2001) and a discussion on the role of the National Clinical Assessment Authority (NCAA). The HSJ describes the body as 'Tackling the problem early arresting the damage before it gets to the steps of the GMC'. Through the promotion of these and other means, the role of the conduct committees within professional self-regulation should become less frequently used and required only when all other options have failed.

This section has considered the systems underpinning professional self-regulation. The case for the use of clinical governance as a mechanism for influencing accountable practice can be seen through the reforms within the regulatory framework. If professional bodies are to change their roles and functions in line with policy and legislation, then other means of accountability will become increasingly important. The chapter moves on to explore a final key concept in accountability, i.e. the political drivers in the form of the modernisation agenda.

THE MODERNISATION AGENDA

Policy issues are widely discussed in other parts of this book; therefore, the aim of this brief section is to locate the concept of modern accountability within the policy context. To do this it is important to consider the emergence of the modernisation agenda and how it has affected both health- and social-care providers. This will include discussions about partnerships, working with the people who use services and quality. Understanding the development of new structures for accountability at a service level is essential to a clear view of the relationship between accountability, professional self-regulation and clinical governance.

Within health, the discussion begins with a consultation paper from the NHS Confederation in 1997: *Towards the 21st Century – A Way Forward for the NHS*. Section four of this document addresses the issues of accountability and governance. Key recommendations within this include the development of a clear and consistent framework that opens up every part of the service to scrutiny. This document also suggests that accountability should be developed within the existing frameworks.

Using consultation documents such as these, the government produced the first blueprint for the modernisation of the NHS with *The New NHS: Modern, Dependable* (Department of Health 1997). Concern with accountability can be seen at many levels within this document. *The New NHS: Modern, Dependable* sets out a vision for the

development of national standards. This is a crucial development in service delivery, as laying down these means that there is a commitment to delivery of those standards. This essentially creates an overarching system of accountability.

The publication of the *National Service Frameworks (NSF) for Mental Health* (Department of Health 1999a), *Older people* (Department of Health 2001b) *Coronary Heart Disease* (Department of Health 2001c) and others all build upon the ideals set out in the 1997 document. There is a consensus that the frameworks are based upon evidence-based practice. For both the commissioners and deliverers of service it is essential that such frameworks be based upon identifiable evidence. In terms of accountability, evidence-based practice creates a link between theory and practice that allows confidence and certainty in service development and the standards professionals are being measured against.

Each of the NSFs contain key statements, for example: 'sets national standards and defines service models; puts in place underpinning programmes to support local service delivery and establishes milestones and a specific group of performance indicators against which progress will be measured' (Department of Health 2000a). The implementation of these structures has significant implications for accountability. There is now a national framework around which performance measures are set. This means that for the first time, both commissioners and providers of services, as well as individual practitioners, are accountable against minimum standards with clear structures and lines of accountability.

Another aspect to consider in *The New NHS: Modern, Dependable* (Department of Health 1997) is the way it addresses relationships between the health authorities and other structures, such as the then primary care groups. Page 39 states: 'there will be accountability agreements between primary care groups and health authorities – in addition health authorities and primary care groups will agree targets for improving health, health services and value for money'. Whilst many of these organisations no longer exist the principles still apply.

From 1997 there has been a range of developments in the delivery of the National Health Service Act (1999b). Accountability can be seen, for example, through the implementation of section 18 of the Act: the duty of quality. In addition, *The NHS Plan* (Department of Health 2000a) sets out key objectives for taking forward the modernisation agenda that complement the emerging themes of partnership and empowerment.

Within the consultation document on the review of workforce planning, *A Health Service for All Talents* (Department of Health 2000b), some key professional issues are addressed. The restructuring of the education consortia into Workforce Development Confederations urges that new roles and practice development be taken into account when considering workforce development. This provides a crucial link between the previous discussion on the professional role and accountability and the new agenda. Also, within this, the consideration of the non-statutory providers and the impact that this has on the workforce is addressed for the first time. Similarly, social services are for the first time included. Appendix three of this document lays out the suggested arrangements for the commissioning of education and training, and shows the relationship between the National Workforce Development Board and the substructures. Once again this is in the framework of a performance management structure, demonstrating clearly that accountability is pervading all parts of the system.

Against this, new systems for practitioner preparation are emerging with an emphasis on partnership and clinical competence. The *Making a Difference* (Department of Health 1999c) document sets out the future for the preparation of nurses. New medical schools are emerging and an emphasis is being placed on multi-professional learning opportunities.

In the summer of 2001, *Shifting the Balance of Power* (Department of Health 2001d) was published. Using the 1997 proposals for the streamlining of health authority functions, this key document sets out the future relationships between the NHS trusts, the primary care trusts, local partnership boards and the new Strategic Health Authorities. These proposals were accepted into statute in the form of the National Health Service Reform and Health Care Professions Bill in November 2001 (Department of Health 2001a).

Within the social care arena, it can be seen that there are similar modernisation issues. The publication of *Modernising Social Services* in 1998 (Department of Health 1998a) mirrors some of the changes seen within the health service. The review of social services is as far reaching as the healthcare modernisation agenda. The key drivers within the white paper fall into three areas: promoting independence, improving protection and raising standards. Each of these carries with it issues of accountability. Social work structures and training are also under scrutiny, new systems of practitioner preparation, e.g. the new social work degree are taking account of this emerging agenda.

This focus on new ways of working is of concern to all health- and social-care practitioners. As previously stated, both *Modernising Social Services* and *The New NHS: Modern, Dependable* set the agenda for the development of the key themes underpinned by partnership and participation. A cornerstone of the modernisation agenda is the development of partnerships between different professional groups, disciplines, agencies and those who use services, the purpose of which is to ensure a seamless and consistent approach to service delivery.

A key policy initiative is the involvement and participation at all levels of the people who use services. In relation to accountability, this involves all stages of delivery being open to scrutiny by those who are, perhaps, the most concerned, that is the users of that service. Service providers have always been accountable to users, and evidence shows that consultation and involvement of this group have always formed part of the policy-making process (Ham 2001).

However, what is emerging is a political driver that puts the users of services and their local representatives on an equal footing with the professionals who develop and deliver local services. For all professional groups this kind of working is relatively new.

THE QUALITY AGENDA

As with the key themes of partnership and participation, current policy is underpinned by another important driver – the quality agenda. *The New NHS: Modern, Dependable* once again lays the foundation. This document was rapidly followed by *A First Class Service* (Department of Health 1998b). This document outlined the way in which the NHS would account for the quality of the services in the future. It is from this that many of the clinical governance issues have emerged. *A First Class Service* has been superseded by the policies outlined in the section above, each of which have strong elements of quality in them.

Current policy initiatives focus upon establishing internal reporting mechanisms and external scrutiny that supports the delivery of a quality service. An example of this is the 'annual survey of patient experience' (Department of Health 1998b, 2000a). There are also mechanisms such as the Commission for Health Improvement (CHI) (Department of Health 1997, 2001a) who have, in the NHS Reform and Health Care Professions Bill of November 2001, had a new range of statutory duties placed upon them as amendments to the 1999 NHS Act. Section (2c) of the Health Bill (Department of Health 2001a) states:

> ... the function of conducting reviews of and making reports on the quality of data obtained by others relating to the management, provisions or quality of health care and access to health care for which the NHS bodies or service providers have responsibility, the validity of conclusion drawn from such data, and the methods used in their collection and analysis.

Whilst written in legal terms this paragraph extends the role of the CHI in to being able to scrutinise, not only the evidence, but also the methods used to gather this evidence which is a very powerful tool for external accountability.

EMERGING STRUCTURES AND SYSTEMS

In order to develop quality services that are accountable a range of new structures are necessary. An earlier part of this chapter focused on the development of the new structures for professional regulation. However, these need to be seen within the context of new service driven structures around which the strategies for accountable practice are hinged. This will form the basis of the first half of the next section, whilst the second half will give a brief overview of the systems for monitoring and reporting that support accountable practice at both an individual and organisational level.

April 2001 saw the first stage Primary Care Trusts (PCTs) become a reality. These organisations are accountable to local people in terms of the commissioning and delivery of local healthcare needs. The key issue here is that the PCTs, whilst being accountable, are also accessible. This is through individual access but, more importantly, through the involvement of local lay representation at board level. Within social care the development of the Social Care Trusts are closely linked to the same philosophy.

The development of Local Strategic Partnerships (LSPs) is seen as being crucial to the modernisation agenda and it is through these and the development of Health Improvement Programmes (HImPs) and Joint Investment Plans (JIPs) that the government is urging complex local issues to be tackled. These are not merely confined to health and social care but, for example, include housing, transport and employment. The *Local Strategic Partnerships – Government Guidance* (Office of the Deputy Prime Minister 2001) has a section on accountability that states: 'Individual partners will remain accountable and responsible for decisions on their services and resources' (p. 22).

Delivering the LSPs' common goals will, therefore, depend on their ability to demonstrate to individual partners that they can help them to achieve their individual goals. This sort of joint working is seen in the HImPs where local authorities contribute to a number of centrally driven goals. The guidance goes on to say that LSPs need to operate within robust and transparent frameworks of local accountability. This means that LSPs are able to build upon existing accountability frameworks within each component partner's arena. For those delivering services, this means that partnership working involves each partner remaining autonomous and accountable within its existing mechanisms, yet there are also new and emerging lines of accountability that need to be worked upon.

The development of the Patient Advice and Liaison Service (PALS) in 2001 is again evidence of the policy makers commitment to the needs of service users, their families, carers and friends. PALS are another mechanism for the external scrutiny of health and, in some cases, social-care delivery. However, unlike the CHI, PALS are non-affiliated and non-professional in their dealings.

In addition, organisations are charged with the development and implementation of internal monitoring systems. The UKCC in *Professional Self-Regulation and Clinical Governance* (1999) describes the process of clinical governance as underpinning:

> *... quality improvement initiatives such as risk management, clinical audit, standard setting and monitoring, evidence based practice, critical incident reporting, complaints procedures and*

> *clinical supervision (p. 1 of the clinical governance section).*

The recent health and social care reforms place these elements at the heart of the modernisation agenda and it is through an exploration of these in practice that the challenges for the modern practitioner emerge. Other mechanisms can be seen as being driven by policy and these form the basis of much of the next section on the development of best practice and the introduction of benchmarking as a concept for quality service delivery.

Activity 9.3

Using the models of accountability discussed above how do you think the current policy initiatives support the need for accountable practice?

It can be seen that the key themes of current health- and social-care policy thinking are driven by concepts of partnership, user and carer involvement and quality. Each of these and every part of the current health- and social-care reforms are driven by accountability. New ways of working are emerging and there are many issues that face the modern practitioner within today's health- and social-care system. Section four moves on to explore some of the real life issues that face practitioners on a day-to-day basis.

CLINICAL GOVERNANCE, BEST VALUE AND ACCOUNTABLE PRACTICE – BRINGING THE CONCEPTS TOGETHER

Within this book there is much written on clinical governance and best value and its underpinning structures and systems. The aim here is to explore how the different aspects of accountable practice can be enhanced through the modernisation agenda. The section begins by bringing together the concepts of accountability, clinical governance

Table 9.1

	Accountable to who?	Accountable for what?
Professional	Regulatory body of relevant profession	Actions carried out in the day-to-day function that are commensurate with competence of practitioners within that profession.
Employment/contractual	Employer	Carrying out the role and function of the job as specified in job description and appraisal.
Legal	Through the law and the judicial system	Acts and omissions that result in harm to individuals. These can include systems failure where the individual is responsible for the system and acts of delegation to an incompetent other.
Moral/personal	Self	Asking the question – have I done all that I can?
Societal/political	People who use the service, organisation	Providing the most competent and up-to-date service possible within resources.
Organisational – a corporate accountability in which the practitioner is accountable through employment	People who use the service, commissioners of the service, local PALS and other representative groups	Fiscal accountability, acts or omissions by individuals within the organisation. Organisational direction.

and best value. It then goes on to explore some of the key features of current professional practice. These are best practice and the dissemination of best practice, working with people who use services, lifelong learning and continuing professional development, as well as issues for leadership and management.

Clinical governance and best value allows any situation to be unpicked and analysed in a constructive and non-punitive manner. To adopt clinical governance and best value, an organisation must be able to explore and analyse all levels of service delivery. That is, from the action of an individual practitioner to the way in which teams function, from leadership and management and how the organisation relate to the wider policy issues.

Exploring different dimensions of accountability through a framework is a useful approach to the application of the modernisation agenda.

Activity 9.4

Using the following categories:

- professional
- employment/contractual
- legal
- moral/personal
- societal/political
- organisational.

What do you think are the main issues of accountability in relation to clinical governance and best value?

Table 9.1 identifies some of the issues you may have considered.

SHARING BEST PRACTICE – THE CHALLENGES FACING ACCOUNTABLE PRACTITIONERS

The development of practice that is underpinned by an evidence base is a key way of developing competent, safe and accountable practice. The modernisation agenda demands that best practice is disseminated and there are numerous ways in which this can occur.

The Department of Health has recently promoted a benchmarking project and this should be developed in conjunction with clinical governance and best value. The first attempts at setting clear standards for aspects of care fundamental to the quality of the service users' experience were established through the publication of *The Essence of Care* (Department of Health 2001e). This document identifies that benchmarking involves:

- The identification of aspects of care delivery where comparisons and sharing best practice can be made – these include the softer aspects traditionally difficult to measure.
- Joint user and practitioner involvement.
- The identification of structures that support a user-focused outcome.
- The identification of good evidence that forms the benchmark.
- Using stepping stones to build the benchmark.
- Use of good evidence for comparison and sharing.

Activity 9.5

What benchmarking projects are happening in your area of practice? How can you disseminate information about the good practice that you are involved in to other people?

Traditional methods of dissemination continue to be important. Journal articles and papers at conferences remain a useful tool in sharing best practice. Some areas are thinking creatively about such activities and the way in which they are pitched. For example, best practice symposia appear to be a relatively new way to allow practitioners to come together to share best practice initiatives.

The issue of best practice raises two particular questions:

- how is best practice validated?
- how do we address issues of poor practice in an equally open way?

Once again clinical governance and best value must hold the key.

Case study

Davina and Rob work together as part of a drug rehabilitation programme that has been funded through health action zone money. Davina is a trained social worker with an interest in addictions; Rob is a community psychiatric nurse. They have developed a project in which they have worked together with the local Connexions network (Connexions is a government sponsored initiative to support young people on a range of issues). The work also involves local police and probation services. The project has involved a rehabilitation programme working with sympathetic local employers who have been willing to take on a young person and give them a chance. At the moment there are three people on placement. It is hoped that, through this intensive work, future health- and social-care problems may be avoided. Davina and Rob are aware that they have created something unique.

Both Davina and Rob are keen to share their work but each have managers who, whilst wholeheartedly supporting the project, wish to take the credit for their own organisation. They are blocking every attempt to spread the word.

Activity 9.6

What are the issues of accountability in this case study?

Thinking back to the discussion on strategic local partnerships, practitioners who work across traditional boundaries remain accountable to their own employers. Developing evidence-based and best-practice initiatives are key to any professional development. In this case it appears that Davina and Rob have fallen foul of difficulties in partnership working. Particularly as there are often some problems when bringing together different organisational systems, cultures and management styles.

How could clinical governance and best value help?

Rob should be familiar with clinical governance and best value through his own employment and this could be his first port of call for examining the reasons for his managers' reluctance to support extra development around the project. For Davina the system may be different. In social services, governance systems are linked to supervision and through her own reflection she could also use governance to consider the barriers. Both must engage in a process of problem solving. There are many models around that can help with this. Using governance systems can support this problem solving approach.

For me, this case and the problems are symptomatic. The issues really lie in the development of partnership working that allows the different partners to find the common ground yet respect differences. In this case, what should happen is that the partners should focus upon identifying mechanisms for exploring the next phase of the project. What no-one must do is to lose respect for the three individuals who are on placement. Perhaps working with these young people, a solution may be found that allows them to share the outcomes of each other's best practice. The case study also describes lots of other agenciesinvolved and the friendly employers. A collective response to dissemination should arise from using an analysis of the problem.

In joint initiatives such as this, the governance system should be part of the project development. This would allow a shared approach to the management, not only of the project, but also of the enhanced work involved. Using governance systems to analyse the issue would allow Davina and Rob, the young people on placement and their managers to have collective ownership of the good practice.

From this case study it can be seen that there are real challenges in the development of systems that support partnership working. Projects such as this demand openness and understanding from all those involved. Often this incorporates a significant amount of learning for some people, in such circumstances support is essential. Using personal reflection to support such developments and to implement the principles underpinning clinical governance and best value can aid practitioners in the process of beginning to think differently.

WORKING WITH THE USERS OF SERVICES, THEIR FAMILIES AND FRIENDS

Earlier discussion identified the importance of working with the people who use services, their carers, friends and families both in terms of general accountability and in relation to the underpinning political drivers. This section builds upon this discourse by exploring some of the real life situations that practitioners experience. At an individual level, the relationship between the practitioner and the carer is built upon mutual trust and respect. The understanding of this relationship, whilst not easily evaluated, can be monitored by the success of proposed interventions and the carer's willingness to continue engaging with that relationship. However, it is far more difficult to evaluate this experience at either a service or an organisational level. Equally difficult is the challenge of involving the public within strategic decision making, particularly in a meaningful way that can be classified as equitable.

A particular challenge has arisen within the National Health Service with the abolition of the Community Health Councils (Department of Health 2001a), though advocates of the act would argue that these organisations had been replaced by the creation of an independent patients' forum for every NHS and Primary Care Trust in England. The aim of these fora is to perform inspection and represent patient need. With these and similar structures appearing, the challenge to professionals is to ensure that they are able to work with users and carers as equals. Whilst this is undeniably a complex agenda, a number of structures and systems exist that may support the successful achievement of this goal. This may include an exploration of complaints using a clinical governance mechanism to help to highlight deficiencies within the organisation in terms of the general culture towards service users.

Of importance is recognition of the different needs of people who use services; single representation is not adequate. Similarly, there are marked differences between the aspirations of service users and their carers.

The following is an example of how clinical governance can be used to develop an inclusive approach to service delivery.

Case study

John has Down's syndrome and at the age of 45 was diagnosed as having early-onset dementia. This is not uncommon in older people with Down's syndrome and often results in rapid and marked effects upon health and well-being. John has had a series of chest infections and is having difficulty breathing. His GP has arranged admission to the local district general hospital. This is done through a busy admissions unit that is already feeling a pressure on beds as a result of a recent flu epidemic. John's sister has come along with him, as his mum, who provides most of his day-to-day care, is herself unwell and, at 80 years old, finds the situation daunting. John's sister Mary explains to the doctor that John has both diabetes, controlled by tablets, and needs to take his epilepsy medicine three times a day. Mary also gives this information to the staff nurse, Simon, who admits John. He is careful to write down all the special requirements John needs to help him to eat and drink. Mary checks the details and when satisfied she leaves to collect her children from school. Before leaving Mary lets Simon know the

name and contact details for the community team that helps her mum with John, explaining that they may be able to help as well. When Mary returns later that evening she finds that John has had an intravenous infusion prescribed by the doctor, and a new member of staff, Louise, explains that this is because he is dehydrated and needs to have antibiotics. John also has oxygen through a nasal cannula and seems quite settled and happy.

The next day, however, when Mary visits, she finds that his lunch and his tablets are left on the bedside table. Mary is concerned and explains to the staff that John cannot feed himself and needs help with his tablets. Louise, the staff nurse, appears to Mary to be in a rush and very disinterested in the situation, and more or less tells her to see to him herself. Upset yet not feeling that she can do anything Mary proceeds to do just this, ensuring that John has some food and his tablets. Mary visits again the next day to find that not only has the same thing happened with John's tablets, but also that he has been incontinent and his skin is very sore. She makes a formal complaint.

Activity 9.7

What do you think the issues are regarding the accountability of the nursing team in the case study above?

Professional issues – the individual practitioners

Simon – he was very careful in the quality of the admissions process and demonstrated good practice through checking out with Mary that the information was correct. It appears, however, that the quality of follow up information exchange could have been better. Either Simon failed to hand over the information to the remainder of the team, and specifically to the next nurse to provide care and support to John, or the nurse to whom he gave that information either misunderstood the data presented to her or chose to ignore it. In order to ensure his accountability, therefore, Simon should have not only communicated John's needs and wants to the appropriate staff, but also ensured accurate interpretation of the information. Simon cannot be held responsible for someone choosing to ignore information he has given, assuming he knew the information was correctly understood. However, Simon is accountable for ensuring the person he hands responsibility for care to is competent to undertake the appropriate roles and functions. In addition, Simon is responsible for ensuring that the medical and nursing staff were aware of the eating, drinking and medication problems. Simon demonstrated good practice in his own accountability of the admissions process, but appears not to have succeeded in following that through to handing over care.

Louise – demonstrates good practice by explaining to John's sister why there is an intravenous infusion, but became defensive and rude when Mary challenged her about the food and tablets. This resulted in a serious relationship problem that adversely affected both John's and Mary's experience. On a personal level, Louise must be accountable for her attitude, which does become a professional issue as it effects both John and Mary, and the quality of care delivered. In this context, Louise has some real issues to deal with in relation to the way that she views the role of family carers.

Medical practitioner – assessed John's immediate priorities but failed to take account of long standing underlying healthcare needs. This practitioner is accountable for the failure to help John to have his medical needs met.

Professional issues – systems, management and leadership issues

In addition to the professional issues identified above it is important to consider the organisational accountability within this case study. Analysis of

the information highlights a number of crucial areas for any organisation. These include:

- Shared values and approaches to working with people who use the service and their families across the team.
- Staff confidence and understanding of people who have special needs.
- Adequacy of the admissions process with respect to people who have complex care needs.
- Effectiveness of the hand over process.
- Care management processes and their effectiveness.
- Clinical supervision of all staff – could Simon's poor communication and Louise's negative approach have been prevented through supervision?
- Responsibility for ensuring that people on the ward are competent to carry out the tasks required in their job, for example, basic feeding, drinking and hygiene.
- Supervision and accountability for those staff carrying out the designated tasks that constitute care delivery.
- Organisational accountability for staff working within their own competence and ensuring help is sought when appropriate, for example, ensuring that they use all available help when caring for John and others like him, such as the community team for people who have a learning disability.
- Support for John's family network.
- Involving John in decisions about his care.
- Ensuring effective interagency working.

Exploring these areas will inevitably lead to further questions and, subsequently, to staff development and training needs. These may fall into a category of job competence or may be in the area of values and attitudes. The latter are not as easy to address through education and training, and will require effective analysis and reflection both by individuals and also by the organisation. For this to occur, it is important that the clinical governance agenda, often perceived as only relevant to individuals and their immediate team, is developed to an organisational level. This demands that some key structural questions are explored and resolved. These include a focus upon resources and management, and an organisational culture, particularly in relation to developing inclusive and equitable health care.

CONTINUING PROFESSIONAL DEVELOPMENT AND LIFELONG LEARNING – A VEHICLE FOR DEVELOPING ACCOUNTABLE SERVICES

Currently, there is a great emphasis on the use of continuing professional development and lifelong learning as a tool for the development of competence in the workforce. There have never been as many opportunities for professional development, however, there are still difficulties in resourcing such opportunities with the subsequent implications for the accountability of professional practice. Changes in the education commissioning systems means that clinical governance should be recognised as a means of influencing the opportunities that are provided for continuing professional development. Whilst many service providers criticise the formal education offered within higher education, clinical governance and the development of new partnerships means that managers can more clearly articulate the educational needs and expectations of their organisation. In order to meet these needs education providers need to be more flexible and responsive.

Activity 9.8

What are your continuing professional development needs? How do these fit with the needs of your colleagues? How do you inform key players in your organisation of your development needs? How are these communicated to key strategic organisations such as Workforce Development Confederations and Learning and Skills Councils?

Again the responsibility for professional development and lifelong learning is collective. There is accountability on behalf of the individual practitioner and, as a part of the professional role, there is an expectation that practitioners keep up to date. There is also an organisational and managerial element, which involves developing a system of personal review and personal development plans, along with a realistic and achievable programme of professional development through a range of mechanisms. These should then be used to inform training needs analysis, service development plans and a whole range of other structures and systems particular to individual organisations.

LEADERSHIP AND MANAGEMENT

Current health- and social-care organisations are undergoing a drive to develop and to provide leadership that enhances practice. The concept of leadership is well explored in the nationally sponsored Leading in Empowered Organisations (LEO) programme. One of the models presented discusses the concept of leadership as involving facets of drive and vision, as well as skill, knowledge and competence (University of Leeds 2001). Accountability has clear links with leadership and the underpinning framework for the programme is based on authority, accountability and empowerment. As such, every professional needs to be aware of their own leadership role within practice.

CONCLUSION

At the start of this chapter, accountability was presented as a complex and potentially problematic issue. Through the development of the discussion, different dimensions of accountability have been presented. To enhance the accountability process, new systems and political drivers have emerged. Not least the changes to the regulatory bodies means that there are some significant issues with regard to the system of professional self-regulation requiring the attention of both professionals and organisations. Health- and social-care are complex systems; frameworks such as clinical governance can be harnessed to meet the need of the practitioners, users of services, their families and other partners in the development and sustainability of practice built on accountability. The modernisation agenda provides a platform for practitioners to work in new and interesting ways. However, with this comes the one thing that accountability is designed to minimise: risk. Without these drivers the risk would be that the service would never develop and complacency would dominate service delivery.

Consequently, the challenge for today's practitioner is to find ways to capture the ethos of these emerging structures and to use them to enhance the quality of the service that is provided. The structures inherent in clinical governance and best value can make this a reality. This is, however, dependent upon the appropriate structures and systems being put in place to support individual practitioners such as supervision and review systems, which allow professionals to develop the skills underpinning clinical governance and best value.

REFERENCES

Audit Commission 2000 Annual report 1999. HMSO, London.

Bristol Royal Infirmary 2001 The inquiry into the management of the care of children receiving complex heart surgery at the Bristol Royal Infirmary 1984–1995. Chair: Professor Ian Kennedy. HMSO, London.

Clothier C 1994 The Allitt Inquiry: independent inquiry relating to deaths and injuries on the children's ward at Grantham and Kesteven General Hospital. HMSO, London.

Davies C 2000 The demise of professional self-regulation – a moment to mourn. In: Lewis G, Gerwitz S, Clarke J (eds) Rethinking social policy. Sage, London.

Department of Health and Social Security 1972 Report of the Committee on Nursing. Cmnd 5115, Briggs Report. HMSO, London.

Department of Health 1983 Mental Health Act. HMSO, London.

Department of Health 1993 NHS and Community Care Act. HMSO, London.

Department of Health 1997 The new NHS: modern, dependable. HMSO, London.

Department of Health 1998a Modernising social services. HMSO, London.

Department of Health 1998b A first class service – quality in the new NHS. HMSO, London.

Department of Health 1999a National service frameworks – modern standards and modern services: mental health. HMSO, London.

Department of Health 1999b The National Health Service Act. HMSO, London.

Department of Health 1999c Making a difference – strengthening the nursing, midwifery and health visiting contribution to health care. HMSO, London.

Department of Health 2000a NHS plan. HMSO, London.

Department of Health 2000b A health service for all the talents – consultation document on the review of workforce planning. HMSO, London.

Department of Health 2001a The National Health Service Reform and Health Professions Bill. HMSO, London.

Department of Health 2001b National service frameworks – modern standards and modern services: older people. HMSO, London.

Department of Health 2001c National service framework for coronary heart disease. HMSO, London.

Department of Health 2001d Shifting the balance of power. HMSO, London.

Department of Health 2001e The essence of care – patient focussed benchmarking for health care practitioners. HMSO, London.

Department of Health 2002 National Health Service Reform and Health Care Professions Act. HMSO, London.

Dimond B 1995 Legal aspects of nursing. Prentice Hall, Hemel Hempstead.

General Medical Council 1999 The duties of a doctor registered with the General Medical Council. GMC, London.

Hallett C 2002 Nursing Times monograph – Accountability. EMAP Publications, Hemel Hempstead.

Ham C 2001 Health policy in Britain, 4th edn. Macmillan, Basingstoke.

Health Service Journal 15th November 2001, editorial comment. EMAP Publications, London.

Home Office 1974 Health and Safety at Work Act (HASAWA). HMSO, London.

Moloney Margaret M 1986 Professionalization of nursing current issues and trends. Lippincott, Philadelphia.

NHS Confederation 1997 Towards the 21st century – a way forward for the NHS. HMSO, London.

Office of the Deputy Prime Minister 2001 Local strategic partnerships – government guidance. HMSO, London.

Seedhouse D 1995 An ethical perspective – how to do the right thing. In: Tingle J, Cribb A (eds) Nursing law and ethics. Blackwell Science, Oxford.

Stacey M 1995 Medical accountability in whistle blowing in the health service. In: Hunt G (ed.) Accountability, law and professional practice. Edward Arnold, London.

Tingle J, Cribb A 2002 Nursing law and ethics. Blackwell Science, Oxford.

Tschudin V 1992 Ethics in nursing – the caring relationship. Butterworth-Heinemann, Oxford.

University of Leeds 2001 LEO Programme. University of Leeds Press, Leeds.

United Kingdom Central Council for Nursing, Midwifery and Health Visiting 1999 Making the connection: professional self-regulation and clinical governance register. UKCC, London.

United Kingdom Central Council for Nursing, Midwifery and Health Visiting 1992 Code of professional conduct. UKCC, London.

Walsh M 2000 Nursing frontiers. Accountability and the boundaries of care. Butterworth-Heinemann, Oxford.

Young Ann P 1994 Law and professional conduct in nursing, 2nd edn. Scutari Press, London.

USEFUL RESOURCES

The following is a selection of useful reading and reference points for information:

The Department of Health as a search engine on the website, this can be found at opengov.doh/search*** – this allows links through key words to all parts of the website and can be used to link to other organisations.

Professional Self Regulation and Clinical Governance – UKCC Information Pack (October 1999) – the aim of the pack is to illustrate the many aspects of self-regulation that impinge on clinical governance. Available from UKCC, 23 Portland Place, London W1N 4TJ. Tel: +44 (0) 121 6377181

Exploring New Roles in Practice (ENRiP) implications of development within the clinical team 1999 ScHARR University of Sheffield, SPS, Bristol and the Kings fund London. A research project exploring how practitioners in nursing and other healthcare professionals can develop advanced practice roles. Alongside this is the Mike Walsh 2000 publication Nursing Frontiers – Accountability and the boundaries of care.

The Essence of Care, Department of Health 2001. This is the information pack for the clinical benchmarking project; it contains the eight fundamental activities and their standard, offers advice on the development of practice through benchmarking and contains a presentation and information guide.

10

Risk, clinical governance and best value: restoring confidence in health and social care

Andy Alaszewski

KEY

♦ Disasters – indicate underlying systemic
  failures in health and social care,
  especially failures of foresight,
  communication and risk management

♦ High trust organisations – should
  effectively manage risk to minimise
  harm and maximise user and public
  confidence

♦ Key definition of risk – importance of
  open, broad and inclusive definition as
  opposed to narrow hazard and
  exclusive expert approach

♦ Inside the black box of decision making –
  trust can only be enhanced if users and
  the public are convinced of the sincerity
  of decision makers.

INTRODUCTION

The current drive to modernise public services
including health and social care is intended to
restore public confidence and create 'high-trust'
organisations (Department of Health 2000). The
government wants to restore the trust in these
services and those professionals who deliver them

and reverse the recent decline in public confidence in services such as the NHS. A situation which it believes was eroded during the 1980s and 1990s. Central to this modernisation strategy are improvements in the quality of decisions with improved reporting of 'warnings' or critical incidents and the overall reduction of risks (Secker-Walker 1999, p. 77). The government intention was to improve the quality of decision making, reduce risk and increase public confidence through clinical governance and best value combined with improved professional self-regulation:

> *Clinical governance will be the process by which each part of the NHS quality-assures its clinical decisions ... Professional self-regulation provides clinicians with the opportunity to help set standards.* People need to be confident *that the regulatory bodies will exercise rigorous self-regulation over the standard and conduct of health professionals and will act promptly and openly when things go wrong (NHS Executive 1999, pp. 2–3, [emphasis added]).*

Risk is also seen to be 'at the very heart of the social services department' (Williams 1998, p. 23). Risk has been a feature of the NHS and social services departments since their formation; uncertainty about the outcome of professional decisions is not a recent phenomenon. However, in the early stages of the development of the health and social services there were defensive mechanisms that masked the importance of risk. For example, clinical autonomy and crown immunity protected the NHS and meant that the nature of risk, and the ways in which it was managed, was not seen as a government concern. The first part of this chapter will consider the various disasters which underpin the development of the current government's concern with risk. This chapter will then consider government responses to these disasters and the risk-management strategy proposed in order to prevent them. In the third part

consideration is given to the limitations of the proposed approach, and in the final section ways are identified in which the current approach can be strengthened and developed.

DISASTERS AND THE USE OF RISK TO ALLOCATE BLAME

As Douglas (1990) notes, the meaning and function of risk has changed over time. In the 17th century risk was associated with chance and probability; the study of probability and statistics developed out of an interest in gambling. Increasingly, risk is associated with negative consequences and harm, and risk is a way of identifying sources of harm either prospectively to reduce harm or retrospectively to allocate blame. Risk is used 'forensically' to identify and counteract the dangers that threaten individual and collective safety. An important part of this process is the investigation of disasters when safety measures have failed to protect individuals and groups from unacceptable levels of harm.

In many industries, such as the railways, where dealing with hazardous situations is a regular occurrence, there have been man-made disasters (Turner & Pidgeon 1997). These often result in a cycle of disaster, inquiry and new safety measures. A similar pattern is evident in health- and social-care services, though the changing nature of disasters has influenced changing responses.

The first major disasters in welfare services occurred in the late 1960s and early 1970s, and mainly involved the failure of the health- and social-care agencies to protect vulnerable individuals. In this context, there were examples where these agencies failed to protect children from being harmed, as well as failing other vulnerable groups, such as older people and people who have learning disabilities. However, these failures were not primarily seen in terms of the professionals and risk management, but more in terms of organisational or managerial failures. The following quote reinforces this issue:

> *The reports demonstrate that problems can arise where there is lack of clarity about the different contributions of the various agencies and individuals involved ... there are problems of overlap where particular functions are held in common by more than one agency ... when many people have duties in relation to one family, for responsibility to become blurred and decisions avoided and for vital information to be lost sight of or overlooked (DHSS 1982, pp. 5 & 17).*

The linkage between risk as a hazard is also evident in the ways in which risk management evolved in the NHS in the late 1980s and early 1990s. In 1984 there was a major health and safety issue at Stanley Royd Hospital in which more than 450 patients and staff were infected by salmonella bacteria and 19 patients died. The committee of inquiry, which reported in 1986, found that NHS management was complacent and had failed to put measures into place to effectively manage such hazards and to prevent a repetition of this situation. As a result of the inquiry the government removed one of the measures which had protected the NHS: it removed crown immunity in relation to breaches of environmental health (Edwards 1993, pp. 108–109). As the 1993 NHS Management Executive guidance on risk management acknowledges, this was a major stimulus for the development of explicit risk-management strategies (NHS Management Executive 1993). A further stimulus came in 1996 when the NHS Litigation Authority was created. Trusts that wanted to gain the protection of the authority's clinical negligence scheme needed to assure the authority that they met its risk-management standard (Ferguson 1999, p. 110).

In the 1990s the emphasis shifted from the vulnerability of individuals to their dangerousness. This included increased concerns about dangerous patients, such as individuals with enduring mental health needs who harm themselves and others, for example Christopher Clunis who killed Jonathan Zito in an underground station. It also included health professionals who harmed the very people they were meant to protect from harm, for example Beverley Allitt, Harold Shipman and the surgeons at Bristol Royal Infirmary.

Increasingly, these issues were seen in terms of risk and the relevant inquiries all recommended improved systems of risk assessment and management. For example, the Committee which inquired into the care and treatment of Christopher Clunis recommended that:

> *[All violent mental health patients should have] an assessment ... as to whether the patient's propensity for violence presents any risk to his own health or safety or to the protection of the public (Report of the Inquiry 1994).*

While the disasters in the late 1960s and early 1970s affected mainly vulnerable individuals being cared for within the low tech sectors of health- and social-care services, the welfare disasters in the 1980s and 1990s increasingly affected patients/ clients being treated in the high-tech environment of the acute hospitals.

For example there were disasters in cervical screening, breast screening, histopathological diagnosis and gynaecology (Lugon & Secker-Walker 1999, p. 1). The defining event in this series took place at Bristol Royal Infirmary. In this situation 35 babies were killed by the acts of cardiac surgeons; whilst this indicated incompetence on the part of professionals, it also suggested a systemic failure in the organisation. Whilst the report looking at the deaths in Bristol indicated that some parts of the service were either adequate or more than adequate, this did not alter the fact that a small number of professionals in the hospitals were aware of the harm being caused. It would appear that some nurses referred to the operating theatre as the 'killing fields'.

During this period one anaesthetist tried to alert the senior management in the trust and wider NHS to the harm being caused. Despite this, operations continued and parents were unaware of the unacceptable risks to which they were exposing their children.

The problems at Bristol Royal Infirmary are seen as a watershed by many, including journalists. For example, the editor of the BMJ writing on the consequences of Bristol, entitled his commentary 'All changed, changed utterly' (Smith 1998). The final report of the Bristol inquiry identified a culture of dangerousness and poor risk management at the hospital that had persisted despite some individuals voicing their concerns:

> *The story of the paediatric cardiac surgical service in Bristol is ... an account of people who cared greatly about human suffering, and were dedicated and well-motivated. Sadly, some lacked insight and their behaviour was flawed. Many failed to communicate with each other, and to work together effectively for the interests of their patients. There was a lack of leadership, and of teamwork ... It is an account of a hospital where there was a 'club culture'; an imbalance of power, with too much control in the hands of a few individuals (Learning from Bristol 2001).*

It is clear that following this situation the government and the public no longer trusted the medical profession to provide a uniform standard of care. Variations in the standard of care were now considered to be 'totally unacceptable' (Homa 2000, p. 2). Professional autonomy, the control of decision making and management of risk which had so conspicuously failed at Bristol, was to be replaced by clinical governance, the external inspection of decision making and management of risk, the aim being to 'restore the trust that society and patients historically had in medicine' (Lugon & Secker-Walker 1999, p. 1).

CLINICAL GOVERNANCE AND BEST VALUE: CONTROL, REGULATION AND RISK AVOIDANCE

While it is clear that clinical governance and best value are concerned with the quality of decisions and the effectiveness of risk management, the precise relationship is not clearly defined. There are different ways of assuring decisions and managing risks. Indeed, Hood and colleagues, in discussing risk management, have identified at least seven different areas in which agencies can make strategic choices about the ways in which they manage risk (Hood et al. 1992, Alaszewski et al. 1998, pp. 46–53). Thus, it is important to explore how risk is being defined and the type of choices that are being made. This will enable us to examine the extent to which clinical governance and best value are likely to succeed in their main aim, restoring public trust in the health- and social-care services.

Like many key concepts in health and social care, it is possible to define risk in different ways. As Douglas (1990) makes clear, originally risk was associated with chance or probability, but increasingly risk is being seen in terms of danger or hazard. Alaszewski et al. (2000) found competing approaches to risk in health and social care. The dominant approach was risk as a danger or hazard and, therefore, creating a negative phenomenon that needs to be identified and avoided or negated. One can refer to this as the default or common-sense approach in that it is both the generally accepted lay approach and, therefore, the one that is likely to be used unless an alternative is explicitly identified and justified.

However, we were able to identify other approaches that were less dominant. The most radical of these alternatives emphasised the positive aspects of risk, particularly the benefits of risk taking. Professionals who used this approach argued that risk taking is a part of everyday life that is important for personal learning and development. They felt that vulnerable people, such as people with learning disabilities, should have the right to experience the risks of everyday life, and that concerns with safety were used to justify depriving these people of such opportunities. An alternative and intermediate approach recognised both hazards and opportunities, and saw risk in terms of balance between these two dimensions.

Activity 10.1

Which of the two definitions of risk outlined above underpins your own and your organisation's approach to managing risk?

Since there is little explicit discussion of this in the various policy statements associated with clinical governance and best value, it appears that the common sense, risk as a hazard approach, underpins the current modernisation agenda. For example in the white paper, *The New NHS: Modern, Dependable* (Department of Health 1997), clinical governance and best value is seen as underpinning a 'quality organisation' and it is clear that the defining characteristics of such an organisation is the minimisation of harm. For example, a quality organisation will ensure that:

- risk reduction programmes of a high standard are in place
- adverse events are detected, and openly investigated, and the lessons learned are promptly applied
- lessons for practice are systematically learned from complaints made by patients/clients
- problems of poor performance are recognised at an early stage and dealt with to prevent harm to patients/clients (Department of Health 1997, p. 47)

Given this approach to risk, it is hardly surprising that the strategy underpinning clinical governance and best value is one of risk avoidance in

which regulation and control are prominent features. As Klein notes, the reforms are 'intended to make the NHS more quality conscious by means of more central direction and control' (1998, p. S52). The system that has been established has many of the features of classic bureaucracies in which rules and regulations are used to minimise uncertainty and avoid risks to the organisations (Alaszewski et al. 1998, pp. 46–48).

Activity 10.2

What systems and structures have the government and your organisation put in place to manage risk?

The NHS variant is based on a number of linked elements. At the centre of the system is the National Institute for Clinical Excellence and National Service Frameworks. The role of the institute is to collect evidence identifying best clinical practice, which can then be used as the basis for guidance and for National Service Frameworks that provide a structure for clinical practice and decision making. At a service level, it is the responsibility of the Chief Executive and professionals to ensure that clinical guidelines are implemented and used as the framework for clinical decisions. The main source of evidence for compliance is the outcome of clinical practice. *The New NHS: Modern, Dependable* (Department of Health 1997) sees outcomes as the key to establishing public confidence and places it at the centre of the NHS relationship with users. In *The New NHS* the government made a commitment to produce a new NHS charter that would 'place greater emphasis on the outcomes of treatment and care…focus on things that really matter' (Department of Health 1997, p. 66). These outcome measures will be used to identify potentially dangerous practitioners. It is suggested that these will be rapidly identified from the data collected around the outcome measures established for different areas of practice, and action will be taken when necessary to minimise harm.

The final component of the system is the Commission for Health Improvement. This organisation is responsible for checking the performance of individual trusts and services against established outcomes, to ensure that they all meet national standards. It also identifies trusts in which performance is unacceptable and in such circumstances recommends remedial action to the secretary of state. This may include removing trust chairs and executive and non-executive directors where there is evidence of systematic failure (Department of Health 1997). The public is informed of the performance of local services through the traffic lights system:

All NHS organisations ... will for the first time annually and publicly be classified as 'green', 'yellow' and 'red' (Department of Health 2000).

The implication of this coding system is clear. The public can have full confidence in green-coded services. Amber-coded services are not completely satisfactory and need to be treated with caution, while red-coded services are potentially dangerous and need remedial action. This system will be linked to the commission's inspections. Organisations with green coding will be given a degree of autonomy while:

Organisations rated as 'red' under the Government's system of 'earned autonomy' will be subject to more frequent, two-yearly Commission for Health Improvement inspection (Department of Health 2000).

When the Department of Health published the first league table of hospital trusts in 2001 it used a star system rather than traffic lights. Given the investment that is taking place in the development of this system, I will examine in the next section whether it is likely to achieve the stated objective of increasing public confidence in health- and social-care services.

WILL THE MODERNISATION AGENDA INCREASE USER, CARER AND PUBLIC CONFIDENCE IN SERVICES?

There are a number of ways of considering the likely impact of the modernisation agenda. It is possible to assess whether clinical governance is likely to be effective and, therefore, change the way in which practice based decisions are made. Should this be the outcome then public confidence in the welfare service should improve. However, should clinical governance and best value not achieve the desired effect, then alternative approaches may need to be introduced.

Activity 10.3

Look at the ways in which clinical governance and best value are being addressed in your organisation. How much is this affecting decisions made in practice and how much more are patients/clients and carers involved in this process?

The impact of clinical governance and best value will depend on how effective it is in regulating and controlling the decision making of practitioners. Accumulated evidence on bureaucratic mechanisms for controlling behaviour is not very encouraging about the likelihood of success. These mechanisms are based on formal structures and controls in which front-line workers are treated as passive implementers of procedures and processes.

This approach disregards the ability of this group of staff to resist formal control and scrutiny through informal networks. The importance of these informal relationships were first recognised by psychologists examining the effects of the working environment on productivity. They noted a paradox now known as the Hawthorne Effect. Both positive and negative changes to the working environment increased productivity. This effect drew their attention to the key role of informal groups and their leaders (Roethlisberger & Dickson 1939). As McKinlay (1975) has pointed out:

> *It appears, from considerable field research, that in reality formal organizations are influenced (perhaps even controlled) from the bottom, as well as, or instead of, from the top (p. 349).*

This observation is particularly pertinent to risk management. In the mid 1990s Alaszewski et al. (1998) undertook a study of the ways in which nurses and social workers managed the risks associated with providing support for vulnerable adults in the community. They found that practitioners had little awareness of organisational policies and only cited these when they felt that such policies could be used to justify the decisions they wanted to make. The main justification of their decisions were the interests and needs of individual patients/clients. It was noted that:

> *Respondents presented themselves as operating with an altruistic and professional orientation to risk management which left little room for defensive, self-interested decision making ... Front-line workers (88 per cent) cited the service user either alone or in combination with other parties as the subject of concern in the overwhelming majority of decisions (Alaszewski et al. 1998, p. 80).*

Clinical governance and best value may make front-line workers more aware of agency risk policies, but it seems unlikely that it will shift their prime orientation especially if clinical governance and best value are seen in organisational terms, e.g. protecting agencies from litigation. It is also not clear that such a shift would be desirable. As with many aspects of risk the relationship between harm reduction and increased confidence is not as straightforward as it first appears. If expert measurement of risk in terms of harm is the same as public or lay perceptions of risk, then harm reduction should increase confidence. However, there is evidence that expert assessment and lay perceptions are very different.

Calman et al. (1999) used psychological research to identify a range of 'fright factors' that heighten public sensitivity to risk. These include whether the risks are a product of new and unfamiliar technology, and if there is a lack of information or conflicting information about the risk. Psychological research which compares objective assessment of risk with subjective perceptions indicates that, generally, individuals tend to overestimate the probability of high-consequence/low-probability events, (e.g. lightning striking) and underesti-mate the probability of low-consequence/high-probability events, (e.g. the common cold) (Pidgeon et al. 1992).

In modern society there is often an inverse relationship between objective and subjective assessments of risk. This inversion can be seen in 'the fear of flying'. According to objective assessments of risk, flying in a scheduled airline is a relatively safe form of transport, yet it is perceived to be more dangerous and provokes more anxiety than other forms of travel. This inverse relationship is also evident in food panics when there appears to be an exaggerated response to what are often low probability risks (Reilly 1999). This apparent inversion underpins what Taylor-Gooby (2000) has called the paradox of timid prosperity in which increased security is associated with increased anxiety:

> *Material levels of security in the western world are higher than ever before ... However, the sources of uncertainty and the mechanisms available to most people to deal with them have changed, leading to the paradox of timid prosperity – growing uncertainty amid rising affluence (Taylor-Gooby 2000, p. 3).*

The problem associated with this paradox is that those measures which objectively increase security, may not be reflected in an individual's own sense of security, particularly if they are achieved through mechanisms which the public do not understand or feel that they own. With regard to clinical governance and best value, one of the government's key strategies to increase public confidence in welfare services, there is little evidence that the public understands or feels ownership of this agenda. Thus, it seems unlikely that clinical governance and best value in its current form will markedly increase public trust and confidence. If this is the case, it is important to consider how trust can be increased and the next section explores this issue.

IMPROVING TRUST IN HEALTH AND SOCIAL CARE SERVICES: COMMUNICATION AND BEYOND

Trust and risk are linked concepts. Risk deals with uncertainty and is often associated with negative outcomes, whereas trust is a process by which an individual can manage uncertainty and the associated anxieties. It is a 'protective cocoon' that filters out the 'potential dangers impinging from the external world' (Giddens 1991, p. 244). In traditional societies this protective cocoon was provided by religion and magic. In modern society it is provided through impersonal expert-based systems such as the NHS and personal social services (Lupton 1999, pp. 2–4).

In the United Kingdom the high point in the development of expert systems for dealing with risk came in the late 1940s and early 1950s with the development of the welfare state, which included profession based health and welfare systems to protect citizens from such threats as disease and poverty. Both governments and the public appeared to place unconditional trust in the professions. For example, *The NHS Plan* argues that in 1948 there was unconditional trust as 'deference and hierarchy defined the relationship between citizens and services' (Department of Health 2000, p. 6).

It is clear that the government no longer has 'unconditional trust' in professionals and the services they provide. For example, the government notes that the NHS 'falls short of the standards patients expect' (Department of Health 2000, p. 2). While in its review of social services, the government noted the failure of social services to protect vulnerable individuals and stated that:

> The government will act to protect vulnerable people who are put at risk by poor services, and it will ensure that it has the statutory powers at its disposal to do this (Department of Health 1998).

It is, however, important to note that government's distrust is not necessarily shared by the public and users of these services. For example, the Department of Health undertook a consultation exercise as part of the process of developing *The NHS Plan*. The results of this exercise are included in an annex to the plan entitled 'The public's concern about the NHS today'. This may indicate an overall interpretation of the evidence, however, while the public may be critical of some parts of the service, the criticism does not appear to extend to distrust of the professionals providing it. This is evidenced in the following summary:

> People trust, value and admire the dedication, expertise and compassion of staff who work day-in and day-out for patients. Ninety per cent of the public are satisfied with the way doctors do their jobs, 96% are satisfied with the way nurses do their jobs. They are the most trusted professions in the country (Department of Health 2000, p. 136).

However, in view of the stated government objective of increasing confidence in health- and social-care services, it is necessary to consider how trust in these services and the professionals that provide them can be maintained and enhanced.

Activity 10.4

What do you and your organisation do to foster trust between yourselves and the people who use the service? What could you do to improve this situation?

The starting point for this must be trust and the factors that enhance or diminish this; however, trust is an elusive concept (Alaszewski et al. 2000). It is about relationships and, particularly, the confidence that one party can accept information, advice or statements without the need for checking and additional questioning or obtaining additional evidence. Giddens has defined it as:

The vesting of confidence in persons or in abstract systems, made on the basis of a 'leap into faith' which brackets ignorance or lack of information (Giddens 1991, p. 244).

If this is the case then a strategy, such as clinical governance and best value, which depends on collecting more information to question or check decisions will not increase trust. For example information was not the problem at Bristol Infirmary, as they were 'awash with data' from the late 1980s (Dyer 2001). Trust is embedded in relationships especially in the communications between professionals and the users of their services. For example, a more detailed analysis of situations such as the Bristol Royal Infirmary indicates that, while parents were upset about the outcomes, they felt their trust was betrayed by the concealment of information. For example, Michael Parsons, whose daughter Mia died following cardiac surgery at Bristol Royal Infirmary, has said that:

Had we known of the real statistics we would never have accepted the referral … When I signed the consent form I believed I was doing the best thing for Mia. However, in retrospect I know that I did not. I maintain that my consent was obtained by giving me false information. This is in my view criminal (cited in Boseley 1999).

The inquiry report highlighted the importance of effective communication in the development of trust and the failures which underpin events in Bristol:

We were left in no doubt that one of the principal lessons from Bristol is that parents wish to be treated with respect. They want their particular knowledge of their child to be valued, and they wish to be included in the process of caring for their child. Parents are entitled to nothing less, and good practice now reflects this. Our experience of receiving the evidence of parents, 238 of whom gave formal written statements to the inquiry, is that they do not, for the most part, expect healthcare professionals to have all the answers. What they do expect is that their concerns as parents will be addressed. As Jean Simons, Head of Bereavement Services, Great Ormond Street Hospital for Children, points out, parents become angry or frustrated when a healthcare professional unilaterally decides which topics are 'too difficult' for them to deal with. Making such assumptions, or avoiding certain issues altogether, are not good practice. Healthcare professionals caring for children should be trained in the particular skills necessary to communicate with parents. There needs to be a willingness on the part of the healthcare professional to be more open with parents about difficult issues, and to assess to what degree the parents want to discuss them (Public inquiry 2001).

The importance of communication in the development of trust and the effective management of risk has been acknowledged by Calman and colleagues in the following way:

Communication with cancer patients represents a paradigm case, both in the disease's exceptionally high 'dread factor' and in the need to weigh up the risks of different treatments or none. It is a poignant footnote to the founding of the NHS that Nye Bevan should have died of cancer without ever having been told of the diagnosis. From a situation in which this was normal practice, there has been a swing toward honest and careful discussion about the disease and its treatment … This is not something that can be dictated in detail from the centre.

Nevertheless it can and is being encouraged. In the specific case of breast cancer, the need for good communication with patients features strongly in the guidance offered to purchasers of services (Calman et al. 1999, p. 109).

While communication is important, it is not considered appropriate for the Department of Health to directly investigate or interfere with this. As a result it would appear to this author, that there is a 'black box' at the centre of clinical governance. While the department is willing to investigate the outcomes of the decision-making process it is not willing to look inside the box and directly examine the decision-making process and the relationship between users and professionals in making decisions. This avoidance can only be justified if there is strong evidence that users are closely involved in and participate in decision making. However, currently there is little evidence to support this.

Hallowell (1999) studied communication in an area in which professionals are sensitive to the importance of effective communication about risk, that is, counselling women about hereditary breast/ovarian cancer. She notes that the stated aims of such counselling are to provide 'information about individuals' genetic risks, and the available risk management options and the costs and benefits of genetic testing in both a neutral and non-directive manner' (p. 267). However, she found the communication was not neutral and information was provided in a way that shaped women's decisions:

Genetic counselling for these types of cancer is not neutral, but can be seen to be overtly and covertly prescriptive. The analysis of genetic consultations indicates that the clinicians suggest that the risk of cancer is manageable, and that individuals have a responsibility to act to manage their risks in particular ways. It is observed that the selective presentation

of the different risk management options potentially limits the risk management choices that are available to at-risk women (Hallowell 1999, p. 267).

Other studies of communication also indicate that there are serious deficiencies. Mohanna and Chambers conducted a study of the ways in which 15 General Practitioners (GPs) communicated about risk. They found there were four distinctive approaches to communication, and while GPs could and would use more than one, they tended to develop their own distinctive approach. Most of the GPs had their favourite way of describing a specific risk, and when it formed part of a consultation they used a standardised routine or pattern. A second common approach was to present information in such a way as to steer the patient towards the 'right' decision. Some GPs interpreted risk for patients. They made an assumption about what and how a patient understood risk and tried to explain it using what they felt was the patient's language, for example, avoiding technical numerical formulations and using descriptions. The fourth and final approach was to avoid a discussion and refer the patient on to a specialist who can provide information. While there is pressure for more openness and provision of information for patients, it is difficult to see any of these approaches meeting the criteria of full open communication, and, therefore, providing the basis of informed decision making by patients. There is a strong element of paternalism. For example, one General Practitioner who is described as an interpreter of risk provides the following account of communication:

I have already read the evidence, done the thinking and can give them a potted version of it. Patients don't want details and sometimes it's hard to get them involved in the discussion. They are quite willing to do what the doctor thinks is best (Mohanna & Chambers 2001, p. 23).

If the government is serious about increasing public confidence in health and social services, then it cannot concentrate solely on evaluating decisions in terms of the outcomes. It needs to consider the process as well as the outcome. In order to successfully achieve this, it will be necessary to consider the process underpinning decision making, not just the outcomes. In exploring the process, it is also necessary to ensure that effective communication is taking place and that people who use the services and the public are full participants that are genuinely engaged in the decision-making process.

CONCLUSION: MANAGING RISK AND INCREASING SECURITY

Traditionally, risk management was left in the hands of health and social services professionals. The government, people using the services and the public were happy to rely on professional

altruism as a safeguard to the decision-making process.

The high profile events of the 1990s have changed this. The government is no longer willing to accept professional reassurance without hard evidence of 'safe' outcomes. As such, clinical governance and best value is the cornerstone of a new regulatory process. However, as discussed in this chapter, it is not clear that clinical governance and best value will enhance trust without a better understanding of the impact of risk management from the perspective of opportunity and benefits to patients/clients. Subsequently, while it may lead to objective evidence that safety has improved, it is not clear that it will genuinely increase the public's sense of security. To do this, the government needs to support professionals to make their decision-making process more open and transparent to all on the receiving end. Implicit within this is the need for professionals to effectively communicate with the users of their services and the public.

REFERENCES

Alaszewski A, Harrison L, Manthorpe J 1998 Risk, health and welfare. Open University Press, Buckingham.
Alaszewski A, Alaszewski H, Ayer S, Manthorpe J 2000 Managing risk in community practice. Baillière Tindall, Edinburgh.
Boseley S 1999 Father 'given false information' over girl's operation. The Guardian, 18th March 1999, p. 6.
Calman KC, Bennett PG, Coles DG 1999 Risks to health: some key issues in management, regulation and communication. Health, Risk and Society 1: 107–116.
Department of Health 1997 The new NHS: modern, dependable, Cm 3807. The Stationery Office, London.
Department of Health 1998 Modernising social services, Cm 4169. The Stationery Office, London.
Department of Health 2000 The NHS plan, Cm 4818-I. The Stationery Office, London.
Department of Health and Social Security 1982 Child abuse: a study of inquiry reports. HMSO, London.
Douglas M 1990 Risk as a forensic resource. Daedalus, Journal of the American Academy of Arts and Sciences 119: 1–16.
Dyer C 2001 There's no incentive to admit error, only to cover it up. The Guardian, 24th July 2001.

Edwards B 1993 The National Health Service: A manager's tale. The Nuffield Provincial Hospitals Trust, London.
Ferguson A 1999 Legal implications of clinical governance. In: Lugon M, Secker-Walker J (eds) Clinical governance: making it happen. The Royal Society of Medicine Press, London, pp. 107–115.
Giddens A 1991 Modernity and self-identity: self and society in the late modern society. Polity Press, Cambridge.
Hallowell N 1999 Advising on the management of genetic risk: offering choice or prescribing action? Health, Risk and Society 1: 267–280.
Homa D 2000 Commission launch heralds new era for NHS standards, News Release, Commission for Health Improvement, January–September 2000.
Hood CC, Jones D, Pidgeon N et al. 1992 Risk management. In: The Royal Society Study Group (eds) Risk: analysis, perception and management. The Royal Society, London.
Klein R 1998 Can policy drive quality? Quality in Health Care 7: S51–S53.
Learning from Bristol: the report of the public inquiry into children's heart surgery at the Bristol Royal Infirmary 1984–1995. 2001 Command Paper: CM 5207. The Stationery Office, London.

Lugon M, Secker-Walker J 1999 Introduction. In: Lugon M, Secker-Walker J (eds) Clinical governance: making it happen. The Royal Society of Medicine Press, London.

Lupton D 1999 Risk. Routledge, London.

McKinlay JB 1975 Clients and organizations. In: McKinlay JB (ed.) Processing people: cases in organizational behaviour. Holt, Reinhart and Winston, London, pp. 339–378.

Mohanna K, Chambers R 2001 Risk matters in healthcare: communicating, explaining and managing risk. Radcliffe Medical Press, Abingdon, Oxon.

NHS Executive 1999 Clinical governance in the new NHS. Health Service Circular, HSC 2000/065. Department of Health, Leeds.

NHS Management Executive 1993 Risk management in the NHS. Department of Health, Leeds.

Pidgeon N, Hood C, Jones D et al. 1992 Risk perception. In: The Royal Society Study Group (ed.) Risk: analysis, perception and management. The Royal Society, London.

Public Inquiry 2001 Learning from Bristol: the report of the public inquiry into children's heart surgery at the Bristol Royal Infirmary 1984–1995, CM 5207. The Stationery Office, London.

Reilly J 1999 'Just another food scare?' Public understanding and the BSE crisis. In: Philo G (ed.) Message received. Longman, Harlow Essex.

Report of the Inquiry into the Care and Treatment of Christopher Clunis 1994 HMSO, London.

Roethlisberger FJ, Dickson WJ 1939 Management and the worker: an account of a research program conducted by the Western Electric Company. Hawthorne Works, Little, Brown, Chicago, MA.

Secker-Walker J 1999 Clinical risk management. In: Lugon M, Secker-Walker J (eds) Clinical governance: making it happen. The Royal Society of Medicine Press, London, pp. 77–91.

Smith R 1998 All changed, changed utterly. British Medical Journal 316: 1917–1918.

Taylor-Gooby P 2000 Risk and welfare. In: Taylor-Gooby P (ed.) Risk, trust and welfare. Macmillan, London.

Turner BA, Pidgeon NE 1997 Man-made disasters. Butterworth-Heinemann, Oxford.

Williams J 1998 Drawing the boundaries of risk and regulation: perspectives from the public sector. In: Allen I (ed.) Best value, risk and regulation. Policy Studies Institute, London, pp. 23–32.

Structured approaches to care delivery

A key focus for delivering high quality care, particularly in NHS services has been the introduction of structured approaches to care delivery. On the one hand, this includes development such as managed care, an approach that is discussed by Elaine Morris and Brian Foottit and is potentially of greatest interest to those working in the NHS. On the other hand, however, this section discusses Integrated Care Pathways, an approach that can have its greatest successes when developed across agencies, as well as being an approach that is applicable to all groups of people who receive welfare services.

11

Structured care

Elaine Morris
Brian Footitt OBE

KEY ISSUES

◆ Clinical governance and its impact upon service delivery

◆ Managed care in the USA and the UK

◆ Building and implementing care pathways

◆ Care pathways and their relevance to the clinical governance agenda.

INTRODUCTION

This chapter reflects on the clinical governance agenda and provides an overview of the relevant issues for healthcare professionals. It examines some of the different processes currently used in the UK and the USA to structure care and their relevance to clinical governance.

Different methods used to structure care are examined and evaluated in terms of their potential to secure the clinical governance agenda and the aspects they are likely to secure. Practical examples are used to illustrate this discusion and pinpoint criteria likely to influence their success.

CLINICAL GOVERNANCE

In 1998 the government's modernisation agenda was underpinned with the launch of a new document, *A First Class Service – quality in the new NHS* (Department of Health 1998).

Unlike previous government directives, this particular document proved difficult for professionals to ignore as Trusts were charged with the production of annual reports on clinical governance issues. In addition, chief executives were made accountable on behalf of the Trust Board for assuring the quality of the service. Clinical involvement is secured by the requirement that a designated senior clinician should take responsibility for ensuring that systems for clinical governance are in place and their effectiveness monitored. Not only does this establish clear lines of accountability, but the initiative places quality at the heart of the agenda for Trust Boards, and emphasises that quality reports on clinical care should be given the same importance as financial reports in the aims and management of the organisation.

Whilst chief executives have clearly been given the responsibility for the quality of care delivered, this is at an organisational level. In order to monitor standards in relation to quality a number of national organisations and structures have been established. The inter-relationship between some of these organisations is identified in Figure 11.1.

The establishment of the Social Care Institute for Excellence (SCIE), the National Institute for Clinical Excellence (NICE) and the production of National Service Frameworks (NSFs) are the tools by which standards for much of clinical care will be set effectively throughout the country. The Commission for Health Improvement (CHI) and the National Care Standards Commission (NCSC) are the bodies that will monitor the implementation of these standards.

Engaging with the document, *A First Class Service* (Department of Health 1998) is, therefore, a necessity within health care, as is its integration

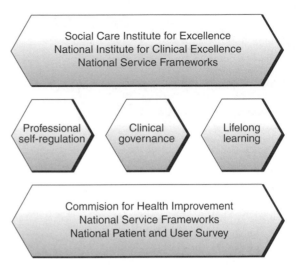

Figure 11.1 Inter-relationship between current policy developments and clinical governance.

within a Trust's strategic activities (as ensured via the chief executive, the designated senior clinician and the annual report). For many professionals reflecting on the developments since 1998 they may question the impact of these changes on clinical care delivery. Conversely, activity at a strategic level appears to be frantic, particularly in relation to establishing structures and processes to integrate financial control, service performance and the targets set in the NSFs, the NHS plan and other documents.

Whether care delivery is driven by the core quality activities of clinical governance, e.g. evidenced-based care, risk management, audit etc, is debatable. To put quality at the heart of the organisation, these processes need to be in place at every level in the management of health and social care, not just those areas covered by policy documents. It is questionable just how far trusts have gone down the quality road. Indeed, delivering a quality service requires not only changes in the way professionals work, but also in the culture and the way they think. The enormity of this task is noted by Scally and Donaldson (1998 pp. 61–65): 'the idea (clinical governance) could inspire and enthuse', but they recognise that the 'challenge for professionals is to turn the concept into reality'.

Activity 11.1

Consider how this agenda will impact upon how you think about the care that you deliver. What does this mean you as an individual need to do differently and what systems, structures and processes will you need in place as a team?

At the core of care delivery will be quality improvement processes, evidenced-based practice, clinical audit and research, and clinical risk management to name but a few, and all this will be supported with quality data with which to review, analyse and improve care. The umbrella for sheltering and containing this activity is the ethos of patient/client-focused, cost-effective care and the need for professionals to work together to develop standards of care which apply throughout the country.

Given the relatively short time-scale since the introduction of clinical governance, it is not surprising then that not all professionals have engaged with this agenda. Given the enormity of the task, what is surprising is that so many good initiatives have been implemented. However, again it is individual professionals in the main and their teams that have been responsible for these developments. For some professionals life goes on as usual and clinical care delivery is a traditional activity, impacted here and there with the slow uptake and implementation of research with proven benefit to patients and clients. This defeats the aims of clinical governance as a proponent to join up quality initiatives to achieve a quality agenda within welfare services.

In this busy working environment professionals have neither the time nor the energy to reinvent the wheel, and the search is on for a framework that can be used to facilitate the transition into the care clinical governance agenda. This approach needs to be compatible with contemporary care delivery, particularly in relation to the involvement of those people who use the services.

The tool that is being promoted as being potentially useful is the concept of managed care which is inherent in the USA healthcare system. One of the structures that is seen as being able to deliver on the promises of managed care is that of care pathways. This approach is becoming increasingly popular in the UK, particularly as a consequence of the demands of the clinical governance agenda.

Activity 11.2

Consider the terms 'managed care' and 'care pathways'. What do these concepts mean to you? Discuss your ideas with your team.

Kongstevedt (1995) defines managed care as a system of care delivery that manages the costs, the quality and the access to welfare services. Care pathways, a tool within managed care, provide a detailed outline of care for a particular episode or disease and communicating this information to patients/clients informs them of what they can expect from their care experience. In a managed care organisation, this level of detail is used to manage resources, including contracting staff, and to monitor cost and quality issues.

Confusion also exists over the many terms used to describe care pathways; these include care maps, integrated care pathways; multidisciplinary pathways of care, anticipated recovery paths, critical care pathways. Then there are a plethora of labels, such as care protocols, care guidelines and clinical algorithms. To differentiate, very simply, those care process that coordinate and structure care, outline it in the patient/client document and use it on a day-to-day basis to record the care given and any variations, are from the care pathways group. The protocols group broadly defines care that is not usually incorporated in the patient, client document and variations are not recorded.

MANAGED CARE IN THE USA

The 1980s saw an escalation in hospital costs in the USA, a growth in the number of new hospitals opening each year and a payment system which reimbursed hospitals on a dollar for dollar basis for the care they provided. There was little incentive to consider cost containment as hospitals were paid for whatever care they delivered, whether that care was deemed necessary or not. The growing number of people without insurance or the means to finance health care became a problem, and in a country where health and welfare provision depends on the ability to pay, insurance is the primary way of accessing care. People without insurance or the means to pay for care can be in a difficult position should they become ill.

As a response to this situation the government in the USA changed the system of reimbursement and launched a payment system around diagnostic-related groups. Hospitals receive a single negotiated fee for each person dependent upon the diagnosis. This single fee is paid no matter how long the person is in hospital and no matter what care they receive. In order to benefit from this system hospitals now needed to manage resources and care in order to make sure that people only receive the tests and care needed within as short a stay as possible. Managed care organisations grew in an effort to control costs and retain a good standard of care. In theory, these organisations offer basic quality care at a reduced cost and, subsequently, opened up cheaper insurance to those members enrolling with them. This resulted in the potential for more people on lower incomes to access care.

The use of managed care in the USA is now well established and organisations are claiming wide-ranging benefits from the process. Initial studies in the USA suggest that it integrates clinical and business objectives by addressing quality issues as well as reducing costs through the efficient use of resources (Hart 1992). However, the initiative is not popular with all healthcare professionals and research on the topic is inconclusive and gives no definitive answer from which to make informed judgements on potential benefits. Robinson and Steiner (1998) give a good account of evidence from their study in their book *Managed Health Care*. What is evident is that managed care hospitals and community services cost less to run, they can deliver to a named standard and offer a less costly alternative to the population of the USA when they are looking to insure for health care.

In addition, industry, the second main purchaser of health care in the USA, is also looking for cheaper alternatives to ever-increasing healthcare costs. They purchase health care for their employees through insurance, and in order to minimise spending, make use of the power of the competitive marketplace, in particular, through encouraging employers to enrol with insurers offering discounted managed care alternatives (Rosenstein 1994).

The concept of managed care in the USA is synonymous with efficient care provision. Costs are potentially more controllable through planning, coordination and the astute management of professional input and treatment for an episode of care (Zander 1988).

Activity 11.3

What do you think the advantages of a managed care system may be?

Activity 11.4

Think about the differences between the healthcare system in the USA and that in the UK. What are the major differences and what do you think the response of the UK public would be to the USA approach?

You may have thought about this question on a number of different levels and from the perspective of a number of different people. For example, some politicians may like the idea of managed care as it has the potential to shift the cost of welfare services from taxation to insurance, making health- and social-care issues less of a political agenda. Professionals may view the issue differently, some believing it would be a good way forward, others feeling it would undermine the basic principles of the welfare system in the UK. Meanwhile the views of the general public will also be varied as some people will focus on the opportunity to reduce taxation, whilst others will respond emotively as this would be seen as the destruction of the welfare system.

CARE PATHWAYS AND MANAGED CARE

Critical pathways were developed as a project management tool in the 1950s to map process flows in order to detect 'bottlenecks' in the production industry and to identify the relationship between processes and whether the achievement of one target affected the achievement of another (Bryant 1987, McCloskey 1994).

Pathways, often called care maps, are widely used in the USA as a managed care tool to inform the hospital about the resources, tests and treatment necessary for a particular episode of care. In the mid west, Washington and California, over 80% of patients are cared for using care maps and, overall, 60% of hospitals in the USA use pathways (McKie et al. 1994).

The pathway process as part of a managed care initiative is described as a method which organises care delivery with the emphasis on communication and coordination among healthcare teams. The process ensures that care is organised and coordinated with written criteria to guide care and a tool to track progress. Patients/clients report feeling less anxious because the process informs them of what to expect each day and the care is seen to be well organised (Mosher et al. 1992). They also report improvements in communications (Rasmussen & Gengler 1994, Stead et al. 1995). The improvements are said to be the result of the multidisciplinary approach to planning care and from professionals understanding their colleagues' input and delivering the same care plan.

The move to develop pathways is seen by some as being influenced by the move to total quality management (TQM) (Lumsdon & Hagland 1993). At first sight, pathways are simply charts showing the key events that typically lead to the successful treatment of people in certain homogenous populations. Yet they have changed the way patients/clients are managed. When care is planned, given, documented and evaluated using pathways a reliable dynamic process evolves that is said to fit the TQM concept in several areas:

- It defines quality outcomes.
- It is consumer/patient/client orientated.
- It focuses on work processes.
- The documentation of problems, variations and corrective action provides a proactive, preventative system for the management of patient/client care.
- The ongoing review of the pathway and variations provides a process for continuous improvement.

Hospitals see the benefit of pathways within the context of continuous improvement as enabling experienced care givers to set the standard of care and then analyse any variations and outcomes. In addition, the data can be used to update the pathway to achieve the best outcomes possible for individuals (Lumsdon & Hagland 1993).

Using pathways facilitates the standardisation of care and, unless standards of practice are uniform, efficiencies and quality issues will never be achieved (McEachern 1995). If standardisation in practice is not achieved, care and support may be so diverse as to make quality issues unattainable and service efficiencies impossible to attain. Patients/clients are often the recipients of varying standards of care depending on the unit, or hospital they visit. Pathways are described as a useful process to standardise clinical practices and they address quality issues because they are agreed and written by all those responsible for delivering that particular episode of care.

Activity 11.5

Identify the ways in which care pathways can support the clinical governance agenda in the UK. What are the strengths and the difficulties of this approach?

The claims for care pathways as a quality tool fits the current clinical governance agenda as they offer a means to set and improve standards of care in welfare services throughout the country. However, it is a mistake to think that in implementing pathways you are implementing a managed care system. It is more likely that you are utilising one of the tools used within a managed care environment.

Managed care organisations in the USA not only utilise tools such as care pathways, but also organise their finance and purchasing systems, management, skill mix and workforce planning around the care they offer. As such they are able to define the cost, the inputs and standard for each episode of care. Whereas in the UK doctors define and give the care they deem necessary for their patient/client, in the USA additional inputs of care are charged and require the payee's, e.g. patient's/client's or insurer's approval before it can go ahead.

Most of the cost-saving claims associated with managed care organisation come from the revamping of the materials management and purchasing

systems, and reductions in lengths of stay. Care pathways are used to map details of everything that should happen for a patient/client at a given point in time, including what supplies are needed. Outcomes are identified, standards set and care is coordinated and continually assessed. Clinical protocols are used and often included in the pathway. Managing the care process in this way ensures the patient's/client's journey is smooth and reduces the likelihood of care being duplicated or omitted.

However, using cost reductions created from decreasing lengths of stay is not necessarily a useful index for effectiveness and efficiency (Shirkiar & Warner 1994). When decreasing the lengths of stay, people will not necessarily use less resources; they may in fact use the same amount in a shorter period of time. The impact of this would be an increase in the cost per day. However, identifying and stabilising lengths of stay presents an opportunity to maximise resource use per day which should ultimately see a decrease in costs. If the volume of patients/clients increase with reduced lengths of stay then costs per case could be expected to decrease at a faster rate.

Activity 11.6

Consider measures used in your organisation to maximise cost efficiencies. Compare these with the managed care approach and identify the advantages and disadvantages to this way of delivering welfare services.

The benefits identified with the managed care process in the USA clearly fall into the cost, quality arena and it is easy to see with the introduction of clinical governance why the sudden surge of interest has occured in the UK. The next section examines the transportation of the process to healthcare establishments in the UK.

MANAGED CARE IN THE UK

If the criteria for managed care is that it permeates everything an organisation does, then this concept does not yet appear to exist within the UK. Many NHS Trusts have taken managed care tools such as care pathways and applied them to care delivery in parts or throughout their organisation.

People entering the healthcare system in the UK do not appear to have access to the detail about their care that their counterparts in the USA receive. Within the UK different professionals may often give different accounts regarding what will happen to them. Some are told they are likely to be in hospitals for 4 days, others 6 days; for patients/ clients this is not very helpful when planning their home life or return to work. Individuals talking with friends often find it disturbing to learn that people with similar illnesses are receiving different treatments, operations, advice and care. While this in itself may not be a problem, when people are not given an adequate explanation or choice of treatments, they often feel they have received inappropriate care or worse, an inferior standard of care.

Regional variations make the issues more acute and result in people, rightfully, querying the standards of care delivery within welfare services. Most people have a clear perception regarding the quality of the care they receive. However, this is often only judged either when things go wrong, or in the context of the way in which professionals communicate and treat them.

Care pathways are frequently being seen as the solution to this difficulty. However, within the UK there is insufficient rigorous systemic evaluation of care pathways to advocate their unequivocal use. The research studies that have been carried out point to some benefits, but again are statistically insufficient in number to provide conclusive evidence. The Clinical Resource and Audit Group (CRAG) (1999) evaluated 103 pathways in two hospitals in Scotland and found copious, consistent and statistically significant evidence to support the effectiveness of care pathways in almost all the areas they evaluated.

Unfortunately, in the days of evidence-based practice, much of the contemporary literature is anecdotal; nevertheless, it points to significant perceived benefits from using pathways. Pathways are seen to provide individuals with a forecast of their treatment (Scott & Cowen 1997) both in relation to interventions and projected timescales. Defining the parameters or standards for practice in this fashion addresses the issues of what should be done and to what standards. The evidence for care pathways, both anecdotal and research based, points to several areas in which the care pathways process can be used to benefit patients/clients, professionals and welfare organisations.

RISK MANAGEMENT

Care pathways offers a process approach to manage and integrate care by identifying the patient's/client's needs in a given area (Wilson 1997). The pathway is the staged plan which outlines the appropriate care and timing of procedures in order to enhance the effective delivery of services (Wilson 1997). In this fashion the process can also be used to secure the best outcomes for people. In devising the pathway, professionals and managers communicate the process of care they expect for the patient/client. This dialogue provides an opportunity to identify risks and take relevant action, however, providing this information does not necessarily result in appropriate action. For this to occur there has to be both an awareness and ownership of the risks. The pathway process provides an opportunity to coordinate and manage care, thus creating the opportunity for awareness and ownership to develop, a situation that potentially reduces the margin for errors.

In devising the pathway, clinicians agree preplanned actions of care/treatment to a relevant standard. The importance of getting every stakeholder on board cannot be overemphasised as their agreement sets a collective standard for an episode of care. Moving from individual practices to this professionally agreed collective standard ensures a consistency throughout a person's experience of care.

In terms of minimising risk, pathways can help to reduce variations in standards and facilitate the continuous improvement of care through increased coordination (Wilson 1997). Consistency in practice with reduced variations is important, particularly in decreasing opportunities for multiple standards of care provision within the same organisation (Wilson 1997).

Recording and analysing the variations in each individual's care indicates any changes or omissions for each person. The collection and analysis of these data provides information about a patient's/client's progress and response to the care outlined in the pathway, and about the smoothness or efficacy of the process of care delivery.

EVIDENCE-BASED CARE

A multidisciplinary approach to developing a pathway opens communication channels for professionals and agencies working together. It also creates opportunities that facilitate the examination and incorporation of evidence within care delivery. Herring (1999) believes that this process creates a positive environment for developing 'research based practice'.

However, creating the environment is often not enough; evidence-based care has to be on the agenda of the professionals in order for it to be on the agenda of the pathway. Evidence-based care was introduced as part of the NHS Research and Development strategy back in 1991, and reinforced as a key part of the clinical governance agenda. However, the literature suggest there is still a long way to go before all professionals are adequately engaged with the issue (Clinical Standards Advisory Group 1988, Walshe & Ham 1997, Grange et al. 1998). Strategies for change

management need to interface with the process of developing care pathways in order to engender an evidence-based or best-value approach to care delivery.

In addition, the pathway can be used as a tool to monitor care. Recording and analysing variations provides an opportunity to gather data about the effectiveness of the care delivered. Finally, acting on the data to action improvements offers a cycle to continuously review and monitor evidence-based care.

AUDIT

The way care pathways are developed and implemented provides an opportunity to develop a system of working which parallels the audit cycle. Professionals can use the document on a day-to-day basis to record the care given and any variations. These variations provide data about every patient/client and their progress in the care system. Analysing these data gives details of the positive and negative aspects of care. This process illustrates the way that care is delivered, examined, reviewed, updated and then, where necessary, fed back into the pathway document that subsequently leads to improvements in care delivery (see Fig. 11.2).

The key is for professionals to be aware of this aspect of the process and to incorporate the audit cycle into their way of working. The literature

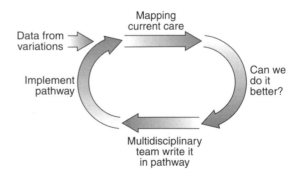

Figure 11.2 Pathway process.

cites pathways as an audit tool and one which has brought significant improvements to patient/client care.

The level of detail outlined in the pathway and the fact that all professionals write in the document and record the same details makes pathways an audit-friendly tool. Auditors tell grim tales of the problems associated with collecting meaningful data from client's/patient's notes. Most professionals record what is important to them so there is no consistency in what is written in notes and, as such, this presents a problem in retrieving accurate and consistent data. That is why an audit will often involve devising and filling an audit sheet containing the information required. The audit paperwork structures the information and asks every professional to record the same details. Data can then be collected from such paperwork to start the audit process. Using a pathway at this stage provides a tool to incorporate the data required by the audit. The pathway is implemented simultaneously and data retrieval is quick and effective. These data are then fed into the audit process, improvements identified and relevant actions taken.

Case examples

Kitchiner (1997) examined the potential use of care pathways as an audit tool which was demonstrated to have rewarding outcomes for patient care. In the absence of research or evidence, data from the analysis of the variations were used to improve aspects of care for children with cardiac disease. The data became the evidence from which informed decisions were made to develop care.

In one study, pathways were used successfully as an audit tool to record the international prostate symptom score for men with an enlarged prostate. The score aggregates the seven attributes of micturition and is recorded before and following surgery. Improvements in symptoms can

then be quantified and the changes compared over a period of time to similar data in national studies. As the collection of the data is built into the pathway the audit process is assured.

In mental health care, pathways are seen to provide a structural format from which to plan and audit the provision of care (Jones 1997). A common problem for people with enduring mental health problems, with poor levels of social functioning and living skills is the availability of suitable accommodation on discharge from hospital. Collecting data from the variations provides evidence of this problem. The data are a tool to inform and drive a solution.

Merritt et al. (1999) caution the use of pathways and argue that the fast-track uptake implementation of guidelines and care pathways has not been appropriately audited to determine effectiveness in achieving their goals. Following the introduction of care pathways in one hospital for neurology and neurosurgery the process provided a significant amount of valuable data that were fed into the audit cycle. Subsequently, care and patient/client management has been further developed and improved (Baldry & Rossiter 1995).

COST SAVINGS

The introduction of care pathways in the UK has not been associated with cost savings. They have mainly been introduced as a means to improve care and address quality issues. However, it is prudent to scrutinise the costs associated with the implementation of the process before committing resources, though the literature suggests that in some areas the introduction of care pathways can result in cost savings. Cost savings have been identified in the clinical field of orthopaedics through reductions in lengths of stay and reductions in the use of prophylactic antithrombotic drugs (Poole & Johnson 1996). This piece of work also noted, over a period of 3 years, an improvement in clinical outcomes and increased patient/client satisfaction.

The case for cost savings using pathways is not purely based on reduction in the lengths of stay, particularly if this compromises quality and increases readmission rates (Lowe 1998). The ability of pathways to combine process, practice and audit ensures that care is integrated and cost effective.

As a tool to manage resources effectively, and thus produce cost savings, pathways have been identified as avoiding waste and replication by ensuring the process of care for a particular intervention follows an explicit pattern of good practice. Professionals are able to plan a prescribed, logical and orderly intervention that has the potential to improve patient/client outcomes. The improvements may be so impressive that onward referral becomes unnecessary (Edwards 1999). This concept demonstrates that the right care inputs given at the right time can improve patient/client outcomes to such an extent that there is no need for follow-on or repeat care.

In the USA, Zehr et al. (1998) found that standardised care pathways for major thoracic cases reduced hospital costs and maintained the quality of care. Consistency in providing care was found to be an effective way of improving quality, and physician-directed diagnostic and therapeutic plans were shown to be crucial to this process. Using standardised pathways to incorporate and monitor these interventions resulted in a marked reduction in lengths of stay for all the major thoracic patients and a significant reduction in diagnostic testing. Indirect improvements were seen in pain management, mortality rates remained unaffected and quality of care was maintained by using this process.

In a review of six non-randomised studies of acute stroke, Sulch and Kalra (2000) evaluated the success of using care pathways as a method to facilitate quality and cost improvements. Although some benefits were found the evidence was weak and the recommendation was for further research.

In looking for a tool to assist quality and cost improvements, as previously stated, care pathways are cited as having some positive benefits. It is, however, unrealistic to hail a process as the long awaited solution to the cost, quality agenda. Welfare service delivery is complex and multifaceted and depends on so many variables that care pathways alone cannot provide all the answers. What they can provide is a process to bring professionals together to review the way they deliver care, to use an evidence-based approach to make improvements, to record the effect and any variations and then to use these data to further improve care.

In evaluating pathways we should not necessarily be evaluating the process, we should be examining the way the process is implemented and used as it is people that make and sustain change.

PATIENT SATISFACTION AND CARE PATHWAYS

There are several small-scale studies in the UK, which point to increased patient/client satisfaction with the use of care pathways. In particular, the study carried out at St Mary's Hospital NHS Trusts found that care post implementation of pathways was comparable to, and in some instances better than, their previous hospital experience. People felt encouraged to ask questions and indicated a greater level of satisfaction with responses from doctors and nurses, and they were more informed of their discharge date. The findings are similar in other studies, and although statistically insufficient in numbers to be scientifically rigorous, they are heartening from a service users perspective.

CONCLUSION

It is evident from the literature that claims for care pathways as a tool to achieve quality issues are well founded, and in this capacity pathways

Box 11.1   Steps to care pathways

Steps	Rationale
1. Identify area of care to develop. Identify project leader/the team and network. Identify resources required.	To achieve maximum rewards for efforts – high volume, high cost care is a useful starting point. To bring the team onboard and give them ownership of the pathway.
2. Identify the usage of the pathway. Identify how the data from the pathway and variations will be collected and used. Identify how the pathway will be evaluated.	To incorporate NSF, guidelines, risk management, audit. Agree who will collect and collate data. To identify benefits/disadvantages.
3. Map the current process of care. Critically appraise literature, research etc. Consensus agreement on evidence base for the pathway.	To see whole picture of care including patient's perspective. To identify good practice and areas for development. Collective agreement on standards to be used in pathway. Evidence to be adopted by everyone.
4. Each professional group writes their input to the pathway, including patient involvement. Team comes together to review their inputs. Agreement on who does what, when and how and written in the pathway.	To ensure patient-focused, effective coordinated care, with relevant professionals, giving relevant input at the right time. Risks identified and managed. Ownership of the pathway by all professionals.
5. The team implements and pilots the pathway. Project leader to coordinate implementation, monitor compliance and keep team motivated.	To manage the change to ensure its success. To monitor the pathway and compliance.
6. The team reviews the pathway. Data from variations collated and used to develop care and update the pathway. Date set to further review variations and update the pathway.	To see how effectively the pathway is used. To evaluate patient's response to care outlined in pathway. To monitor the efficiency and effectiveness of the process of care delivery.
7. Evaluate the pathway, consider: – impact on patient care, groups of patients, on the ward, unit, department or trust – impact on implement NHF and other guidelines – impact on professional practice, professional culture, skill mix, teamwork, standardising practice.	To evaluate the effect of the pathway. To further develop evidence based care.
8. Sharing good practice via publications, networks, conferences.	To share good practice.

have a place in the healthcare agenda to assist professionals with their efforts to implement the clinical governance agenda. The lack of a significant body of research on this subject is an omission and must be redressed sooner rather than later if the NHS is to avoid missing out on this important catalyst to the modernising of services.

The pressure for a consistent approach to both practice and record keeping is not only being sought by professionals and patients/clients, but is also becoming increasingly relied upon to defend against a more litigious society. Clinical governance, as previously stated, requires consistency not only in the quality and timely delivery of care, but also in record keeping by all health- and social-care professionals. In addition, the further development of care pathways will help professionals manage the blurring of role boundaries and secure consistency in care no matter who delivers it.

Experience leads us to believe that multi-disciplinary care pathways, underpinned by appropriate clinical protocols or guidelines will assist with a much called for progression to exception reporting. Once the emphasis of recording care moves from repetitive or, at worst, ad hoc, listing of everything done to that of exception reporting, the result will lead to a significant release of professionals' time, which they can then spend more appropriately focused on direct interventions. A structured approach to care management is a

pre-requisite for the successful implementation of electronic records and computerised care planning, both of which will improve and speed up communications between professionals and patients/clients.

It is important, however, that we quickly recognise the evidence base of current care-planning practice and the acceptance of a common template if we are not to waste more time reinventing the wheel. The paucity of research supports a cautioned approach to the use of care pathways and the implementation process appears to be key to their success.

From years of practical experience in using pathways, the steps outlined in Box 11.1 are offered as a guide to write and implement a pathway. A rationale is given for each of the steps and the framework is a starting point for teams wishing to start using pathways. More detail relating to each of these steps can be found in Chapter 12.

REFERENCES

Baldry JA, Rossiter D 1995 Introduction of integrated care pathways to a neuro-rehabilitation unit. Physiotherapy 81(8): 432–434.

Bryant S 1987 Management techniques on the critical path. The Health Service Journal (6): 906.

Clinical Standards Advisory Group 1988 The implementation of clinical effectiveness. A summary of the CSAG report on clinical effectiveness using stroke as a marker condition. CSAG report.

CRAG 1999 Clinical audit and quality using integrated pathways of care. Project CA96/01. West Glasgow Hospitals, Glasgow.

Department of Health 1998 A first class service: quality in the new NHS. HMSO, London.

Edwards JNT 1999 A potential role for integrated care pathways in resource management. Journal of Integrated Care (3): 90–92.

Ellis BW, Johnson S 1999 The care pathway: a tool to enhance clinical governance. British Journal of Clinical Governance 4(2): 61–71.

Grange AR, Renvoize EB, Pinder JM 1998 Introducing clinical effectiveness to nursing practice: not so easy! Clinical effectiveness in nursing 2: 98–102.

Hart R 1992 MD-directed critical pathways: it's time. Hospitals 5: 56.

Herring L 1999 Critical pathways: an efficient way to manage care. Nursing Standard 11(13): 47.

Jones A 1997 Managed care strategy for mental health services. British Journal of Nursing 6(10): 564–568.

Kitchiner D 1997 The development, implementation and link to clinical audit with pathways for children with cardiac disease. In: Wilson J (ed.) Integrated care management; the path to success? Butterworth Heinemann, Oxford.

Kongstevedt PR 1995 Essentials of managed health care. MD Aspen Publication, Gaithersbury.

Lumsdon K, Hagland M 1993 Mapping care. Hospitals and health networks (20): 34–40.

McCloskey JC 1994 Nursing management innovations: a need for systemic evaluation. Nursing Economics 12(1): 35–44.

McEachern S 1995 Cardiac integrations means facing heart hitting realities. Health Care Strategic Management 13(8): 19–23.

McKie D, Morris E, Nelson S 1994 Report on a study tour to Canada and the USA. April, Northern Regional Health, unpublished.

Merritt TA, Gold M, Holland J 1999 A critical evaluation of clinical practice guidelines in neonatal medicine: does their use improve quality and lower costs? Journal of Evaluation of Clinical Practice 5(2): 69–77.

Mosher C, Cronk P, Kidd A, McCormack P, Stockton S, Sulla C 1992 Upgrading practice with critical pathways. American Journal of Nursing 92(1): 41–44.

Poole P, Johnson S 1996 Integrated care pathways: an orthopaedic experience. Physiotherapy 81(1): 28–30.

Rasmussen N, Gengler T 1994 Clinical pathways of care: the route to better communication. Nursing 24(2): 47–49.

Robinson R, Steiner A 1998 Managed health care. Open University Press, Buckingham.

Rosenstein A 1994 Cost effective health care: tools for improvement. Health Care Management Review 19(2): 53–61.

Scally G, Donaldson J 1998 Clinical governance and the drive for quality improvements in the new NHS in England. British Medical Journal 317: 61–65.

Scott E, Cowan B 1997 Multidisciplinary collaborative care planning. Nursing Standard 12(1): 39–42.

Shirkiar MS, Warner P 1994 Selecting financial indices to measure critical path outcomes. Nursing Management 29(9): 58–60.

Stead I, Arthur C, Cleary A 1995 Do multidisciplinary pathways of care affect patient satisfaction? Health care risk report, pp. 13–15.

Sulch D, Kalra L 2000 Integrated care pathways in stroke management. Age and Ageing 29(4): 349–352.

Walshe K, Ham C 1997 Who's acting on evidence? Health Service Journal 107(5547): 22–25.

Wilson J 1995 Multidisciplinary pathways of care: a tool for minimising risk. Journal of Health Care Management 1(14): 720–722.

Wilson J 1997 Integrated care management. Nursing Management 4(7): 18–19.

Zander K 1988 Nursing case management: strategic management of cost and quality outcomes. Journal of Nursing Administration 18(5): 23–30.

Zander K 1992 Total quality management: the health care pioneers. In: Melum MM, Sinioris MK (eds) Total quality management: the health care pioneers xvi 338. American Hospitals Publishing Incorporated, America.

Zehr KJ, Dawson PB, Yang SC, Heitmiller RF 1998 Standardised clinical care pathways for major thoracic cases reduce hospital costs. Annals of Thoracic Surgery 66(3): 914–919.

12

Integrated care pathways

Their contribution to clinical governance and best value

Jeanette Thompson
Sharon Pickering

KEY ISSUES

- Identifying the problem or need

- Gathering support

- Establishing the team

- Reviewing practice

- Identifying best evidence

- Writing an integrated care pathway

- Piloting

- Evaluating, monitoring and reviewing

- Implementing the integrated care pathway.

INTRODUCTION

The benefits of care pathways have been discussed within a variety of healthcare settings for a number of years. More recently, care pathways have become part of the toolkit not only for quality care delivery, but also for achieving the outcomes identified within both the NHS plan and more broadly within clinical governance. Whilst very little discussion has taken place in relation to care pathways and the best value agenda within social-care settings, it is arguable that they could and should have similar benefits for such areas of care delivery. The concept of care pathways is briefly discussed in Chapter 11. Within this, a number of definitions are offered, along with discussion around some of the potential uses of care pathways and the ways in which they are able to support the clinical governance agenda.

It is the intention of this chapter to further reinforce this link with clinical governance, discuss the approaches and strategies involved in developing a care pathway as well as consider the relevance of integrated care pathways (ICPs) within social care. In addition, consideration will be given to the issues relating to the development of care pathways both across and within agencies.

Chilcott and Hunt (2001) define care pathways as 'structured multidisciplinary care plans which identify the essential steps and expected outcomes in the care of patients who have a specific clinical problem or are undergoing a particular surgical procedure'. Wilson (1992) defines them as a 'multidisciplinary process of patient-focussed care which specifies key events, tests and assessments, occurring in a timely fashion to produce the best prescribed outcomes, within the resources and activities available for an appropriate episode of care'. Hounslow and Spellthorne Community & Mental Health NHS Trust, Riverside Mental Health Trust (1996) define care pathways as 'A process approach to clinical care which is multidisciplinary and focuses on the interventions, procedures, and tasks that must occur within a specified time to ensure a prescribed outcome is achieved'.

As can be seen, these definitions focus upon clinical care delivery in healthcare settings. However, this does not mean that care pathways do not have relevance for other areas of welfare service delivery. This is clearly demonstrated when considering the aims of care pathway approaches as identified by Campbell et al. (1998), these include:

- the facilitation of the introduction of guidelines and systematic audit into practice environments

- the improvement of multidisciplinary communication
- the reaching and exceeding of existing standards for practice
- the reduction of unwanted variations in service delivery
- the improvement of communication between those delivering services and those in receipt of them
- improved client satisfaction
- the identification of research and development questions.

It is difficult to envisage anyone disagreeing with these fundamental principles as goals for welfare services of any description. It is by focussing upon these issues and the values that underpin the development and delivery of care pathways, that this chapter will demonstrate their validity to a range of settings, including social care. The key principles discussed within this chapter include:

- an emphasis upon real issues as experienced within practice settings – it is this that forms the basis of an ICP
- developing research-based/evidence-based practice that meets best value and clinical governance agendas
- multi-professional approaches
- multi-agency approaches
- involvement of both those who use services and their carers
- teamwork
- the ability to audit service delivery.

In addition to discussing these key principles, ICPs can be seen to have a number of key characteristics that are important as part of the development process, these are as follows:

- ICPs are locally developed
- have a clear user focus

- are developed and owned by the team
- are outcome/goal oriented
- are task, intervention and procedure specific
- are time specific
- monitor and record variations from the pathway (Thompson & Saunders 1999).

MODELS OF CARE PATHWAYS

According to Turley et al. (1994) three models of ICPs have been identified. The first and most commonly described of these models is characterised as reactive. Such approaches are frequently designed around acute and emergency care settings and require a project manager whose role is to monitor, evaluate and record variations from the pathway. As such, the project manager takes on the role of policing the implementation of the pathway. Although this model has the potential to reduce variation over the long term, it tends not to produce effective team and user/carer involvement. It could be argued that this reduces the potential within this approach for sustainable change.

The second model also involves the concept of a co-ordinator, but is much more interactive in its approach. Pathways developed from this perspective usually have active multidisciplinary team, and user and carer involvement throughout. This can be seen as increasing the potential for success within the implementation of the pathway. In this context, variance tracking and outcome measurement are captured and compared with the pathway in order to provide useful information regarding the continued development of the pathway. The third approach is a proactive or radical outcome method and was developed by Turley et al. (1994). This model attempts to anticipate both problems and opportunities for accelerating health gain. In doing this it attempts to upgrade the pathway design to meet the needs of the individual who is using the service as each person engages with the pathway. Within this approach both the team and user involvement allow the patient/client to improve on the outcomes set by the system.

Irrespective of which of the above approaches is utilised, a number of key benefits can be articulated. These include:

- The promotion of effective multi-disciplinary team working, with the role and unique contribution of each team member clearly identified.
- Improved communication and understanding between team members, clients and carers.
- The promotion of quality care by incorporating local and national standards and research findings.
- The existence of written and timely reminders for staff of what tasks should be completed at what point in time.
- Facilitation of discussion and communication that is user focused at information handover points.
- The planning of work schedules by staff based upon data contained within ICPs. This can facilitate the effective use of staff skills, competencies and expertise.
- The induction of new staff, using ICPs as a teaching aid.
- Measuring outcomes.
- Defining problems to ensure fast efficient follow-up actions are initiated.
- Ensure inefficient and unsafe practices are identified and eliminated (Thompson & Saunders 1999).

Analysis of these outcomes allows us to clearly place them into a number of broad categories. These include research, teamwork and communication, quality, skills and competencies, and, last but not least, the client as the focus of care delivery, all of which can be seen as fundamental principles upon which clinical governance and best value are based. The value of these underpinning structures to the successful development and implementation of a care pathway is discussed later in this chapter.

STAGES IN DEVELOPING A CARE PATHWAY

Before continuing any further with this chapter it is useful to consider what the actual process of developing and implementing an ICP might involve. Box 12.1 explores these stages.

It is the intention of the following section to explore these issues in more depth in order to assist the reader in designing and implementing a care pathway.

Identify the problem or area of need

Selecting the area of practice that will be the focus of an ICP is crucial. A number of factors may inform this process. Muir Gray (1997) notes the value of regularly scanning the literature to identify developments in best practice and the research evidence to proactively inform changes within care delivery, any of which could form the basis of an ICP. Whilst this may have some significant benefits in prompting professionals to consider where their practice is not as current as it may be, this approach does not always create local ownership and, consequently, support for any proposed changes.

Other factors prompting the development of an ICP may include, for example, an area of interest within a team, the existence of research evidence, evidence from audit activity, feedback from users of the service, new service developments and complaints. More specifically, they should include areas:

- that are of concern to either patients/clients, carers or staff
- where there is a debate as to what constitutes best practice

- where there is a high volume and/or high cost involved
- where a wide variation in practice and/or outcome exists.

It is important to remember that whatever the driver for an ICP, the process of identifying the problem is a fundamental stage (see Chapter 6 for a more in-depth analysis). Particularly as this forms the basis of a whole sequence of work activity which will either prove useful or otherwise depending upon the effectiveness of this part of the process. To this end, it is crucial to ensure the problem or area of practice that becomes the focus of this work is both the real problem and one that is of importance to people who use the service.

Activity 12.1

How could you involve people who use your service in identifying possible areas for the development of an integrated care pathway?

Whilst we as professionals have now developed significant skills in involving people within the delivery of their own care, we have not been as successful in involving people who use the service in the development and evaluation of care delivery and/or ICPs. There are, however, a number of approaches that can be utilised when involving those who use services in developing a pathway. The most obvious of these is direct consultation. This can be achieved by the use of satisfaction surveys, structured interviews and questionnaires. Whilst these approaches are relatively easy, cost effective and can gain a snap shot of opinion on a range of issues there are significant disadvantages. These include the risk of poor response rates, the quality, or otherwise, of the data returned, but most importantly it means the person using the service is only consulted on the issues identified by professionals and service

Box 12.1 Developing a care pathway

Stages	Actions
1. Identify the problem or area of need	Ensure problem is a real problem Ensure resolution will benefit people who use the service Involve service users in problem identification
2. Gather support for the development of the pathway	Identify key stakeholders and include within discussions Identify those people who will make the project succeed and those who may hinder its implementation. Identify appropriate actions to work with those people who will hinder progress
3. Establish the development team	Pull together key people who will contribute to the development of the ICP Ensure you have an appropriate skill mix within the team Identify project management requirements and develop a project plan Identify resources required within the team
4. Review current practice	Audit existing practice Identify issues relating to the infrastructure required to support the development of ICPs, e.g. the existence or otherwise of multi-professional notes
5. Identify key elements of current best practice	Undertake a literature search Check National Service Frameworks (NSFs), National Institute of Clinical Excellence (NICE), Commission for Health Improvement (CHI) and Social Care Institute for Excellence (SCIE) for good practice guidance Review policy areas Benchmark against other similar services
6. Agree the evidence base for the pathway	Arrange a stakeholder meeting at a convenient time (including for carers and users of the service)
7. Write the draft ICP	Ensure local involvement Identify intended format and layout
8. Pilot the draft ICP	Identify pilot area Communicate necessary information to pilot site, including education and training needs Identify objectives Establish clear timescale Identify expected outcomes Analyse variations to the pathway
9. Evaluate the pilot and update the ICP	Ensure local involvement Communicate key outcomes to the wider team Identify any education and training needs
10. Introduce the ICP into area(s) of practice	Ensure clear start date Remove any previous methods of recording data relating to the area of the ICP
11. Monitor, review, evaluate the pathway to ensure continuous quality improvement	Utilise the skills and expertise of people in audit roles Ensure areas noted in analysis of variance are acted upon Engage with those who use the service to ensure changes meet their needs and expectations
12. Identify learning and share information	Via team meetings, newsletters, publications, web sites, conferences etc.

providers, and is therefore only involved in one part of the process.

The use of unstructured interviews and focus groups can help with the resolution of some of these difficulties in that they provide an opportunity for people who use the services to identify their own priorities and issues. However, unless these approaches are utilised at regular stages during the development of an ICP, they run the risk of only involving people at one stage in the process once again. To utilise them at key stages during the process can prove very worthwhile, particularly regarding the richness of the information gained to inform the development of the ICP. A caution here, however, is the resource intensive nature of such an approach; if this strategy for inclusion and consultation is to be utilised it must be adequately resourced from the outset. Failure to do so can lead to significant frustration for those involved in developing the pathway.

In addition, when addressing problems in practice environments, it is also important to consider whether the problem that you are about to focus your time and energy on is a genuine or real problem. It is also crucial that there is clarity about who perceives the situation as a problem. On occasions, we embark upon lengthy pieces of work aimed at developing practice only to find that the problem that has been resolved, whilst being valid from a professional perspective, was not perceived as an issue by those using the service. We would argue that whilst some changes that create benefits for practitioners are valid, in a world of finite resources it is important to ensure that any change will ultimately result in improving outcomes for clients or patients.

Consideration of this aspect, therefore, introduces an additional dimension into the process of problem identification that may necessitate some work in order to ascertain the views of those in receipt of services. This can be achieved through a number of different approaches including patient or client satisfaction surveys, focus groups and audit etc. Care must, however, be taken, whatever the approach, that the questions being asked are such that they will illicit unbiased and useful information. It is not unusual to see satisfaction surveys and audit questionnaires which ask questions that are of crucial importance to the staff team, but not to the client or patient.

A further issue to consider is whether the problem that you have identified is the right problem. Whilst this may sound ridiculous, many teams have invested inordinate amounts of time and resources in resolving a particular issue only to find that they have not been focusing their attentions on the real problem.

Essentially, therefore, when considering all the above information and identifying the problem that you need to work upon, it is important to ask yourself a number of key questions. These include:

- What is of concern to patients/clients or carers who use the service?
- What is of concern to you?
- What is of concern to your colleagues?
- What is of concern to your managers?
- What is the focus of current policy?

Whilst the process of checking out the area of practice or problem that will form the basis of an ICP may appear tedious and unnecessary, it is actually crucially important as clear identification of the problem will influence the future direction and management of the whole development process. Failure to undertake this stage of the process will make the act of gathering support less focussed and less effective.

Gathering support

Gathering support is crucial for the effective development and successful implementation of ICPs. Within this, it is essential to identify key stakeholders and ensure that they are adequately represented throughout both the development and implementation of the care pathway. Meadows et al. (1993) identify stakeholders as individuals and/or groups who are affected by change and are capable of influencing it either positively or negatively. They suggest three main categories of stakeholder:

- Key individuals within an organisation or team.
- Key groups within an organisation or team.
- Key external individuals or organisations.

Within this, it is important to consider not only the immediate team of people with whom you work, but also the management structure, particularly the executive team and people from outside the organisation, especially if the ICP will impact on other organisations and you need their support for the pathway to be successful. In addition to noting the role and influence of different members of the above groups, it is also important to identify the less obvious stakeholders and ensure their inclusion in the process. With ICPs key, but often not obvious, groups are carers and those who use the service and non-professionally qualified staff.

In addition to identifying those key stakeholders whose support is essential for the success of your pathway, it is important to consider those who may make efforts to hinder the success of your proposed changed, for whatever reason. Kuhlman and Jones (1991) offer a framework (shown in Table 12.1) to aid you in dealing with this issue.

Completing Table 12.1 will help provide clarity regarding the most effective way to utilise your time and energy when engaging in the crucial task of gathering support for the successful introduction and development of your project.

When considering the process of developing an ICP, the enthusiasm of getting on with the work can often mean that insufficient time is spent on the earlier stages of the process, particularly gathering support. On occasions this may be to the detriment of the successful implementation of the pathway.

Establish a development team

Effective teamwork is crucial to the successful development of an ICP, particularly a care pathway that will result in improved outcomes for those who use services. There are three important aspects that impinge upon the success of this part of the process; the skill mix of the team, project management skills and resources required. As already stated, it is crucial that the team has the 'right' make up. In this circumstance it is important that the team has the appropriate knowledge, expertise, skills and competencies within it.

Activity 12.2

Think about your area of practice and an ICP that you use or are involved in. Who was included in the development team? What skills, knowledge, expertise and competence do they bring to the table? Is this skill mix appropriate in terms of what the team is trying to achieve? Are there any obvious gaps? Where are you likely to find the skills that are missing in your team?

In considering the above exercise, it is important not only to have on board those affected by the development, but also individuals who have the relevant expertise of practice, project management, education and training, and information and communication skills. Wherever possible the team should also include people who use the service, as well as carers. It is only through working with

Table 12.1

Key player	Not committed	Let happen	Help happen	Make happen

Reproduced from Kuhlman S, Jones M 1991 Managing radical change. MHNA Publications, York, with kind permission of APLD Publications, York.

this group of individuals that genuine change will be possible for those using the service.

Equally important when establishing the team that will develop and implement the ICP, is the need to ensure all people forming the team do so on the basis of equality of responsibility and involvement. This will create a variety of challenges for the different practice areas for which ICPs are relevant. For example, in an acute hospital setting the consultant may either feel they have greater knowledge and expertise or be granted this position by other members of the team. This will create its own difficulties in relation to the effectiveness of the team. Within learning disability services, for example, difficulties may arise in relation to making information accessible for people who have a learning disability. The inability to do this successfully will create a power imbalance for those people who use services in that setting. This context requires that the whole process of developing an ICP is managed using a systematic approach and that good project management structures are put into place.

Project management

Good project management and prospective planning are essential elements of a successful ICP and can facilitate their implementation into routine practice and care delivery (Wilson 1997). As a systematic approach to change, project management approaches fit well with the concepts of clinical governance and best value, as they support the achievement of the key goals of improving the quality of care delivery. As such, a well-planned project will ensure the identification of the following:

• project benefits
• achievements
• early problem identification.

The purpose of project management is to ensure that individuals are aware of what their responsibilities are, and what the completion date for their

actions is. In addition, it provides a basis for measuring progress and achievement. Alongside this, a good project management approach will identify the vision collaboratively and inclusively with the team. It can also facilitate the setting of achievable and acceptable objectives for both the team and the service user. In order to achieve this, there are a number of simple rules in relation to project management that should be followed. These are:

• keep the scope and objectives clear
• build a comprehensive product and activity breakdown
• ensure a rigorous communication and dissemination system
• have realistic expectations
• have clearly defined criteria for success upon which to measure and report back to the steering group.
• monitor and evaluate

In order that everyone is clear as to the plan, it is essential that each stage within it is explicitly articulated. As such, a project plan should include the following:

• a route map – a working document that should be continually updated
• a series of tasks and responsibilities for the project team
• information about resources.

Resources

Whenever project managing any change or developing an ICP, one of the first things to address is any resource implications. These may include financial costs – often the quickest to be acknowledged – but equally important are the resource implications relating to staff time and effort, or staff disenchantment. When considering the development of ICPs it is important to note that the implementation of new ways of working are a possible outcome and, as such, will have resource implications, particularly in respect of staff time. It is, therefore, important that this aspect of ICP development is acknowledged at the onset of the change process, and support is gained from senior management for this time investment. In the context of a multi-professional or multi-agency ICP this may mean the support of more than one manager or organisation. One way of ensuring the most effective use of the resources available is to ensure the effective management of the project.

Activity 12.3

With regard to the pathway that you are working with or interested in developing, consider the resources that you think you will require to ensure its effective development and the subsequent implementation of the pathway. Discuss this list with both the team in which you work and your manager. Consider whether or not the resources that you have identified are realistic and also what you need to do to get them.

In the above exercise you may have thought about not just staff and the time that they will need to develop the pathway, but also access to library facilities and the education and training that may be needed. You will also need to consider the resources required for the piloting of the pathway and the collation and analysis of the results. In addition there may be a need to have new equipment, for example, information technology, to deliver more effective care. The first major call on the team's resources is likely to be the process undertaken to review current practice.

Review current practice

When reviewing current practice most of us instantly think in terms of reviewing care delivery around a specific aspect of our work. As has already been noted, if pathways are to help in the process of changing outcomes, as is explicit within the concept of clinical governance and best value, then it is important to consider issues from the perspective of people who use the services. However, there is another area of practice that it is also important to consider in relation to the successful implementation of ICPs, that is the infrastructure into which they are being introduced. This will be the focus of this section of the chapter and will particularly focus upon the importance of multi-professional notes and the challenges associated with this approach.

In order to maintain standards, or before making any changes, it is essential to understand the way in which things work now (National Health Service Executive 1998). It is this process of reviewing current practice – through whatever methodology – that can form the basis of the team discussions about what constitutes the essence of the ICP, what gaps exist and what further research or data collection is required. The real challenge within this and within any audit approach, lies in its application to complex service systems where there are real world pressures, resource difficulties, complex workloads, and interpersonal and multi-professional or multi-disciplinary issues. However, the relationship between audit and ICP is helpful in this context. Rather than discuss audit in detail the reader is referred to Chapter 8. In this chapter the author outlines a complex but integrated approach to audit that involves service users as an integral part of the process at all stages, and the inclusion of a variety of other mechanisms, such as risk management, benchmarking and evidence-based care delivery. Within the audit chapter these are presented as a range of influences upon the process of audit; in the context of ICPs these issues are an integral part of the preliminary work informing the development of the ICP.

Supporting infrastructure

When reviewing current practice in relation to the supporting infrastructure it is important to consider a number of areas. These are described by McSherry and Haddock (1999) as:

- professional development and education and training
- audit, quality and risk management
- management and information systems
- research and practice development.

Professional development, education and training. Implicit within the development of any care pathway is a change in practice. Therefore, in order for the successful implementation of the pathway it is necessary to ensure that all staff are provided with the appropriate development opportunities. This may include training and education relating to issues such as best value\clinical governance and the ethos underpinning care pathways. In addition to this, it will include the need to provide education and training around the specific focus of the care pathway. This education and training needs to take place at all levels in the team, including managers.

Audit, quality and risk management. As already stated, audit, quality and risk management as subjects are well documented in other parts of this text (Chapters 8 and 10); consequently this section will not address these issues. However, what is important in the context of this chapter is the inter-relationship of each of these areas within individual organisations and the existence, or otherwise, of appropriate structures. These are important in relation to both ICPs and the clinical governance and the best value agenda.

Activity 12.4

Identify the structures in your organisation in relation to:
   audit
   quality
   risk management.

How do you engage with these issues and their organisational structures?

Do you need to do anything else to ensure you contribute to the clinical governance and best value agenda?

It may be the case that such structures or departments already exist within your organisation. However, the difficulty may be the level to which many practitioners are able to engage with each of these departments. The reasons why engagement can be difficult are wide ranging but may include the capacity of both members of these departments and members of the practice teams to engage in relevant activities associated with audit, quality and risk management. With the focus on clinical governance and best value, it is important to maximise the existing organisational resources in order to minimise resource implications for yourselves. This is obviously an issue in relation to ensuring the right skill mix exists on any development team.

Management and information systems. In the context of ICPs and the infrastructure that supports them, it is important to consider the issues that surround the management of knowledge. These include: access to libraries, appropriate information technology and approaches to record keeping.

When considering this infrastructure, it is important to know whether your organisation has access to library facilities, and whether within these facilities, you are able to utilise information technology to access the variety of web sites and electronic journals that are clearly outlined in Chapter 7. If this is not the case, then it is important to consider how the ICP development team will resource such activities.

In addition, effective record keeping is crucial to the successful implementation of ICPs. Within this, multi-professional notes are often cited as a prerequisite. The value of multi-professional notes is apparent from both the perspective of good ICP data and clarity when analysing variations, as well as from the client perspective. However, a number of difficulties are also apparent. Some of these issues are technical or practical ones in relation to ease of access to notes both in terms of inserting and extracting information. This issue can become particularly problematic when considering ICPs that cross organisational boundaries. However, it is important to note that just as these issues create difficulties, effective electronic notes or client-held records can actually help to resolve them. The most contentious issue, however, in relation to multi-professional notes, is often the issue of confidentiality, as many practitioners find it difficult to entertain the concept of sharing information about those who use the service. In reality, there is no legal or ethical reason as to why client/patient notes cannot be multi-professional; however, many practitioners perceive that there are many practical reasons as to why such approaches to information sharing are not common practice.

Research and practice development. A culture of dissemination of information about research evidence and practice development in an organisation and a team is fundamental with regard to continuous quality improvement, and, therefore, key to the clinical governance and best value agenda. As with audit quality and risk management, the issue here is whether the infrastructure exists within your organisation to support this issue and whether your team has the appropriate links with that department.

Developing an ICP

The process of developing an ICP includes identifying the key elements of best practice, agreeing the evidence base for the pathway, as well as writing, piloting and evaluating the draft. Key details relating to acquiring information that forms the evidence base for your pathway can be found in Chapter 5. Whichever of the aforementioned stages you are engaging in one of the crucial aspects that must be considered is that of local involvement in the process of writing, piloting and evaluating the pathway.

Local involvement

ICPs should always reflect the context of the service(s) in which they are to be delivered. Local involvement in the development of care pathways creates strength and, as such, they are likely to become more effective because this is instrumental in ensuring a strong sense of ownership. In addition, this process for developing care pathways also facilitates a shared understanding of the aims of the ICP within and across the service(s). The benefit of local involvement is that it ensures agreement about key outcomes within the team(s) and can reduce uncertainty and confusion about care delivery and, as a result, there are real benefits for the person who is using the service.

Additional outcomes relating to the development of ICPs from within the service and with teams is the real and quantifiable implications for the wider organisation. For example, developing an ICP may well prompt changes with regard to organisational structure, training and development, information management and dissemination of best practice. Within this agenda one can never underestimate the impact of the personalities involved, their personal politics and the historical development of the service. Irrespective of all these difficulties, ICPs can provide a route that facilitates an effective and equitable approach to change management.

Writing an ICP

One of the first things that may need to be considered, alongside the evidence base of the ICP, is the format and layout of the pathway documentation. Whilst there is currently an agenda that appears to dictate that all things are the same in different parts of any organisation, this is not necessarily the case for ICPs. In reality it is generally more successful if the ICP documentation is agreed within the team that is developing and using the pathway. This way the format and layout of the documentation can be tailored to the actual needs of the area. This does not, however, mean the process is completely haphazard, as there are specific characteristics that need to be included within any documentation. To some extent these are informed by the team decision about whether they wish to operate on the basis of stages and/or guidelines. Almost irrespective of this, there is a need to consider practical issues, such as how to identify where a care pathway belongs; this might necessitate information, such as the name of the organisation and of the unit being included on the pathway documentation. This is important in circumstances where the care pathway may move with the service user across departments and organisations. This issue is becoming more and more pertinent with the development of patient- or client-held notes.

The need to adhere to standards of record keeping is also important and, to this end, it is necessary to include space for signatures and for the insertion of dates. Other areas of note that should be considered for inclusion in any ICP documentation is a space to identify the projected timescales by which a planned initiative should have taken place.

Piloting an ICP

Once the pathway is established and its format and layout is set, the next crucial stage is to test the pathway out. This part of the process is intended to establish how easy the pathway is to use and how appropriate it is with regard to providing effective care. In planning the pilot it is essential to agree a number of areas. These include:

- the area in which the pilot will take place
- the scope and nature of the pilot

- timescales
- overall objectives
- expected outcomes.

These issues are particularly important to consider when ensuring the success of the pathway that is being introduced.

In addition, the education and training needs of those who are going to use the pathway are paramount. Implicit within this is the need to ensure that all team members understand the pathway and how to use it. Consequently, it is important to design and implement a training package that will meet the needs of the team and ensure the success of the pathway. Once the training and development needs have been addressed it is important that all those involved understand the date at which the pilot will commence, and that the team are all clear with regard to their roles and responsibilities. This is crucial in relation to the monitoring and evaluation of the pathway and the measurement of its effectiveness.

The monitoring and evaluation of this process may take a number of forms. It may include questionnaires and or interviews of those who are using the pathway. Within this, it is essential that the client's or service user's perspective is sought and that their comments on the effectiveness of the pathway are central to the evaluative process. Whatever views result from the pilot, it is important to consider their implications for the pathway. Some outcomes may necessitate changes to the pathway, others to the documentation, and others will indicate training and development needs. Whatever the findings, they will be based upon the questions asked during the pilot and the evaluative process put in place to test out the effectiveness. Potentially the most important part of the data collected will be that relating to the variations from the pathway. Consideration of these will indicate the potential of the pathway to identify weaknesses in the service system and future areas for development.

Analysing variations

A variance or variation from an integrated care pathway occurs when the process of care delivery deviates from that identified within it. As already mentioned, any documentation to support the pathway includes a section for recording this variation and, as a result, the team has an in-built audit tool. For those care pathways that are multi-professional this provides a mechanism for auditing the effectiveness of the team.

Analysis of any variation can be either positive or negative, that is, it will include issues achieved before the scheduled date as well as those achieved beyond the stated deadline. These variations should be analysed to identify how effective care delivery is, and how this measures against best practice in any given area. However, if you have developed a care pathway that is based upon good practice and research evidence, and you and the team in which you work is constantly achieving the targets and goals set within the pathway, then it is necessary to consider if the goals in the pathway need to be more rigorous. A word of caution, however, has to be in the reverse situation; should you constantly achieve goals and targets behind time, then it is not appropriate to instantly consider re-scheduling the pathway. The goal of any pathway has to be to improve the service users' experience and the care delivered to them. Altering any pathway to simply reflect reality or what currently exists is not appropriate. To this end, care pathways also lend themselves nicely to the implementation and monitoring of the achievement of some or all of the standards incorporated within NSFs.

Variations can be caused by a number of factors, these include:

- client-focussed issues, e.g. people not turning up for appointments
- organisational issues, e.g. the work of other departments impacting upon your pathway

- service and professional agendas, e.g. recruitment of speech and language therapists or other professional groups affected by skill shortages.

Whilst it is often helpful to break down the cause of variation into the above categories, it is also important to maintain data in a format that can be analysed within broader categories whenever relevant and helpful.

Implementation

When implementing the final version of the pathway it is crucial that members of the project team are available to support and advise those who are charged with the responsibility of taking the change forward and making it a reality. In this context, it is important to ensure that any new staff are inducted into using the pathway appropriately. In addition, the audit process will ensure that ongoing team members stick to the pathway as it was intended.

The successful inclusion of an audit process alongside care delivered, as within a pathway, will ensure a continuous quality improvement that also includes service users and their carers in the process.

CONCLUSION

We have outlined a number of crucial stages when embarking upon the process of developing an ICP. The early stages include identifying the problem and gathering support, two stages that are easy to bypass, however, failure to effectively address these issues can affect the success of the ICP. Other important areas discussed include local development and the involvement of people who use the services with the process. As can be seen from discussions within this chapter, developing a genuinely inclusive approach to the implementation of ICPs, particularly one that includes the people who use our services, is a time-consuming and complex process. However, we would argue that the potential within ICPs to generate real change from the perspective of those receiving services, and the ability of this to deliver quality services and subsequently to contribute to both the clinical governance and best value agenda, indicates that such an investment is worthwhile.

REFERENCES

Campbell H, Hotchkiss R, Bradshaw N, Porteous M 1998 Integrated care pathways. British Medical Journal 316: 133–137.

Chilcott J, Hunt A 2001 Nurse friendly integrated care pathways. Nursing Times 97(48): 32–34.

Hounslow & Spellthorne Community Mental Health Trust, Riverside Mental Health Trust 1996 A pathway for pathways.

Kuhlman S, Jones M 1991 Managing radical change. MHNA Publications, York.

McSherry R, Haddock J 1999 Evidence-based healthcare: its place within clinical governance. British Journal of Nursing 8(2): 114–117.

Meadows S, Gill P, Hearn P et al. 1993 The people pack, a step by step guide to getting the best from your workforce. Outset Publishing Limited, St Leonards on sea.

Muir Gray JA 1997 Evidence-based healthcare. Churchill Livingstone, Edinburgh.

National Health Service Executive 1998 Achieving effective practice. DOH, London.

Thompson J, Saunders M 1998 Audit in teams: the contribution of integrated care pathways in services for people who have a learning disability. APLD Publications, York.

Turley K, Tyndall M, Roge C et al. 1994 Critical pathway methodology: effectiveness in congenital heart surgery. Annals of Thoracic Surgery 58: 57–65.

Wilson J 1992 An introduction to multi disciplinary pathways of care. Northern Regional Health Authority, Newcastle.

Wilson J 1997 Introduction to integrated care management – introducing multi disciplinary pathways of care into an organisation through project, risk and change management. In: Wilson J (ed.) Integrated care management, the path to success. Butterworth Heinemann, Oxford.

13

Evaluating and adapting practice guidelines for local use: a conceptual framework

Ian Graham
Margaret Harrison
Melissa Brouwers

KEY ISSUES

◆ Evaluating and adapting existing
   practice guidelines for local use should
   be an iterative process

◆ An organisation must first identify an
   area in which to promote best practice

◆ Establishing an interdisciplinary
   guideline evaluation group or task force
   is the next step

◆ The group must establish a guideline
   appraisal process that is systematic,
   rigorous and transparent

◆ The major issues in the guideline
   appraisal process are: searching and
   retrieving guidelines, assessing the
   quality of identified guidelines using a
   guideline appraisal instrument, and
   undertaking a content analysis of the
   specific guideline recommendations

◆ After reviewing the quality of the
   existing guidelines and comparing
   the content of the recommendations
   and the levels of evidence supporting
   each, the group can make decisions
   about which recommendations to
   adopt

◆ Once the adaptation of the existing guideline(s) has been drafted as a local guideline, it is sent out for external review by practitioners, policy makers and others

◆ Once the feedback is incorporated in the local guideline and the guideline modified as necessary, the next step is its official endorsement by the organisation

◆ The last step in the guideline evaluation and adaptation cycle is scheduling review and, when necessary, revision of the guideline to ensure that new evidence that might impact on the recommendations is incorporated as it becomes available.

INTRODUCTION

This chapter describes a framework for evaluating and adapting existing practice guidelines for local use by organisations and groups. The framework presents the major issues related to guideline adaptation and breaks them down into manageable steps. Helpful suggestions are offered about how to develop a rigorous, systematic guideline evaluation process.

The development of practice guidelines appears to be a growth industry. With the ever increasing number of guidelines becoming available, professionals and managers are confronted with numerous, sometimes differing, and occasionally even contradictory guidelines from which to choose (Lewis 2001). This situation is further complicated by concerns being raised about the quality of available guidelines (Ward & Grieco 1996, Graham et al. 1997, Sudlow & Thomson 1997, Varonen & Makela 1997, Littlejohns et al. 1999, Shaneyfelt et al. 1999, Grilli et al. 2000, Graham et al. 2001). Indeed,

adoption of guidelines of questionable validity can lead to harm to patients/clients, inefficient use of scarce resources or ineffective interventions (Feder et al. 1999, Woolf 2000).

Practice guidelines are 'systematically developed statements to assist practitioner and patient decisions about appropriate healthcare for specific clinical circumstances' (Field & Lohr 1990). They are intended to offer concise instructions on how to provide services (Woolf et al. 1999). The most important benefit of practice guidelines is their potential to improve both the quality of care (the process of care) provided by professionals, and patient outcomes (Grimshaw et al. 1995). However, their beneficial effects are contingent on a guideline development process that is methodologically rigorous and incorporates the best evidence available and the successful implementation of the resulting guideline (Grimshaw & Russell 1993, Worrall et al. 1997, Thomas et al. 1999).

Producing valid and reliable practice guidelines can be costly, time consuming, and require considerable content and methodological expertise. It has been estimated that it can take up to 3 years and between $100 000 and $800 000 US to develop a guideline. For many organisations, especially those at the regional and local level, the cost of such an undertaking is prohibitive, and makes the using of existing well-developed guidelines appealing.

At the same time, for an organisation wishing to adopt best practices, determining which existing guidelines are quality products worthy of adoption can be a daunting task. Every effort should be made to identify existing guidelines that have been rigorously developed and adapt them for local use (Feder et al. 1999). However, organisations and practitioners should be discerning users of guidelines and must scrutinise the methods by which they were developed (Shekelle et al. 1999) as well as the content of the recommendations. Even guidelines developed by prominent professional groups or government bodies should not be exempt from this scrutiny, as it has been shown that the quality of guidelines developed by even these organisations may be less than optimal (Grilli et al. 2000).

This chapter elaborates a conceptual framework that we developed to assist organisations to systematically evaluate the quality of existing practice guidelines and adapt them for local use. The framework, referred to as the Practice Guidelines Evaluation and Adaptation Cycle (Graham et al. 2000a), was derived from our experience developing provincial oncology practice guidelines in Ontario, Canada (Browman et al. 1995), from our

efforts to assist Canadian provincial and a regional healthcare organisation select and/or adapt existing guidelines for endorsement and use, and from a review of the literature on appraising the quality of practice guidelines (see Fig. 13.1).

STEP 1 – IDENTIFY AN AREA IN WHICH TO PROMOTE BEST PRACTICE

The first step is for the organisation to select the area in which it wishes to promote best practice. This involves an exercise in priority setting.

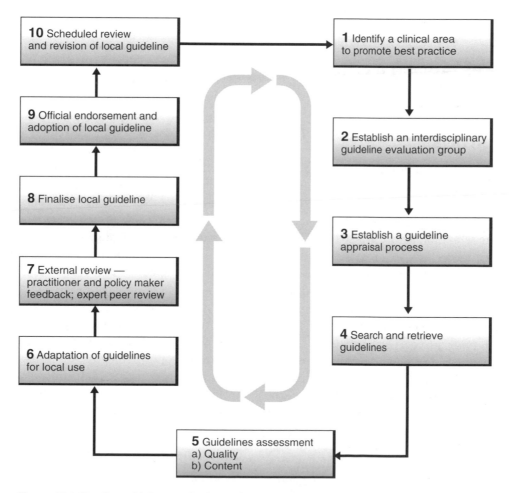

Figure 13.1 Practice guidelines evaluation and adaptation cycle.

The same criteria that have been suggested for prioritising and selecting topics for practice guidelines development can be used to select areas for best practice (Evidence-Based Care Resource Group 1994a, 1994b, Feder 1999, Shekelle 1999). These criteria typically include prevalence of the condition, associated burden of illness, concerns about large variations of practice patterns, costs associated with different practice options, and the likelihood that a guideline will be effective in influencing practice. One other obvious consideration is the existence of relevant evidence-based guidelines. An organisation's quality process, strategic direction or priority setting may also be used to pinpoint areas that might benefit from the implementation of a practice guideline.

STEP 2 – ESTABLISH A LOCAL INTERDISCIPLINARY GUIDELINE EVALUATION GROUP OR TASK FORCE

Group membership

The group should include local individuals from key provider stakeholders who will be affected by the selection of a guideline for local use. Including patients or individuals from the community along with managers can also be desirable. An interdisciplinary group is particularly important if the guideline addresses trans-disciplinary issues, such as referral criteria and treatment issues, that impact several provider groups or require changes in the behaviour of more than one professional carer group (McNicol et al. 1993). Another advantage of using an interdisciplinary group to evaluate existing practice guidelines is that it reduces the potential for bias that might result if only one provider group were involved in evaluating and selecting a guideline for local use. For example, some individuals might unconsciously or systematically favour a guideline that had been developed by their own professional group. While it has not been studied in relation to

the simultaneous appraisal of numerous guidelines, there are studies that show that when presented with the same evidence, a single specialty group may reach different conclusions than a multidisciplinary group, with the single specialty group favouring the performance of procedures in which it has a vested interest (Coulter et al. 1995, Kahan et al. 1996, Shekelle et al. 1999). Others have also suggested that multidisciplinary involvement in guideline development is desirable and probably promotes valid, reliable and implementable practice recommendations (Bond 1995, Petrie et al. 1995, Eccles et al. 1996). There is little reason to doubt these observations would not apply equally to interdisciplinary groups evaluating practice guidelines.

Roles

Similar to the roles required within guideline development groups, guideline evaluation groups should include a group leader, members with practice expertise, members with methodological expertise (e.g. literature searching, guideline appraisal skills), consumers, technical support and administrative support (Shekelle et al. 1999). Increasingly, consumers are participating in guideline development groups. The involvement of consumers on guideline evaluation groups ensures that the perspective of consumers/patients are represented. They are also able to attest to others that the evaluation process was transparent, comprehensive, systematic and fair. The group leader's task is to ensure that the group functions effectively and achieves its aims. This role requires someone with both clinical acumen and group process skills who can guide the group without dominating it.

Consensus development process

Informal as well as formal group processes, such as the Delphi or nominal group techniques

(McGlynn et al. 1990, Jones & Hunter 1995a, 1995b, Wortman et al. 1998) may be helpful to reach consensus. Some groups may find formal group processes artificial and cumbersome, while others may find the structure helpful. Our experience using informal group discussion to reach consensus has been positive, as it emulates the way decisions are often made in organisations.

The value of using a local group

A major advantage of having a local group evaluate and adapt regional, national or international guidelines for local use is the potential future impact on the use of the guideline resulting from the stakeholder's involvement in the process of adaptation. While the involvement of local clinicians in the development and introduction of guidelines does not guarantee their use (Grimshaw et al. 1995), it is widely believed that the greater their involvement in the process of guideline adaptation, the greater the sense of 'ownership' in the resulting guideline and willingness to use it (Burns et al. 1992, McNicol 1993, Brown et al. 1995). This sense of ownership, which may be critical to successful implementation of the guideline, develops as the group modifies an existing guideline to local practice contexts and providers, and identifies strategies to overcome potential barriers to use of the guideline (Karuza et al. 1995).

STEP 3 – ESTABLISH A GUIDELINE APPRAISAL PROCESS

Selecting a guideline appraisal instrument

Guideline appraisal instruments are intended to be used to systematically assess and compare guidelines on the same criteria. They typically consist of a number of quality criteria or items that are used to assess the extent to which each guideline meets these criteria. To date, several appraisal instruments have been developed

(Graham et al. 2000b). They differ in the number and content of items, and in terms of the extent to which they have been subjected to reliability and validity testing. Given the different appraisal instruments available, the selection of an appraisal instrument should be guided by the needs of the evaluation groups.

We have found the Appraisal Instrument for Clinical Guidelines (Cluzeau et al. 1997) greatly facilitates guideline appraisal. This instrument has been shown to be relatively easy to apply and has acceptable reliability and evidence of validity (Cluzeau et al. 1999). A revised version of this instrument known as the Appraisal of Guidelines Research and Evaluation Instrument (AGREE 2001) will replace the Appraisal Instrument for Clinical Guidelines (AGREE Collaboration 2003). The AGREE instrument was developed and evaluated by an international group of researchers and guideline developers from thirteen countries. The instrument has been endorsed by the World Health Organisation.

The AGREE instrument consists of 23 Likert-scale items organised in six domains. Each domain is intended to capture a separate dimension of guideline quality. The quality domains assessed are scope and purpose (three items), stakeholder involvement (four items), rigour of development (seven items), clarity of presentation (four items), applicability (three items), and editorial independence (two items). Each guideline assessed is given a standardised dimensional score ranging from 0 to 100. To ensure that all questions are interpreted consistently, the instrument comes with a user guide.

Establish criteria for selecting guidelines to review

Prior to searching for any guidelines, the group should decide on the criteria that will be used to select the particular guidelines that will be subjected to the evaluation. For example, the group may wish to restrict the evaluation to evidence-based guidelines; or national or international guidelines; only include ones that have been developed or updated in the past 2, 3, or 5 years or since the publication of important study results; only include systematic reviews; or, finally, only ones that have been published in peer-reviewed publications. The groups may wish to review only guidelines published in a specific language(s) or may want to focus only on guidelines dealing with management or prevention of the topic of interest. Whatever the criteria, they must be documented in order to ensure reproducibility of the process by which the group selected the specific guidelines to review.

STEP 4 – SEARCH AND RETRIEVE GUIDELINES

A systematic search for all relevant guidelines is necessary so that guidelines that members of the groups may not be aware of are not overlooked. This can be done electronically searching MEDLINE (http://www.ncbi.nlm.nih.gov/pubmed) and/or EMBASE. Search terms (MeSH headings) and text words that can be used are: practice guideline, practice guidelines, clinical practice guideline, clinical practice guidelines, standards, consensus statement, and consensus (Grilli et al. 2000). Practice guidelines as a publication type can also be used to search for guidelines in MEDLINE (Feder 1999). Chapter 7 gives useful tips and guidance in search techniques.

Increasingly, guideline developers are posting their guidelines directly on the web. This avoids delays in waiting for journals to publish guidelines, permits rapid updating of the guidelines and reduces dissemination costs. When guidelines are posted directly to the web, there is a greater chance that they may not be indexed in commonly consulted bibliographic databases such as MEDLINE or EMBASE. For these reasons, it is now prudent to also search the world wide web for guidelines. We

Box 13.1	Selected meta-crawlers – meta-search engines
Ask Jeeves	http://www.askjeeves.com/
Copernic	http://www.copernic.com/
Dogpile	http://www.dogpile.com/
Google	http://www.google.com/
Metacrawler	http://www.metacrawler.com/index.html/
Pandia Q-Cards	http://pandia.com/q-cards/
ProFusion	http://www.profusion.com/
Search.com	http://search.com/

have found meta-search engines or meta-crawlers useful in conducting searches of the web. Box 13.1 provides some examples of such search engines.

Important sources of rigorously developed guidelines in the UK include the Scottish Intercollegiate Guidelines Initiative (SIGN), the Clinical Resource Efficiency Support Team (CREST), and the National Institute for Clinical Excellence (NICE) among others. NICE has been given the mandate by the NHS to enter into partnerships with professional colleges and professional associations to develop national clinical guidelines. Box 13.2 provides a list of website databases of practice guidelines that we have compiled as we have searched for guidelines on various topics. This compilation is intended to be a starting point and not an exhaustive list. The list is divided into websites that primarily function as guideline clearinghouses and guideline developers.

A useful source of information on the quality of evidence-based healthcare websites (including practice guideline websites) is the Evidence-Based Medical Practice website of Department of Family Medicine, University of Laval, Quebec, Canada (http://www.medecine.quebec.qc.ca/default.htm).

Practice example

When a home-care authority searched for guidelines on the care of leg ulcers, 19 potential guidelines were located (Graham et al. 2000a). Fourteen of the guidelines were identified by MEDLINE, four by a search of the web, and one by a colleague.

Box 13.2   Listing of selected practice guideline websites

Country	Organisation	Website
Practice guideline clearing houses or listings		
Canada	Canadian Medical Association Guideline Infobase	www.mdm.ca/cpgsnews/cpgs/index.asp
	Queen's University (Kingston, Ontario) Clinical Practice Guidelines – index of guidelines published in the medical literature by month	http://post.queensu.ca/~bhc/gim/cpgs.html
Finland	Evidence-Based Medicine Guidelines	www.ebm-guidelines.com/index.html
UK	Medic8.com	http://www.medic8.com/ClinicalGuidelines.htm
	National Pathways Association	www.the-npa.org.uk/
	TRIP Database	www.tripdatabase.com/publications.cfm
USA	National Guideline Clearinghouse	www.guideline.gov/index.asp
	Medscape Women's Health	http://womenshealth.medscape.com/
	Medscape Multispecialty: Practice Guidelines	www.medscape.com/
	National Institutes of Health (NIH)	www.nih.gov
	NLM Health Services/Technology Assessment	http://text.nlm.nih.gov/
	University of California San Francisco Guidelines	http://medicine.ucsf.edu/resources/guidelines/index.html
Practice guideline developers/programmes		
UK	British Cardiac Society Guidelines	www.bcs.com/
	British Society of Gastroenterology Guidelines	www.bsg.org.uk/
	British Society of Hypertension Guidelines	www.hyp.ac.uk/bhs/resources/guidelines.htm
	British Thoracic Society Guidelines	www.brit-thoracic.org.uk/guide/guidelines.html
	Center for Health Services Research, University of Newcastle upon Tyne (North of England)	www.ncl.ac.uk/
	Clinical Resource Efficiency Support Team (CREST)	www.crestni.org.uk/publications/pubsah.asp
	Core Library for Evidence-Based Practice	http://www.shef.ac.uk/~scharr/ir/core.html
	Equip Guidelines and Protocols	www.equip.ac.uk/cgi/equip/documents.php3?mode=1
	National Institute for Clinical Excellence (NICE)	www.nice.org.uk/
	Prescribing Guidelines	http://medweb.bham.ac.uk/gp/mpg/
	Royal College of General Practitioners	www.rcgp.org.uk/rcgp/clinspec/guidelines/index.asp
	Royal College of Nursing	www.rcn.org.uk
	Royal College of Obstetricians & Gynaecologists Guidelines	www.rcog.org.uk/guidelines/eb_guidelines.html
	Royal College of Physicians London (RCPL)	www.rcplondon.ac.uk
	Scottish Intercollegiate Guidelines Network (SIGN)	www.sign.ac.uk
	Well Close Square	www.wellclosesquare.co.uk/
Australia	Medical Journal of Australia	www.mja.com.au/
	Monash University Centre for Clinical Effectiveness	http://www.med.monash.edu.au/healthservices/cce/evidence/

(continued)

Box 13.2 *(continued)*

Country	Organisation	Website
Canada	Periodic Task Force on Preventive Health Care	www.ctfphc.org/guide.htm
Alberta	Alberta Medical Association	www.albertadoctors.org
British Columbia	British Columbia Council on Clinical Practice Guidelines	http://www.hlth.gov.bc.ca/msp/protoguides/index.html
	BC Cancer Agency	www.bccancer.bc.ca/pg_g_04.asp?PageID=21&ParentID=4
Ontario	Cancer Care Ontario Practice Guidelines Initiative	www.cancercare.on.ca/ccopgi
Denmark	Danish College of General Practitioners	www.dsam.dk
Finland	Finnish Medical Society Duodecim	www.duodecim.fi/english
France	Agence Nationale d'Accreditation et d'Evaluation en Sante (ANAES)	www.anaes.fr
	French Federation of Comprehensive Cancer Centres (FNCLCC)	www.fnclcc.fr
Germany	Abeitsgemeinschaft der Wissenschaftlichen Medizinischen Fachgeselleschaften (AEMF)	www.datenbahn.de/
	Compliance Network Physicians/ Health Force Initiative	www.cnhfi.de/index-engl.html
Italy	Agency for Regional Health Services (ARHS)	www.assr.it
The Netherlands	Dutch Institute for Healthcare Improvement CBO	www.cbo.nl
	Dutch College of General Practitioners (NHG)	www.artsen.net
New Zealand	New Zealand Guidelines Group (NZGG)	www.nzgg.org.nz
Sweden	Swedish Council on Technology Assessment in Health Care (SBU)	www.sbu.se
Switzerland	Swiss Medical Association (SMA)	www.fmh.ch
USA	Agency in Healthcare Research and Quality (AHRQ)	www.ahrq.gov
	Allergen Immunotherapy Parameters	www.jcaai.org/param/
	American Association of Clinical Endocrinologists	www.aace.com/clinguideindex.htm
	American Association for Respiratory Care Clinical Practice Guidelines	www.rcjournal.com/online_resources/cpgs/cpg_index.html
	American College of Cardiology Guidelines	www.acc.org/clinical/statements.htm
	American Medical Association	http://www.ama-assn.org/
	CDC Prevention Guidelines Database	http://wonder.cdc.gov/wonder/prevguid/prevguid.shtml
	Institute for Clinical Systems Improvement (ICSI)	www.icsi.org
	US Preventive Service Task Force (USPSTF)	www.ahrq.gov/clinic/uspstfix.htm

Web addresses were up to date as of 10 February 2003.

Two of the guidelines not identified by MEDLINE were among the eventual five guidelines the group extensively evaluated. Indeed, high-quality evidence-based recommendations from both these guidelines were eventually incorporated into the local leg ulcer protocol. This case illustrates that relying solely on MEDLINE to identify guidelines can result in good-quality evidence-based recommendations being missed. Research is needed to determine whether this observation is generalisable to guidelines for other conditions.

STEP 5 – GUIDELINE APPRAISAL

Systematically assessing the quality of selected guidelines using a guideline appraisal instrument

Once the search has identified all the possible guidelines of interest and the selection criteria has been applied to them, copies of the guidelines meeting the criteria along with the appraisal instrument can be distributed to the members of the group. It may also be necessary to obtain any supporting documents that provide the details of the development process and supply these to the appraisers as well. Although there are no hard and fast rules, each guideline should be appraised by at least two, and preferably four or more, individuals as the reliability of the assessment increases with the number of appraisers (AGREE Collaboration 2003). It is also preferable that the appraisers have different professional and specialty backgrounds. Depending on the explicitness of the guideline appraisal-instrument user manual that explains how appraisal items should be interpreted, and the skills and experiences of the group members in critically appraising guidelines and evidence, it may be helpful to devote some group time to reviewing the appraisal instrument. It is important that group members are comfortable with this part of the assessment process and that the group comes to a common

understanding about how to interpret the items comprising the instrument and how each is to be scored.

Depending on the appraisal instrument, a total score or scores on groupings of items may be calculated. These calculations can be done by hand, with spread sheet software, or by statistical analysis packages. While there may be a tendency to view the results from this quantitative evaluation as an 'objective' measure of the quality of the guidelines reviewed, it is important to remember that these quality scores are influenced by the extent to which the guideline developers described the methods used to develop the guideline and reach consensus on the recommendations. A guideline that was rigorously developed may score poorly if the process was not well described.

Groups that we have worked with have found this initial screening of guideline quality with a validated appraisal instrument helpful for several reasons:

1. it requires the group members to carefully review each guideline in order to determine whether it meets each quality criteria; often busy practitioners do not have an opportunity to thoroughly review all relevant guidelines on a given topic

2. it systematically focuses the members' attention on specific methodological and context issues

3. by comparing how each member scores each instrument item it is possible to identify where there is lack of agreement in the scoring of items; when this occurs, the group can discuss the reasons for the differences in views and hopefully reach consensus on how the items should be interpreted

4. the overall quality scores can be used to help rank the guidelines in terms of meeting the various quality criteria. This type of assessment reduces the number of guidelines

under serious consideration by revealing those that clearly do not meet methodological standards for rigorous development.

Practice example

Box 13.3 presents some of the quantitative results of an interdisciplinary group's guideline appraisal activities (Ottawa Carleton CCAC Leg Ulcer Protocol Task Force). The group consisting of nurses (community and hospital), physicians (family physician, vascular surgeon, dermatologist, and haematologist), a clinical manager, and

health services researchers assessed five leg ulcer practice guidelines using the Appraisal Instrument for Clinical Guidelines. The group was able to easily identify five guidelines meeting their initial criteria and subject these to the Appraisal Instrument for Clinical Guidelines.

Systematically assessing the clinical content of guideline recommendations

The use of a guideline appraisal instrument will provide little detailed information on the actual

---

Box 13.3 Example of selected results of a quality appraisal process on leg ulcer practice guidelines

	RCN	SIGN	CREST	CNP/HFI	VEINES
Developers	Royal College of Nursing Institute (UK)(RCN Institute 1998)	Scottish Intercollegiate Network (SIGN 1998)	Clinical Resource Efficiency Support Team (Northern Ireland) (CREST 1998)	Compliance Network Physicians/ Health Force Initiative (Eriksson et al. 1999)	Venous Insufficiency Epidemiologic and Economic Studies Task Force (Clement 1999)
Date of release	1998	1998	1998	1999	1999
Date to be updated	2 yearly	2000	2001	Indicates reviewed continuously	Not specified

Results of the practice guideline quality assessments

	RCN	SIGN	CREST	CNP/HFI	VEINES
Standardised quality scores	Mean (95% CI)	Mean (95% CI)	Mean (95% CI)	Mean (95% CI)	Mean (95% CI)
Rigour of guideline development (D1)	72% (62–81)	55% (48–61)	45% (38–52)	35% (23–43)	13 (4–24)
Content and context (D2)	75% (62–88)	67% (58–77)	62% (53–71)	55% (34–77)	33 (12–54)
Application (D3)	45% (34–56)	70% (55–85)	40% (24–56)	25% (7–44)	2 (2–7)
Global rating out of 10	8.4 (7.7–9.1)	8.0 (7.2–8.8)	7.3 (6.5–8.0)	6.6 (6.2–8.1)	3.0 (1.7–4.3)
Global assessment					
Highly recommend	$n = 5$	$n = 5$			
Recommend with modification	$n = 7$	$n = 7$	$n = 11$	$n = 10$	$n = 2$
Not recommend			$n = 1$	$n = 1$	$n = 7$

Adapted from Ottawa Carleton CCAC Leg Ulcer Protocol Task Force 2000 recommendations being advanced by the guidelines. Thus, the next step is to conduct what essentially amounts to a content analysis of the recommendations contained in each guideline. We have found it useful to have one or two clinicians experienced in the content area of the guidelines produce a box comparing each guideline in terms of the specific recommendations it makes and the level of evidence supporting each recommendation. We refer to this box as the Recommendations Matrix or Layout (see Box 13.4 for an example). Using the Recommendations Matrix, the interdisciplinary group can then discuss the content of the various guidelines under consideration and quickly identify when the same recommendation is made by different guidelines or when the recommendations differ. The box also assists the group in easily identifying all recommendations supported by strong evidence. It is not uncommon for a guideline to consist of several recommendations supported by evidence of differing strengths. When this happens the group may want to select recommendations supported by the best evidence from the various guidelines under consideration. The Recommendations Matrix provides the basis for a discussion about the clinical usefulness of the recommendations being considered.

STEP 6 – ADAPTING EXISTING GUIDELINES FOR LOCAL USE

Having assessed the methodological quality of the guidelines using an appraisal instrument and then compared the content of the recommendations and the level of evidence supporting each recommendation, the interdisciplinary group must decide whether there is sufficient justification for the local use of any of the recommendations and, if so, which ones. Assuming the group supports the use of some of the recommendations, the next decision may be to either: adopt one particular guideline with all its recommendations as it is;

adopt one guideline and selectively endorse some of its recommendations (i.e. not endorse recommendations that are not supported by strong evidence or can not be implemented locally); or take the 'best' recommendations from each of the reviewed guidelines and repackage them into a new local guideline. The group leader's diplomacy and mediation skills can greatly facilitate this stage in the process. Our experience has been that as the group struggles with adapting existing guidelines, the local issues that might negatively impact on the use of the recommendations are carefully considered and solutions identified.

Guideline developers are always concerned that local adaptation of guidelines will result in the modification of recommendations to suite the local setting that ignore the evidence. Local adaptation of existing guidelines should never involve changing evidence-based recommendations unless the supporting evidence changes. Whenever recommendations are modified in any way, the rationale for this change should be explicitly stated in the resulting local guideline document.

The group should also keep in mind that it might want to update the evidence base supporting the recommendations if the guideline was not recently released or if group members are aware of recently released study results that might have a bearing on the recommendations. When this is the case, high-quality systematic reviews of the literature should be sought. The Cochrane database of systematic reviews and the Cochrane Controlled Trials Register (http://www.cochrane.org), the NHS Database of Abstracts of Reviews of Effectiveness (DARE) (http://nhscrd.york.ac.ek/darehp.htm), and the York Centre for Reviews and Dissemination (www.york.ac.uk/inst/crd) are good places to identify new evidence (Shekelle 1999).

Practice example

With one group that we were working with (Pressure Ulcer BPG Development Panel 2000),

Box 13.4 Example of a Recommendations Matrix: comparison of selected leg ulcer practice guideline recommendations with level of supporting evidence

	Practice guideline				
Recommendation	RCN+	SIGN	CREST	CNP/HFI	VEINES
Assessment of leg ulcers					
Record features indicative of non-venous disease	III	III	II		
The person conducting the assessment should be aware that ulcers may result from many different causes. If any unusual appearance refer for specialist assessment	III	III	III		
Information relating to the ulcer history should be recorded in a structured format: ulcer site, first occurrence, number of episodes, time to heal, past treatments, previous venous surgery, use of compression hosiery	III	II- current ulcer site only	*	III- current ulcer site only	
The following measurements should be taken: blood pressure, body mass index, urinalysis, and blood work (BW)	III- except BW		*BW only	*BW only	
Doppler measurement of the Ankle Brachial Pressure Index (ABPI)	I	II	I	II	
ABPI should be done by trained staff	II		*		
No routine bacteriological swabbing	I	I	II		*
Serial measurement of the ulcer	III	II	II		
Criteria for specialist referral	III	III	III		

Adapted from Ottawa Carleton CCAC Leg Ulcer Protocol Task Force 2000

I = level I evidence (evidence from randomised clinical trials or meta-analyses); II = level II evidence (evidence from well designed controlled or uncontrolled non-randomised studies); III = level III evidence (expert opinion, consensus statements, guideline developers' recommendation based on clinical experience); * = level of evidence not stated by guideline developers; Blank or empty boxes indicate no recommendation issued; + = RCN definitions of levels of evidence.

Level I = generally consistent finding in a majority of multiple acceptable studies; level II = either based on a single acceptable study, or a weak or inconsistent finding from multiple studies; level III = limited scientific evidence which does not meet all the criteria of acceptable studies or absence of directly applicable studies of good quality. This includes published or unpublished expert opinion.

the members decided on adopting many recommendations from one guideline that was several years old, and felt it was necessary to perform their own review of the literature to identify randomised clinical trials or other strong evidence that may have been published since the guideline was released. These data were incorporated into the guideline the group produced. In this case, the more recent evidence (a recent systematic review) supported the original recommendations, thus the group was not required to modify the recommendations. Additionally, this exercise provided the group with even greater confidence in their recommendations.

Strategies to promote guideline uptake

Once the local recommendations are decided upon, other guideline adaptation activities can also be undertaken to facilitate eventual guideline uptake (Littlejohns et al. 2000). This should involve ensuring that the recommendations are formatted in terms of measurable criteria and targets for quality improvement (Feder et al. 1999). These criteria are sometimes reported in guidelines, but often they are not (Graham et al. 2001). It is important to explicitly identify measurable criteria or outcomes for monitoring guideline adherence, as this ensures that the process of care reflects the guideline recommendations. The organisation's quality monitoring and improvement processes may provide an excellent venue to formalise this activity.

Uptake of the guideline can also be promoted by designing guideline prompts such as reminder systems. This can involve modifying assessment, charting or test ordering forms, or the electronic health record, so as to encourage the gathering of the appropriate data required to follow the guideline. The group should consider these implementation activities concurrently with the guideline adaptation process.

Practice example

After deciding on the recommendations to be included in the local protocol, one group designed a comprehensive assessment form that prompted the professional to collect all the clinical information necessary to make thoughtful decisions about the appropriateness of specific recommendations. The assessment form was designed with practitioners to ensure it met their charting needs,

and was subsequently incorporated into the institution's health record.

STEP 7 – EXTERNAL REVIEW

Practitioner and policy maker feedback on the proposed local guideline recommendations

Once the group has determined which recommendations will likely be included in the local guideline/protocol, the next step is to send the draft recommendations to local practitioners, other stakeholders, and even organisational policy makers for review. The process of seeking practitioner and policy maker feedback on the proposed guideline has several advantages:

1. it ensures that those who are most likely to use the guideline have had an opportunity to review it and offer their feedback; this feedback provides the group with an indication of potential practitioner acceptance of the guideline and it can also identify problems with the guideline or local issues that might inhibit its uptake;

2. it permits policy makers the opportunity to consider the impact of implementing the recommendations on the organisation (e.g. impact on human and financial resources) and to begin preparing for its future adoption;

3. the interdisciplinary group has an opportunity to revise the guideline based on the feedback before the final draft of the proposed guideline is formally put forward to policy makers for their endorsement

4. soliciting practitioner feedback serves as the first wave of dissemination of the proposed guideline.

The results from the practitioner and policy maker feedback process should be documented and any resulting changes to the guideline explicitly described.

Seeking practitioner feedback during the development of oncology guidelines has been an integral part of the Clinical Practice Guidelines Initiative of Cancer Care Ontario's Program in Evidence-Based Care (Browman et al. 1995) and has been shown to be beneficial (Browman et al. 1998). Opening up this two-way communication between those evaluating and adapting guidelines and the recipients of the guidelines has the potential to increase practitioner ownership of the eventual guideline. In addition it identifies controversial issues that might negatively impact guideline adoption, if the guideline developer neglected to proactively address them.

Practice example

With one project, the protocol developed by the group was sent to over 100 family physicians in the region who had patients with the identified condition. The protocol was faxed to the physicians with a questionnaire asking them: to write in any concerns they had about the protocol or implementing it; the extent to which they felt the protocol would be appropriate for their own patients; and to indicate whether the home-care authority should adopt the protocol. The value of undertaking the practitioner feedback was evident when written comments alerted the group to the need for an educational intervention for family physicians as many indicated that they were unfamiliar with how to conduct a particular clinical aspect of the protocol. The group was able to proactively respond to this concern by preparing educational information for physicians on the procedure that would accompany dissemination of the guideline.

Formal peer review

As should be the case with the development of all guidelines, locally adapted guidelines should also receive external peer review to ensure content validity, clarity and applicability (Shekelle

et al. 1999). It is also used to ensure the recommendations from existing guidelines have not been taken out of context or adapted inappropriately. Furthermore, independent review conducted by clinical content and/or methodological experts familiar with the welfare system, but outside the formal guideline evaluation and adaptation process, can enhance the credibility and legitimacy of the local guideline (Browman et al. 1995). Submitting the locally adapted guideline to a journal for publication and the necessary peer review process can also be used to fulfill the requirement for independent review. However, this process may be more cumbersome and time consuming than approaching independent experts directly. The local document should describe the results of the external review.

STEP 8 – FINALISATION OF THE LOCAL GUIDELINE

The local interdisciplinary group should respond to any recommendations from the practitioner and policy maker feedback, and independent reviewers. It should modify the guideline where appropriate. Any changes made to the guideline in response to this feedback should be documented. Similarly, in cases where the group chooses not to modify the guideline despite the feedback it receives, the rationale for this decision should be made explicit.

Practice example

With one group, the feedback process led to substantive changes in the draft guideline. The stakeholders responding to the draft guideline revealed that the original guideline evaluation group should have included more representation from allied professional groups. The reviewers offered specific suggestions about additional recommendations that might be included in the document. These suggestions were reviewed by the group and incorporated into the guideline.

STEP 9 – OFFICIAL ENDORSEMENT AND ADOPTION OF THE GUIDELINE BY THE ORGANISATION

This step involves the proposed guideline (which may have been modified based on practitioner and policy maker feedback or comments from the independent external reviewers) being reviewed by the sponsoring organisation and formally adopted and given official status. This is an administrative step which provides the organisation with its final opportunity to consider the impact of the proposed guideline on its functioning. The formal decision making and procedural process required to endorse a guideline needs to be made explicit and documented by the organisation. Once the organisation provides its 'seal of approval', the guideline is ready for dissemination and implementation.

STEP 10 – SCHEDULED REVIEW OF EXISTING GUIDELINES AND REVISION OF THE LOCAL GUIDELINE

The guideline group should provide an expiry date for the guideline to ensure that the evidence supporting the guideline recommendations is re-examined on a regular basis. Just as research evidence becomes dated or superceded by new research, practice guidelines and the evidence supporting guideline recommendations also become outdated. Situations requiring guidelines to be updated include those when there are: changes in the evidence on existing benefits and harms of interventions; changes in outcomes considered important; changes in available interventions; changes in evidence that current practice is optimal; changes in values placed on outcomes; and changes in resources available for health care (Shekelle et al. 2001). A guideline expiry date ensures that guideline recommendations will not continue to be applied indefinitely. There should also be contingency plans to update the local guideline whenever the guidelines upon which it was based are updated, or when new evidence becomes available that might alter the recommendations. Depending on the extent of the changes in guideline recommendations required by new evidence, the guideline group may want to simply seek practitioner and policy maker feedback on the changes or start the entire guideline evaluation cycle over again. In any case, plans for reviewing the guideline and any changes made to it must be documented.

CONCLUSION

With the ever increasing production of practice guidelines and the cost of rigorously developed evidence-based guidelines, it is becoming more feasible and efficient for local healthcare organisations to adapt existing guidelines for use rather than attempting to develop their own. Unfortunately, not all guidelines are created equally. Some guidelines are not rigorously developed or based on the most current research and their uncritical adoption is not prudent and may even result in harm.

This chapter described the Practice Guidelines Evaluation and Adaptation Cycle, a step-by-step map that both clinical and administrative decision makers can use when considering whether to adopt existing guidelines. A major advantage of using this framework is that it breaks down a fairly complicated process into discrete and achievable phases. It promotes the adoption of the best evidence-based recommendations after consideration of local needs and circumstances. The framework structures the guideline evaluation process so that it is inclusive of the stakeholders (both when evaluating the guidelines and in reviewing the local adaptation of them), rigorous, and systematic. The emphasis on documenting all decisions and reasons for them, as well as the details of the process (e.g. the search strategies, results of the guideline appraisal, content analysis of the recommendations and stakeholder feedback) ensures that the process is transparent and reproducible.

Another advantage of the process is the consensus building that occurs among practitioners, policy makers and others as an organisation works through evaluating and adapting guidelines. The process can also be a non-threatening educational and updating experience for the practitioners involved in reviewing the existing guidelines or commenting on the draft of the local guideline. One other important value of the process relates to the underlying assumption that by engaging an interdisciplinary group of stakeholders in such a process (step 1); ensuring that the resulting guideline is based on the best available evidence (steps 2–5); soliciting feedback on the draft local guideline from practitioners and policy makers, as well as other external reviewers and attending to this feedback (step 7); and considering strategies to promote the new guideline simultaneously with its development (step 6) the eventual uptake of the guideline is being promoted.

REFERENCES

AGREE Collaboration 2001 Appraisal of Guidelines for Research and Evaluation (AGREE) Instrument. http://www.agreecollaboration.org.

AGREE Collaboration 2003 Development and validation of an international appraisal instrument for assessing the quality of clinical practice guidelines; the AGREE project. Quality and Safety in Health Care 12: 18–23.

Bond CM 1995 Multi-disciplinary guideline development: a case study from community pharmacy. Health Bulletin 53(1): 26–33.

Browman GP, Levine MN, Mohide A et al. 1995 The practice guidelines development cycle: a conceptual tool for practice guidelines development and implementation. Journal of Clinical Oncology 13(2): 502–511.

Browman G, Newman T, Mohide A et al. 1998 Progress of clinical oncology guidelines development using the Practice Guidelines Development Cycle: The role of practitioner feedback. Journal of Clinical Oncology 16(3): 1226–1231.

Brown J, Shye D, McFarland B 1995 The paradox of guideline implementation: how AHCPR's depression guideline was adapted at Kaiser Permante Northwest region. Joint Commission Journal on Quality Improvement 21(1): 5–21.

Burns LR, Denton M, Goldfein S, Warrick L, Morenz B, Sales B 1992 The use of continuous quality improvement methods in the development and dissemination of medical practice guildelines. Quality Review Bulletin 18: 434–439.

Clement D 1999 Venous ulcer reappraisal: insights from an international task force. Journal of Vascular Research 39(Suppl 1): 42–47.

Cluzeau F, Littlejohns P, Grimshaw J, Feder G 1997 Appraisal instrument for clinical guidelines. St.George's Hospital Medical School. http://sghms.ac.uk/phs/hceu/

Cluzeau F, Littejohns P 1999 Appraising clinical practice guidelines in England and Wales: The development of a methodologic framework and its application to policy. Joint Commission Journal on Quality Improvement 25(10): 514–521.

Coulter I, Adams A, Shekelle P 1995 Impact of varying panel membership on ratings of appropriateness in consensus panels – a comparison of a multi- and single disciplinary panel. Health Services Research 30: 577–591.

CREST 1998 Guidelines for the assessment and management of leg ulceration. Recommendations for practice. Clinical Resource Efficiency Support Team (CREST), Belfast.

Eccles M, Clapp Z, Grimshaw J, Adams PC, Higgins B, Purves I et al. 1996 North of England evidence based guidelines development project: methods of guideline development. British Medical Journal 312: 760–761.

Eriksson E, Moffatt C, Neumann H, Stark G, Werner K, Wolff K 1999 Guidelines for outpatient treatment. Venous and venous-arterial mixed leg ulcer. Compliance Network Physicians/Health Force Initiative, www.cnhfi.de/index-engl.html.

Evidence-Based Care Resource Group 1994a Evidence-based care: 1. Setting priorities: How important is this problem? Canadian Medical Association Journal 158(8): 1249–1254.

Evidence-Based Care Resource Group 1994b Evidence-based care: 2. Setting guidelines: How should we manage this problem? Canadian Medical Association Journal 150(9): 1417–1423.

Feder G, Eccles M, Grol R, Griffith C, Grimshaw J 1999 Using clinical guidelines. British Medical Journal 318: 728–730.

Field M, Lohr K (eds) 1990 Clinical practice guidelines: directions for a new program. Institute of Medicine ed. Washington, DC: Institute of Medicine, National Academy Press.

Graham I, Beardall S, Carter A, Laupacis A 1997 The state of the art of practice guidelines development, dissemination, and evaluation in Canada. Scientific Basis for Health Services, Amsterdam.

Graham ID, Lorimer K, Harrison MB, Pierscianowski T for the Leg Ulcer Protocol Task Force, Leg Ulcer Protocol Task Force Working Group et al. 2000a Evaluating the quality and content of international clinical practice guidelines for leg ulcers: preparing for Canadian adaptation. Canadian Association of Enterostomal Therapy Journal 19(3): 15–31.

Graham ID, Calder L, Hebert P, Carter AO, Tetroe JM 2000b A comparison of clinical practice guideline appraisal instruments. International Journal of Technology Assessment in Healthcare 16(4): 1024–1038.

Graham I, Beardall S, Carter A, Glennie J, Hebert P, Tetroe J et al. 2001 What is the quality of drug therapy clinical practice guidelines in Canada? Canadian Medical Association Journal 165(2): 157–163.

Grilli R, Magrini N, Penna A, Mura G, Liberati A 2000 Practice guidelines developed by specialty societies: the need for a critical appraisal. Lancet 355: 103–106.

Grimshaw J, Russell I 1993 Effect of clinical guidelines on medical practice: a systemic review of rigorous evaluations. Lancet 242: 1317–1322.

Grimshaw J, Freemantle N, Wallace S et al. 1995 Developing and implementing clinical practice guidelines. Quality in Health Care 4: 55–64.

Jones J, Hunter D 1995a Consensus methods for medical and health services research. British Medical Journal 311: 372–380.

Jones J, Hunter D 1995b Consensus methods for medical and health services research. British Medical Journal 311: 376–380.

Kahan JP, Park RE, Leape LL et al. 1996 Variations by specialty in physician ratings of the appropriateness and necessity of indications for procedures. Medical Care 34: 512–523.

Karuza J, Calkins E, Feather J, Hershey CO, Katz L, Majeroni B 1995 Enhancing physician adoption of practice guidelines. Dissemination of influenza vaccination guideline using a small-group consensus process. Archives of Internal Medicine 155(6): 625–632.

Lewis S 2001 Further disquiet on the guidelines front. Canadian Medical Association Journal 165(2): 180–181.

Littlejohns P, Cluzeau F, Bales R, Grimshaw J, FG, Moran S 1999 The quality and quantity of clinical practice guidelines for the management of depression in primary care in the UK. British Journal of General Practice 49: 205–210.

Littlejohns P, Cluzeau F 2000 Guidelines for evaluation. Family Practice 17(1): S3–S6.

McGlynn E, Kosecoff J, Brook RH 1990 Format and conduct of consensus development conferences. International Journal of Technology Assessment in Health Care 6: 450–469.

McNicol M, Layton A, Morgan G 1993 Team working: The key to implementing guidelines? Quality in Health Care 2: 215–216.

Ottawa Carleton CCAC Leg Ulcer Protocol Task Force 2000 Ottawa Carleton Community Care Access Centre (CCAC) Venous Leg Ulcer Care Protocol: Development, methods, and clinical recommendations. Full Report. Loeb Health Research Institute, Ottawa.

Petrie J, Grimshaw JM, Bryson A 1995 The Scottish Intercollegiate Guidelines Network Initiative: Getting validated guidelines into local practice. Health Bulletin 53(6): 345–348.

Pressure Ulcer BPG Development Panel. Registered Nurses Association of Ontario (RNAO) Best Practice Guidelines. Assessment and management of stage I to IV pressure ulcers 2002 Toronto, Registered Nurses Association of Ontario. www.rnao.org/bestpractices/PDF/BPG_Pressure_Ulcer_Pt1.pdf

Royal College of Nursing Institute 1998 Clinical practice guidelines. The management of patients with venous leg ulcers. Recommendations for assessment, compression therapy, cleansing, debridement, dressing, contact sensitivity, training/education and quality assurance. Royal College of Nursing Institute, London www.rcn.org.uk/services/promote/clinic/clinical_guidelines.htm.

Shaneyfelt T, Mayo-Smith M, Rothwangl J 1999 Are guidelines following guidelines? The methodological quality of clinical practice guidelines in the peer-reviewed medical literature. Journal of the American Medical Association 281(20): 1900–1905.

Shekelle P, Woolf SH, Eccles M, Grimshaw J 1999 Developing guidelines. Western Journal of Medicine 170: 348–351.

Shekelle P, Eccles M, Grimshaw JM, Woolf SH 2001 When should clinical guidelines be updated? British Medical Journal 323(155): 157.

Scottish Intercollegiate Guidelines Network 1998 The care of patients with chronic leg ulcer. SIGN Publication Number 26. Scottish Intercollegiate Guidelines Network (SIGN), Edinburgh www.sign.ac.uk/html/htmtxt26.htm.

Sudlow M, Thomson R 1997 Clinical guidelines: quantity without quality. Quality in Health Care 6: 60–61.

Thomas L, Cullum N, McColl E, Rousseau N, Soutter J, Steen N 1999 Guidelines in professions allied to medicine. Cochrane Library 3: 1–14.

Varonen H, Makela M 1997 Practice guidelines in Finland: availability and quality. Quality in Health Care 6: 75–79.

Ward J, Grieco V 1996 Why we need guidelines for guidelines: a study of the quality of clinical practice guidelines in Australia. Medical Journal of Australia 165: 574–576.

Woolf SH, Grol R, Hutchinson A, Eccles M, Grimshaw J 1999 Potential benefits, limitations, and harms of clinical guidelines. British Medical Journal 318: 527–30.

Woolf SH 2000 Evidence-based medicine. Interpreting studies and setting policy. Hematology-Oncology Clinics of North America 14(4): 761–784.

Worrall G, Chaulk P, Freake D 1997 The effects of clinical practice guidelines on patient outcomes in primary care; a systematic review. Canadian Medical Association Journal 156: 1705–1712.

Wortman P, Smyth J, Langebrunner J, Yeaton W 1998 Consensus among experts and research sythesis. International Journal of Technology Assessment in Health Care 14(1): 109–122.

Organisational culture and the change agenda

SECTION CONTENTS

The impact of the culture of an organisation upon how care is delivered is well documented. Within this section the chapters explore this concept from both an individual and an organisational leadership perspective. In addition, this section explores some of the strategies and approaches that can be put in place to assist with that all elusive outcome of sustainable change which is the cornerstone of achieving the modernisation agenda.

14

Organisational culture

Amanda Ashton

KEY ISSUES

◆ Culture and change

◆ Creating a culture for a learning
  organisation

◆ Leadership

◆ Partnerships within learning
  organisations

◆ Teamwork

◆ Developing effective teamwork

◆ The professional organisation.

INTRODUCTION

From examples such as the Bristol Baby Heart Surgery Inquiry and the Kent and Canterbury Cervical Smear Test Inquiry there is insurmountable evidence that lives have been needlessly lost as a result of poor care. As a direct result of some of these incidents clinical governance frameworks are now a statutory obligation in every care institution and mirror the same legal requirements as corporate governance which covers the finance agenda. As with corporate governance, clinical governance and best value can also be seen to be an enforced system of quality control. Consequently, issues surrounding *control* and *freedom* to practice are central to the success or failure of quality improvement. However, the environment or cultural context within which systems and people work can be viewed as the most important factor in determining success or failure. This chapter will consider issues around culture, leadership, partnerships and teamwork and their contribution to the modernisation agenda.

CULTURE AND CHANGE

Many discussions take place about the culture of the organisations in which we work. We like to think that we have an empowered approach for staff within services. Often we find established ways or systems of management, such as a shared governance philosophy, which give clear frameworks and messages to staff and those who use the service that staff are empowered and able to take decisions at local levels.

However, changes to culture take time to happen: the welfare system is a complex adaptive system, and there are rarely simple answers to complex issues. The need to understand the complexity of the situation is the most important starting point for any leader. Secondary to this is the need to find a way of working effectively with this complexity.

It is worthwhile considering some of the key themes that emerge from an analysis of this area. In doing this, it becomes clear that the paradigm of simplicity and the actual experience of organisational life are important issues to consider. There is a need to understand the vocabulary of the different people involved: the underlying concepts, the grammar, and the staff thinking structures and their application. For example, the interpretation of what is meant when we talk about empowerment, culture and decision making will vary according to each individual.

The key assumption that is often made is that culture needs to change or, indeed, that culture can change into something different. The initial question relating to clinical governance and best value has to be: why change the culture within the welfare services? A subsequent question would be: is it possible to plan this change? Furthermore, if change is necessary or inevitable, what kind of change is envisaged and to what end?

Activity 14.1

Focusing upon your own organisation consider your response to the questions below:

How would you describe the present culture where you work?

How may this affect the implementation of clinical governance within the organisation/department or team where you work?

Does the culture need to change?

If so what sort of change do you envisage should happen?

A word of caution about cultural change (Bates 1999), is that the 'push button' for change action is an elusive concept in itself. Culture is not an objective state, something which can be manipulated and controlled. For example, a hospital has a culture, nursing has a culture, and as such it is not a technical or scientific activity capable of control or tampering.

Any organisation is an excellent example of a microcosm of the wider world, a construct within which, for example, professionals work. As individual professional groups and as a team of people, each have their own myths and stories, rites and rituals, each influencing the other. Altering these cultural factors is difficult and, indeed, the question needs to be asked should they be, or could they be tampered with? It is important to honour the past, live in the present, then work for a future. Consequently, there is the need to look at culture as something that is alive and set within a context, an environment, and multitudes of people; it is not something that exists within a vacuum (Bridges 1980).

In addition, it is difficult to extrapolate culture from strategy, as strategy supplies the context and direction for work. Deciding on what kind of strategy you may have for clinical governance and best value may help with the fusion of culture and change. Bates (1999) describes four types of strategies:

- Conforming – they adapt/perpetuate the existing social construction
- Deforming – they aim to subvert existing states
- Reforming – they aim to remove existing social constructions
- Transforming – they move across from one form of social construction to another.

Activity 14.2

Following from the answers you formulated in the first activity, consider which type of strategy you would adopt in your organisation when implementing clinical governance and best value.

You may need to consider using one or maybe a combination of all four, depending on the organisation/team size and complexity. Remember too that different groups of staff will have different myths, values, rituals and pasts that will need to be recognised and honoured. The importance of the past and associated values is an important feature to consider. Staff often need to be collectively encouraged to express their valued purposes, which, in effect, shaped their visions and enabled them to formulate their feelings and judgements about the way they want their world to be in the future. In this respect culture, strategy and values become the main

levers for change, and understanding how they are interlinked, and at times compliment and also clash with each other, is an important feature to understand (Hill 1991).

So let us use strategy and values to consider how we may attempt to change a culture in keeping with the principles of modernisation. The question now is what needs to change and how would you start to do it?

Bates (1999) provides four different approaches for consideration:

- Aggressive – power coercive, conflict-centred, non-collaborative, win–lose, imposed and unilateral
- Conciliative – group problem solving, win–win, collaborative, emergent, integrative, a joint approach
- Corrosive – political, coalitional, unplanned, evolutionary, networking, the informal approach
- Indoctrinative – normative, re-educative, the training approach.

Activity 14.3

Using Bates' model for changing culture, critically appraise each approach in relation to your own place of work. Consider the staff, the systems established, the context and environment of your workplace. What would be the driving forces of using each approach and what would be the obstacles? Are you able to choose one approach, or do you favour an eclectic approach?

So what is the best way to approach change and culture in the context of the modernisation agenda? The answer is difficult, however, it could be argued that an eclectic approach combining all four approaches might be the favoured option. The work that fuses these approaches for many is that of creating a learning organisation (Senge 1991).

CREATING A CULTURE OF A LEARNING ORGANISATION

An organisation, whether it be a large hospital, a social services department or a health centre, needs to be in 'good shape'. By this I mean a place where there is a no blame culture, there is transparency in practice, there is good communication between staff members and, above all, there is a philosophy of people, either staff or users of the service, being at the centre of practice. It is for this reason that Senge's (1991) work around learning organisations becomes most relevant in respect to determining leadership style and cultural context for changing practice. Within this it is important to create an environment of supported learning and empowerment for all staff.

Fundamental to this idea is the human desire to learn. For example, a child will learn to walk, talk and build a tower from building blocks. On a recent holiday I watched the children on the beach: all possessed an insatiable drive to explore and experiment: 'how can I get my bucket to fill with water? Wait for the wave; don't get caught in the wave, run away quickly'. It took about a minute for a young girl to learn the important techniques required to build sandcastles. Is this how we manage people or teams? Are we leaders who encourage and develop environments to enable people, or do we either knowingly or subconsciously develop places and ways of working to disable teams, patients/clients and their carers?

What did the mother of that young girl on the beach do to help her get her bucket of water? She sat in the shade 15 metres from the seashore, she observed, she nodded and she smiled at the child when the task was completed. The girl's face beamed and she shrieked and jumped with delight – so much so that the water spilled! How can we, as leaders within health care capture these moments in our organisations? The wealth and richness of intrinsic motivation and pleasure

in learning and growing must be seen as a vital resource in times of change. That 'whoop of joy' is measurable in terms of energy. The role of the mother was not one of command or control but, as Senge writes, one of designer, teacher and steward. In short, the mother was responsible for building a place for her daughter where she can continually expand her capabilities to shape her future – as a leader, a mother is responsible for the learning of her child.

As I sat and observed this scene I had a feeling of unease, as I feared the girl could get caught in the wave and without water wings could be in danger. This fear or tension happens in organisations where learning is central. 'Creative tension' between where we want to be (the vision) and the current reality of where we are. Similarly, we need to create a vision, yet still understand and have a clear insight into the realities of the pain and difficulties of letting go of our past, honouring the past and then moving forward into the new: the recognised steps or transitions of change (Bridges 1980). The idea of creative tension becomes an important feature; the question becomes: how can we create it in a positive and productive way?

The need to lead through creative tension is specifically required, as it is different to leading through problem solution. In problem solving, the energy for change comes from attempting to get away from an aspect of current reality that is undesirable. With creative tension, the energy for change comes from the vision, from what we want to create, juxtaposed with current reality. The distinction may be small, but the consequences are not (Flaherty 1999).

Many people and organisations find themselves motivated to change only when their problems are bad enough to cause them to change. This works for a while, but the change process runs out of steam as soon as the problems during the change become less pressing or more often than not in large systems such as welfare services, they are replaced by other problems requiring more urgent attention. With problem solving, the motivation for change is intrinsic. This mirrors the distinction between adaptive and generative learning, the former having more success in achieving sustainable change in terms of behaviours and, consequently, changed outcomes (Senge 1991).

Activity 14.4

Coordinate a group of people who represent all stakeholders in your service including patients/clients/carers. Ask each of these people to share with each other a piece of music or art that expresses how they understand their current reality and their vision for the future of the service and the organisation.

I was inspired by a question posed by a factory owner in Zimbabwe who wished to improve the morale and productivity of his workforce. He asked: 'How can we make the factory really dance?' If you are familiar with African culture you will be aware of how important music, rhythm and dance are within their cultural setting, this question, therefore, has particular poignancy and relevance. To be able to dance you have to understand the rhythm of the music and work with your partner or the team. There has to be some understanding about when to make an entrance and when to stop. However, one of the most important factors is in developing a sense of fun and having a creative tension that is enjoyable. Change and transitions can be painful, yet in creating a separate plain, or a shift in paradigm thinking linking vision with current reality, an excitement that fosters our childlike abilities to develop, learn and create a new environment or culture may be achieved.

One of the most important factors in leading is the ability to understand the myths, legends and stories which underpin the socialisation processes, behaviours and consequent needs of the workforce. In this respect understanding cultural issues

and interconnections of relationships and history become important (Shiemann 1989).

NEW IDEAS FOR LEADERSHIP

I would like to take you back to the beach again. This time it is an Italian scene. Two middle aged men are introducing their respective son and daughter, both in their early 20s, to each other for the first time. The young man is bronzed, long hair in a ponytail with knee length swimming shorts. The young woman is cute, dark and in a respectable light blue bikini. They start off as a foursome talking as they stand close to the water. The conversation pairs off into couples – the two older men and the two youngsters. The two men stay by the shore; the young couple sit down back on the beach towel. Both couples carefully watch each other to make sure all is in order!

The point of this scenario is that the traditional authoritarian image of the 'Papa' – the leader in a traditional Italian family – has been over simplified with myths and legends associated with that culture, just like the 'boss calling the shots' has equally been recognised as being simplistic as well as inadequate in current cultures. However, leadership is intertwined with the development of cultures – shaping their evolution and sustaining viability. Like families, continuity and survival, the sustaining characteristics in a leader are not those of authority, command and control, but those of designer, teacher and steward. The Italian fathers may have looked awesome, but they knew what they were doing and their children were happy with it.

Leader as designer

It is fruitless to be a leader in an organisation that is poorly designed. Design does not refer to a structure and moving around names within a wiring diagram. Social or people architecture is at the heart of design – deciding on what are the governing ideas of purpose, vision and core values by which people will live. Defining and designing how staff wished to *be* rather than what they *do* must be the first task to be completed (Van Maanen & Schein 1979).

Activity 14.5

Take some time out with the team and encourage them to think about the ways in which they wish to work: not what tasks they need to perform, but the ways in which they will perform them.

The success will be in the demonstration of behaviours to underpin this statement: '... and when that happens we will be able to transform our services'. The following principles may well be some ways of working that staff aspire to:

- We will always act in the best interests of patients/clients and carers.
- We will be supportive of our colleagues within the team/practice/service.
- We will act with integrity and respect each other.
- We will build relationships with colleagues outside of our team based on these values.

Leader as teacher

This work relating to design should also be combined with the second role of a leader in a learning organisation – that of teacher. Leader as a teacher does not mean a leader as an authoritarian expert whose job it is to teach people the 'correct' view of reality. It is about helping the team, including yourself, to gain more insightful views of current reality.

Welfare organisations are politically driven: national and local policy and strategy could be viewed as major tools for radical change within the system. Performance management and development against nationally set targets is accepted

practice across services: clinical governance has a very clear direction for healthcare staff, as does the best value initiative for social care. It could be argued that this is a new reality and that setting a vision to reach this goal is a top priority.

Activity 14.6

Take time to measure the performance of your team/organisation against the reality of clinical governance and best value targets and associated expectations. Some questions you could ask include:

- Where are we now against these aspirations?
- Where should we be and in what time scale?
- How are we going to get there?

Benchmarks of current practice and areas of excellence can be shared between different teams and subsequent project plans compiled. These could become your maps for the medium term and provide a sense of direction and purpose during times of change. By encouraging staff to liberate their minds, acknowledging their natural tensions between fear for the future (or opportunity) and present uncertainty (or excitement) becomes an integral part of your personal evolution as a team.

Leader as steward

This is the one component of leadership, unlike the components of designer and teacher, that is almost solely a matter of attitude. It is an attitude critical to learning organisations, where leaders engaged in a learning organisation naturally feel part of a larger purpose that goes beyond their organisation (Greenleaf 1991).

Leaders' sense of stewardship operates on two levels – for the people they lead and for the larger purpose of that organisation. The first type arises from a deep appreciation of the impact one's leadership can have on others. People can suffer economically, emotionally and spiritually under inept leadership. It could be argued that staff working in a learning organisation are more vulnerable because of their commitment and sense of shared ownership.

Activity 14.7

Can you or members of your team think of leaders who have inspired you and have demonstrated the principles of leaders as stewards?

What changes were they able to bring about and, referencing back to Bates' models for cultural change, which category did they fit into?

The principles of a leader for a learning organisation may fit quite well; the task is to try and spread this amongst the team, so an environment for leadership is created which could become self sustaining and embodies learning and empowerment.

PARTNERSHIPS WITHIN A LEARNING ORGANISATION

To work effectively, clinical governance and best value requires partnerships within and between teams, professionals and managers; between individuals and the organisation, staff, patients/clients/carers and the public. Effective involvement of the whole system is essential to ensure that everyone is fully engaged in the drive for quality. Organisations need to be sure that they focus on what matters, that is excellence in care. So *team working*, and finding the *best type* of model for team working for clinical governance and best value is important.

A paradox is presented in that modernisation is a driver for change that is enforced by law, yet at the same time it demands the total cooperation of a diverse group of people. Within this group there are many struggles for power and leadership, freedom to practice as well as the pull to conform and standardise. Institutional mindsets

versus the need to change and the breaking down of traditional hierarchies pose a great challenge in the future.

To discover more let us look at the following issues:

- *Teamworking and group dynamics.* This is all about people working together as a team. Burying professional boundaries and working as one team is essential.
- *Professional interfaces.* This is about power, gender, leadership, the art of war and every single bit of human behaviour we could wish to examine! It is a fascinating insight into the mysteries within organisations and games associated with work dynamics.
- *Leadership.* Clinical governance and best value will not go anywhere without inspirational leadership. With this part, I really want to look for something beyond a textbook. I want to define what the working world of a care environment could look and feel like; for example, what would a hospital look like if we were to build a place of peace to heal the sick and which cherishes those who suffer.
- *Control and philosophies of control.* An external force is compelling organisations to manage a system of enforced quality control, what does this mean for the care environment?

TEAMWORK

So often we read in the newspapers and hear on the news that the people working in welfare services do not care anymore. However, what is the reality of the situation? What does it feel like to be in the middle of such a complex system? Social defences are a part of everyday life within the care setting, and this is not a new part of working life. Work in the 1960s (Menzies 1989) perfectly demonstrated that in order for nurses to survive doing their jobs they chose to depersonalise activities. Caught between compassion and despair, often engaged in tasks that *'by ordinary standards are distasteful, disgusting and frightening'*. By splitting off their sense of personal authority and agency from their own experience and projecting it onto a social defence, they relieved themselves of responsibility for the individual's experience. This context of caring and organisational life forms a backcloth for the exploration of teams and teamworking within the care setting, and is a unique environment for teams to work effectively within.

Any organisation is a big group consisting of small groups and, in this respect, the success of that organisation will be dependent on the diverse group performances. This is why it is so important to understand the effectiveness of groups, teams and group behaviour. The following activity gives some signposts you could use to evaluate teamwork.

Activity 14.8

Why are group and teamworking important to bring about excellence in care?

How can teams be helped to work more effectively and therefore continually improve standards of care?

Are there tensions in the relationship between group performance and individual performance, within different professional groups which detract from teamworking and good quality care?

So why is teamworking so important within modernisation? It is suggested that there are certain conditions when group working is beneficial (Bowey & Conelly 1977):

- When it produces a better end result – maybe in terms of quality, speed or efficiency – than working separately.
- When the joining together of work into a joint task or area of responsibility would appear meaningful to those involved.

- Where the joint task requires a mixture of different skills.
- Where competition between individuals leads to less effectiveness rather than more.
- Where stress levels on individuals are too high for effective activity.

This framework can be used in many situations to measure when there needs to be a set of beneficial group conditions. A&E is a good example to use, as group effectiveness is essential in a crisis or life saving situation. There is no room for ineffective or poor teams in this situation.

Case example

A 5-year-old girl arrives by ambulance 'blue light 999' into A&E. She fell off her swing in the back garden and has banged her head. She has been unconscious for 20 minutes. Her mother is with her, distraught, and as a single mother she has had to bring her second child with her, aged 18 months.

If we were to apply Bowey and Conelly's framework to team working in A&E what could the comments from staff be? You may wish to use the table below to capture your thoughts with regard to what needs to be in place to ensure effective teamworking in this particular context.

End result speed & outcome	Meaningful responsibility	Mixture of skills	Less competition	Stress levels

All of these propositions are relevant and important to introduce successfully a 'whole systems approach' to the different aspects of care and treatment an individual patient and their families require, expect and desire. Modernisation is about pulling all aspects of care into one successful outcome and, in this respect, making sure teams operate effectively is an essential prerequisite.

However, group effectiveness can present a number of problems, which need to be addressed from the beginning. Group effectiveness is about the group being good enough, and organised sufficiently to achieve its task related objectives, i.e. diagnosis, stabilisation and treatment of the 5-year-old child. However, there are two further dimensions to consider: those of the achieve-ment of the external task and group satisfaction, and, secondly, the internal aspects of the group. Both of these dimensions are measured in different ways.

There is an assumption that the individual will judge the performance of the group in terms of fulfilling his/her needs for friendship, develop-ing or confirming a sense of identity, establishing and testing reality, and increasing both security and the sense of purpose. So member satisfaction and inner knowledge of how we are as individuals is important, and may be regarded as a measure to which internal group goals are achieved. Group satisfaction, that is the extent to which a group sat-isfies the needs of its members and is successful in maintaining itself as a working unit, may affect how productive, caring or safe it may be in respect of delivering health care.

The Hawthorne studies (Buchanan & Huczynski 1997) demonstrated that increasing productivity was not dependent on the physical environment of the organisation, but the social cohesiveness of the team of workers. Mayo wrote that the satis-faction of social needs in face-to-face cooperative relationships with fellow workers should become a prime goal of enlightened management. There is a potential for providing better outcomes for those who use the service if there is an under-standing of the needs of the staff within their teams. Basically, if they are able to fulfil their own individual desires, or social support and cooperation, then they may be more able to enter into meaningful relationships with their work, patients/clients and colleagues.

TEAMS AND THEIR EFFECTIVENESS

So what makes an effective team? McGregor iden-tifies eleven features, which distinguish an effec-tive group from an ineffective one (McGregor 1960):

- informal relaxed atmosphere that demonstrates involvement and interest
- full participation by all members with a clear focus on the task
- acceptance by all of the group objective
- members listen to each other and are not afraid to make creative suggestions
- disagreements are discussed and either resolved or lived with
- most decisions are made by consensus
- criticism is frank and frequent without degenerating into personal attack
- people are free to express their feelings about both the task and the group's way of achieving that task
- actions are clearly assigned to group members and are carried out by them
- leadership within the group shifts from time to time and tends to be based on expert knowledge rather than on formal status or position
- the group is self-conscious about its own operation and regularly reviews the way it goes about its business.

What do people at the grass roots level think about teamworking? If you are to understand the local issues then their opinion is of vital impor-tance. In response to the question – 'from your experience of working in an effective team, what do you think makes that team effective?' poten-tial feedback could be as follows:

- complimentary roles in the team
- good leadership

- rewards for effort and achievement
- owning the goals
- job security
- light-hearted atmosphere
- tact
- diplomacy
- sharing responsibilities
- fairness
- openness
- working off each other's strengths.

The message from the staff is similar to the work of the theorists. Language is important; being knowledgeable of, and using, the same words and phrases as the people in the teams may influence their effectiveness. Conflicts can occur when people use management speak and, although the theory and associated words are good for learning purposes, it is important that the classroom is translated into the reality of the healthcare environment if change is to be meaningful.

Bates (1999) talks about the use of border guards within organisations during any period of change. These people know the language of the people of their organisations; they are used as translators and assist staff in understanding the various issues involved when moving to uncharted parts and the ideals of the organisation. We could visualise a team of border guards, who, like chameleons adopt and change to the most appropriate form/use of language to suit the needs/circumstances of the team during times of change. They carry when necessary, they enable, and they let go. In this way they become servant leaders with the organisation.

So what are the possible responses to the question: 'what do you think hinders team effectiveness?':

- narrow mindedness
- lack of communication
- mood swings amongst members

- one member working to their own ends
- leaving unfinished work for others
- looking after your own goals and not the team's
- lack of leadership
- no understanding of roles
- competition for personal advancement.

Activity 14.9

Using the information above how could you increase member satisfaction and, therefore, improve outcomes within the context of clinical governance?

HOW CAN WE DEVELOP MORE EFFECTIVE TEAMWORK?

It could be argued that rather than throwing people together and hoping that they will form a team, managers can take four conscious steps in order to increase the likelihood of effective team performance:

- Step 1: pre-work
- Step 2: creating performance conditions
- Step 3: forming and building a team
- Step 4: providing ongoing help.

Our knowledge of how groups develop through the forming, storming, norming and performance phases and Belbin's (1981) research on group member roles can form the basis for the interventions. However, this investment in learning, that Hackman purports, does pay dividends in terms of improved team performance and team member satisfaction.

Case example

Using a structured approach to creating their team enhanced the success of an Obstetric and

Gynaecology Team for Clinical Governance. A series of timeouts was used to develop an overall value driven vision for their work. A timetable and project plan was created within the team and communication channels were identified to make sure that all staff had the opportunity to comment and become involved with the ideals.

Cohesion is an important factor in keeping a group or a team together. Modernisation is not a 'one day wonder', but a concept which needs to become entrenched into everyone's daily work pattern. Sustainability of groups or teams is very important in this context. However, the question of whether cohesion helps or hinders group effectiveness needs to be considered. What are the factors that keep the team together? What attracts and what repulses? Evidence would support that there are certain indicators which measure group cohesion, such as the degree of trust and support between members, and the amount of satisfaction they gain from their membership. Various theories of group behaviour emphasise the social exchange idea whereby individuals make an evaluative judgement about the gift relationship within the team, i.e. what they put in, in relation to what they get out of it.

Synergy within the group is also vital, that is the ability of the group to 'outperform its best individual member'. Research would suggest that teams which are effective actively look for the points on which they disagreed early on in their discussions, and, therefore, actively encourage proactive approaches to conflict resolution early in the process of working together. Conversely, groups that performed poorly usually focused on completing the task and were willing to accept a common view quickly to see the task completed. Insights into the obstetric team would support this theory. Tensions between the midwives and doctors were high at the beginning of their timeouts and some creative discussions full of healthy tension resulted in a compromise being reached relating to how clinical governance was to be implemented.

However, there are some downsides of group cohesion. Two phenomena include the 'risky shift' phenomenon and 'group think' (Buchanan & Huczynski 1997). The risky shift phenomenon may occur within a group when it makes decisions that are riskier than those that the members of the group would have recommended individually. Associated with this is group polarisation, which is when individuals in a group begin by taking a moderate stance on an issue related to a common value and, having discussed it, end up taking a more extreme stance. Evidence would suggest that decisions made collectively tend to be more risky when compared with individual decisions.

A second potentially negative consequence of group cohesion is group think. Group think may occur when members striving for unanimity override their motivation to appraise realistically the alternative courses of action (Janis 1982). Thus, while group adhesion can make a positive contribution to group productivity and satisfaction, it may also have negative consequences.

Circumstances surrounding the Bristol Heart Inquiry and other similar incidents would infer that 'group think' played a role within the decision-making process. This suggests that people were not willing to break ranks in respect of what they knew as individuals. In this context, the increased mortality rates of one surgeon were ignored for many years. An interesting element of this is the possibility of whether such a thing as enforced group think that is coercive in its intent can exist.

THE PROFESSIONAL ORGANISATION

The professional organisation is unique; it is democratic, disseminating its power directly to its workers (at least those lucky enough to be professional). It provides them with extensive autonomy even freeing them from the need to coordinate closely with their colleagues. So the professional has the best of both worlds: attached to an organisation and free to serve patients or clients, being constrained only by the established standards of the profession.

However, in these same characteristics, democracy and autonomy, lie the problems for the welfare organisations. There is no evident way to correct deficiencies that the professionals choose to overlook. Inherent within this is the endemic issue of overlooking problems of coordination, of discretion and innovation (Mintzberg 1999). This is what led to the original enquiries and the creation of the concept of clinical governance.

It is argued that the professional has two basic tasks: to categorise the client's needs in terms of a contingency, which indicates which standard programme to use, a task known as diagnosis; and to apply or execute that programme (Mintzberg 1999). What frequently emerges in the professional bureaucracy are parallel administrative hierarchies; one democratic and bottom up for the professional, and a second machine, bureaucratic and top down for the support staff (Mintzberg 1999).

Structures are, however, meaningless unless they are considered within the context of the strategy process. It is the development and production of strategy that clearly marked the difference between the environment of professional bureaucracy and what occurs in other models. For example, at the extreme, each professional pursues his or her own product market strategy, often at the expense of a collective approach. In this context, strategies are formed within professional bureaucracies each of which takes cognisance of developing national priorities in the local market. Such professionally based strategies constantly create tension within the welfare system.

The successful implementation of clinical governance is dependent upon the cooperation of the medical staff and other professional groups. Here we can clearly see the tensions between professional bureaucracies and enforced change. The need to adopt the principles of clinical governance in the welfare services will demand professionals and others to work in different ways. The 'what's in it for me' tenet is strong, and previously there were no rewards or sanctions to ensure change and to support people to work in different ways.

I would suggest that a different type of leadership is essential to make this shift: the ambiguity of transformational change, and the need to bring the professionals along with these changes is the key challenge for leadership within clinical governance.

CONCLUSION

So what would we wish to create in our welfare services to implement the key principles of quality improvement?

The first is an *environment for learning*, where staff feel *empowered* to make their own decisions within their own teams. They also feel motivated to be the best and provide excellence in care delivery, where they feel that if things go wrong they will not be blamed but will be helped to put it right and improve next time. The importance of *effective team working* and *devolved decision making* is vital.

Secondly, is the need for *leaders* within the organisation to have an *insight into their own style and way of being* and to be *truly connected* with the major purpose of the business. To hold the appropriate values as the keystone for the work of the organisation with the necessary associated behaviours to make it a reality is the major building block for change. There is an overriding need to stop compartmentalising people dependent upon our professional focus to people who have their lives, feelings, responsibilities and are 'whole beings'. This development moves away from analytical thinking to systems thinking for the treatment, care and support of those who use the services.

Thirdly, is the desire for a greater understanding of the importance of living with *tension and ambiguity*. By this, I mean the necessity to manage the transition of a professional bureaucracy into a more devolved decision-making matrix organisation, balancing and managing the tension of freedom versus control.

The need for accountability and empowerment and the change in the services, which underpins this shift, causes tension and insecurity. This needs to be led and managed at all levels with staff understanding why the 'both, and' concept is so important at this time.

The complexity of welfare organisations as microcosms of the society in which we operate is immense and clearly demonstrates that change of this order is massive. The homeostatic function within welfare services to keep it stable and maintain the status quo is strong. Equally, the need for change is also irresistible. The dichotomy for leadership and management within this often magnetic, gravitational pull is, I believe, one of the most challenging organisational change programmes in any organisation – perhaps nationally, or even internationally. Clinical governance and best value and its implementation in our services will be a significant measure of that successful change.

REFERENCES

Bates P 1999 Strategies for cultural change. Butterworth-Heinemann, Oxford.

Belbin RM 1981 Management teams: why they succeed or fail. Heinemann, London.

Bowey AM, Conelly R 1977 Application of the concept of group working. University of Strathclyde Business School, Glasgow.

Bridges W 1980 Transitions, making sense of life's changes. Nicholas Brearley, London.

Buchanan D, Huczynski A 1997 Organisational behaviour. Prentice Hall, Europe, pp.178–189.

Flaherty J 1999 Coaching: evoking excellence in others. Butterworth-Heinemann, Oxford.

Greenleaf R 1991 Servant leadership: a journey into the nature of legitimate power and greatness. Paulist Press, Mahwah, NJ.

Hill S 1991 Why quality circles failed but total quality management might succeed. British Journal of Industrial relations 29(4): 541–568.

Janis IL 1982 Victims of group think: a psychological study of foreign policy decisions and fiascos, 2nd edn. Houghton Mifflin, Boston, MA.

McGregor D 1960 The human side of enterprise. McGraw-Hill, New York.

Menzies I 1989 Containing anxiety in institutions: selected essays. Free Association Books, London.

Mintzberg H 1999 The professional organisation. In: Mintzberg H (ed.) The Strategy Process. Prentice Hall, Europe.

Senge P 1991 The fifth discipline, the art and practice of the learning organisation. Doubleday Books, New York.

Shiemann WA 1989 Strategy-culture-communication: three keys to success. Executive Excellence.

Van Maanen J, Schein EH 1979 Toward a theory of organisational socialisation. Research Organisation Behaviour 1: 209–264.

15

Achieving change

Helen Chin

KEY ISSUES

- ◆ 21st century services

- ◆ Why do we need to change

- ◆ The nature of change and the meaning of culture

- ◆ Understanding diversity

- ◆ Tilting triangles – dispelling popular myths

- ◆ New ways of thinking – insights from complexity science

- ◆ Models of change

- ◆ Developing the organic learning organisation

- ◆ Organisations that live and learn

- ◆ Creating the environment

- ◆ Providing the framework for learning and change

- ◆ Playing together as a team

- ◆ Structures to support change

- ◆ Support to stay outside the comfort zone.

We must be the change we want to see in the world.

[Ghandi]

INTRODUCTION

This chapter aims to challenge current thinking and practices regarding achieving effective change within the welfare services. It will provide dynamic and workable models and strategies that are based upon contemporary ideas about how our world interacts in reality. In addition, this chapter explores how we might apply these models in developing a truly modernised and synergistic health- and social-care service. These new ways of thinking embrace and seek to understand the nature and complexity of the modern world, its fast pace, constant change and uncertainty, and its inevitable effects on the current context of care. As we begin to understand what is really happening, we can make sense of the chaos and disorder; lose the fear; embrace creativity, innovation and change; and emerge into a world of health and social care which is suited to the 21st century.

21st CENTURY HEALTH CARE

Here I invite you to follow me on a journey into the future …

5th December 2011

I have just returned home after a 15-hour day, which included a 6-hour return drive in appalling weather. It was a normal day in many respects. After such days I usually feel energised knowing that I have made a difference in somebody's life. My work is centred on personal and professional development. It is demanding but incredibly rewarding. This time it is different. I feel awful. I am all at once hot and cold and am coughing up a really nasty substance. I have no energy and I ache all over. My head is pounding. I have probably got the 'flu'. I cannot afford the time to be ill. I will need some sort of medical help. It is 11pm.

I switch on my computer, log on to my GP's network, key in my personal identification number (PIN) and once accepted, swipe my health smart card through the gismo on the keyboard. I answer a set of questions, which takes me about 1 minute and then the video-link to my GP opens up. We go through the normal routine of polite social exchange and then I relate my ailments. Following a question and answer session, I have indeed got the 'flu', but have also acquired a secondary chest infection. I need rest, fluids, paracetamol and a course of antibiotics. I thank my GP, re-swipe my smart card and log off, again using my PIN.

An hour later the mobile pharmacy service is at my front door with my prescription for antibiotics. All of my details have gone directly from the GP's computer to their terminals including my prescription. The pharmacy service asks for my PIN, which they key into a hand held computer. This gives them a code to a secure portable unit, which cannot be opened until my health smart card is swiped through it and a retinal scan is confirmed as mine. Identification and details are verified and I sign for and accept my drugs. The pharmacy service takes a sample of sputum, which will go directly to the lab for analysis. Once the lab has the results, they are sent to my GP's computer, which has the ability to check and see if I have the right antibiotic to cure the chest infection. If not, the computer alerts the GP who will then inform me of a change in treatment by e-mail.

In the space of 1 hour, I have had a professional consultation, received a preliminary diagnosis and interim treatment, all in the comfort and convenience of my own home. The process has been efficient, effective, tailored to my 21st century lifestyle and reassuring …

Back to the present

I could go on here to relate a whole series of events involving my brush with illness and how it could be tailored to meeting my healthcare needs in contemporary life, but I think you already have the picture. An idealistic notion of health care perhaps? Well, no. I actually think that the above scenario, in some shape or form, will become the future reality of healthcare provision and, in some ways, it is already beginning to happen (see Box 15.1). It is something we need to get used to and it will be a significant change from what we already know and accept.

Those who know me well know that I do not 'do' queues. I do not like to wait, nor do I like to sit around in a doctor's surgery after waiting for 3 days for an appointment, by which time I may be in even worse health than I was before. I am not an impatient person, nor am I unappreciative of the hard work and effort which has gone into making our health service one of the best in the world, but like many others these days, I work long hours in a fast-paced environment. My downtime is valuable and special. Anything which saves me time and is also effective is very much appreciated.

In the current system, I could have called out the emergency GP and taken up his precious time. I could have called NHS Direct who would have probably told me to go see my GP or visit my local Walk-in-Centre. I could have gone to the nearest casualty unit and taken up their valuable time and my own. All I needed was antibiotics. The rest I could do myself. How do I know this? Because I am a responsible, well-informed adult, who has access to a plethora of information through mediums such as NHS Direct, patient information systems and, more powerfully, the internet.

Armed with such an array of facts and supporting information, and with a bit of direction and professional consultancy, I am quite capable of having some idea as to knowing what I need, where I can get it, who will provide it, and to what level of efficiency and effectiveness they will deliver it. In this respect, I am no different from any other member of the general population.

> **Activity 15.1**
>
> Think about how you, as a practitioner, see the future. What part do you think you could play in making it happen? In what ways might your thinking and practice have to change to achieve it?

When engaging in the above activity you may have considered many issues. Perhaps the most obvious is the amount of information and the technology that is currently available combined with the speed at which things continue to develop. This can lead to situations in which clients come to you with what they see as solutions to their problems followed by the expectation that you can make it available for them, for example, an experimental drug. In response to scenarios such as this you may have considered the skills you and your colleagues may need to develop, knowledge you may need to acquire and the implications of these changes upon your value base. All of which will require you and your peers to invest time and energy in yourselves.

WHY DO WE NEED TO CHANGE?

We need to change what we do and the way in which we do things because the world in which we live and work is changing around us. Change follows an awareness that something different is happening in our world. The awareness is a warning signal, which alerts us to series of choices:

- ignore the 'something different' and stay in our comfort zone

---

Box 15.1 The mobile phone health check
(By Paul Kendall, Technology Correspondent, from the Daily Mail, Friday, October 12, 2001, with permission)

A mobile phone system that could revolutionise health care has been unveiled by scientists.

The handset is capable of monitoring heart rate, blood pressure and temperature and then transmitting the information.

It means doctors would be able to check the condition of patients living in remote areas.

Research leader Professor Bryan Woodward, of Loughborough University, in Leicestershire, said: 'The idea of using mobile phone technology is that someone who is not confined to a bed can be monitored remotely by a consultant in a hospital.

'For example, someone who lives in the Highlands of Scotland, perhaps a hundred miles from the nearest hospital, could be given a routine check by mobile.' As the technology develops, health chiefs hope it might help to cut waiting times for referrals and administration costs.

Patients would be able to be 'seen' by their doctor without leaving their home.

Professor Woodward added: 'The medical profession is becoming very interested in telemedicine – using telecommunications to transmit medical information – because it can save a lot of time and money.

We think that by using mobile phone technology we will be able to extend the scope of telemedicine significantly.'

For an electro-cardiogram, measuring heart function, electrodes from the patient's chest would be fed into an electronic circuit contained within a holster on the patient's belt.

The holster would also accommodate a standard mobile phone.

The signal from the electrodes is then processed by the electronic circuitry and converted into an infrared signal, similar to that used in a TV remote control.

The signal is then transmitted to an infrared receiver on the phone, which beams it across the mobile phone network to the doctor's computer.

'Modern phones are equipped to receive infrared signals, so no modification is needed,' explained Professor Woodward. 'The challenging part of the work has been to make the interface. It has required immensely difficult software development.'

The data is encrypted – or scrambled – before it is sent over the airwaves, to maintain patient confidentiality, and then descrambled when it reaches the doctor's computer.

Professor Wooward went on: 'A cardiologist wants to see a signal exactly as if it had come directly off the patient's chest.

Fortunately we have been able to reproduce signals very accurately indeed.

The only limitations appear to be those inherent in the mobile phone network – that is losing the signal if you are going through a tunnel, for example.'

- fight against it
- trust in the process, feel the fear and embrace the change in the face of uncertainty.

Change is a movement from one state of being, behaving or practising to another – from here to there. It is a process, which moves us from where we are, to where we need to be in order to fulfil our potential and to succeed (Taylor 1995).

In the world of health and social care, the zone of awareness has come in the form of advances in medical science and technology, and an explosion in the availability and accessibility of information. These developments have taken us to places we never dreamed of and were not really prepared for. We are bombarded daily with new information which has built up around and above us to the point that we can no longer keep up with it (Porter-O'Grady & Wilson 1995). With a more informed, articulate and assertive population we are being asked to provide a more efficient, equitable, evidence-based and, therefore, effective health- and social-care service. The clear message is to provide more and better within existing resources, and in a way that meets the needs of modern lifestyles and expectations (Chin & McNicholl 2000). There really is no option but to change.

For too long the welfare services have been reactive, sometimes resistant and, on occasions, ambivalent to change. This response is understandable from a professional's point of view. In the last 10 years there has been reform after reform. No sooner has one change been implemented, then another one arrives, and so on. The workforce seems exhausted by the pace and breadth of change, and many have become cynical. Indeed, a recent survey which set out to determine the 'unwritten rules' and culture of the NHS amongst senior professionals (Cullen et al. 2000) noted comments from respondents such as:

- change = money and increasing stress
- we all need a siege mentality
- change for change's sake
- we all have to be super-human
- only do something if there's money in it
- everything is changing all the time
- the past was much better.

The reasons for the cynicism are many and varied. Without the need to blame any official body, policy, economic or moral entity, this rapid pace of change coupled with the absence of a period of relative stability, has led health- and social-care employees to constantly manage crisis after crisis so that we find ourselves in permanent 'whitewater'. The result is a stressed workforce, which feels that it is compromising quality and equity, and is faced with a number of highly public incidents that are affecting public confidence.

To help turn around public confidence, improve services and the working environment for employees, and build a first class service, a series of improvement programmes were implemented by the Labour government starting in 1995; initiatives such as clinical governance, best value national service and performance frameworks, professional self-regulation and leadership drives. These initiatives are further supported by the development of bodies such as the Commission for Health Improvement, Social Care Institute for Excellence, and the National Institute for Clinical Excellence, all of which are designed to have a positive impact upon quality, effectiveness, equity, efficiency and accountability (Department of Health 1998).

Six years later, the jury is still out on most of these policy changes and improvement programmes. However, if looked at in a positive way, they do represent a vehicle which provides an opportunity for every health- and social-care worker, no matter what their profession or designation, to lead effective change, take boundaried risks, re-connect with a higher purpose and make a difference to people's lives. In my own opinion, there has never been a more exciting time to work in the health- and social-care sector. The modernisation initiative has provided a clear mandate which invites all employees to contribute to the future of welfare services and which enables them to:

- adopt an entrepreneurial approach to health and social care
- influence changes to front line services
- innovate and create to provide the best possible care and services for clients and their families
- shift the balance of power from the practitioner to the service users
- determine and promote the use of evidence-based care
- act as adults, make decisions and solve problems at a local level and be accountable for the outcomes
- learn and share from mistakes in order to grow and develop
- be professionally accountable through life-long learning and self-regulation
- form partnerships, strategic alliances and promote cross-boundary participation and collaboration
- challenge the status quo, resource misuse and level of bureaucracy
- implement change from the bottom up and regain a sense of purpose, value, ownership and community (Centre for the Development of Nursing Policy and Practice 2000).

Never before in the history of the welfare services has there been such a confidence in the ability and potential of its workforce to implement change from within. We now have a choice. We can contribute to the modernisation agenda or we can stay in our comfort zone. If we do not contribute, we give permission to put the 'Do Not Resuscitate' stamp on services. In this context we would have little justification for complaining that things did not change for the better (Cowper 2000).

THE NATURE OF CHANGE AND THE MEANING OF CULTURE

When we don't understand, we turn to our assumptions

[Anonymous]

Organisations are a collection of individuals, a social structure in which groups of individuals come together in systems to achieve joint objectives, which are led by a common purpose (Weick & Quinn 1999). For example, the common purpose in the NHS is to provide health care. This notion permeates throughout the culture of the NHS and many would argue that this has always been the case, since its inception in the 1940s. The difference now is that the NHS is being asked to move away from traditional modes of care and service provision to those that are modernised and congruent with contemporary life. This situation is clearly replicated in social care as they too are being asked to modernise in a way that matches the expectations of an ever-changing society.

Modernisation itself is a process, which encompasses social, cultural, technical, economic and political paradigms and is an evolutionary transformative state in terms of norms, values, experiences and beliefs of a community or social mind (Dahlan 1992). As such, it impinges upon all individuals and systems it comes into contact with and involves the totality of human experience (Harrison 1988). Unless we begin to understand the nature of change, at both the individual and collective levels, and the elements involved, we will rely on our assumptions, which can be based upon fantasy rather than reality. This is a dangerous place to be and is not conducive to achieving effective change.

Liminality

Change is an entity, which is often bewildering and confusing. It reminds us of our inability to bring it under control, direct it or keep pace with it (Taylor 1995), and it brings about fear, confusion and chaos. We find ourselves in a state of liminality, as being neither 'here nor there' as 'betwixt and between one state of being and another' (Turner 1967). This state of liminality is a transitional period. Here, where we find ourselves passing through an ambiguous realm where our experiences and knowledge are insufficient to guide us through and towards the future. As a consequence of the clinical governance agenda there is now an emphasis upon basing decisions about care, support and management upon the best available evidence (see Chapters 5 and 7).

This change in focus can cause us to lose our sense of familiarity, identity and belonging. This is important in that we begin to feel insecure, out of place and in strange territory. As such, we often subconsciously perceive ourselves to be in fearful and scary places, and not having a sense of belonging (Douglas 1966).

Becoming

The work of Berger and Luckman (1966) suggests that life is a process of 'forever becoming', consisting of a series of transitions from one state of being to another. The suggestion is that states of being do not really exist for long. They change with new information, knowledge and situations, which in turn create new experiences. The knowledge gained during these experiences helps us cope with life at any one time, but becomes inadequate at the point of transition (Louis 1980). Reality shock sets in at this point causing anxiety and distress. We realise that whilst existing everyday knowledge and past experience may assist in part of the transition, it is in fact insufficient to enable untroubled passage into a new phase of life or professional experience.

Culture and ritual

In modern terms, culture can be understood as 'the way we do things around here' (Carson 1999). The 'way in which we do things' stems from values, beliefs and meanings which are shaped by a process of learning and socialisation, which are influenced by history, geography, science, technology, politics and economics, and serve to construct maps of human behaviour and understanding. These webs of meaning, values and beliefs constitute a culture (Geertz 1993).

The clinical governance agenda is focussed upon changing the culture from one which is based upon doing things that way because they have always been done that way, to one which encourages the workforce to reflect on practice and ask the question: 'what is the right thing to do?' This is in terms of:

- the client/patient needs, wants and expectations
- the organisation
- the team
- the individual practitioner.

Within the world of health and social care, the culture is heterogeneous, i.e. there are cultures within cultures. For instance, *doctors'* prime values centre around diagnosis, treatment and cure; *nurses* value care and nurturing; *administration* values order, bureaucratic structure and process; *finance* values cost effectiveness; *social workers* value clients' rights for protection; whilst the *executive board* values outcomes and achieving targets and organisational objectives.

Within these sub-cultures there are often unwritten, set and 'accepted' ways of behaving and practising. These set and accepted ways provide a safe, familiar environment, which promotes the status quo and the notion of tribal membership to one or other group. A sense of belonging to a social grouping is an inherent part of human need and is obtained through complex social and cultural processes, the main vehicle being the use of ritual.

Ritual is a form of prescribed, symbolic behaviour or action, which serves to communicate information about the culture's values and norms. Rituals express and renew certain basic values and norms and define the context in which individuals must interact if the culture and community is to remain coherent and stable (Turner 1982).

Case example

A surgical or medical 'firm' is perhaps a good example to illustrate culture, ritual and tribal membership within the world of health care. Traditionally, doctors place themselves within a pecking order, the consultant being the chief of the firm and the house officer ranks at the bottom of the hierarchy. As a member of this 'firm', most within it learn how the consultant likes certain 'things' to be done. In the case of surgeons, for instance, particular instruments, techniques and types of prostheses may be used by one consultant during an operation, whilst in the next operating theatre, another consultant, carrying out the same procedure will use a different technique, type of prosthesis and will prefer different instruments during the surgical procedure. Those who know the consultants, including all other staff in the operating theatre, will know their 'ways of doing things' (ritual) and will conform to these values and beliefs (culture). By doing so, the status quo is maintained and the sense of tribal membership and belonging is strengthened.

Newcomers to the 'firm' are often wise and will find out how things are done before or immediately after they arrive. They will often seek out an ally, usually somebody at the same or similar level in the pecking order, and familiarise themselves to the culture and the rituals that are preset. Such newcomers are themselves undergoing a period of liminality and are in the process of 'becoming', of gathering new knowledge and experiences as they find themselves in a process of change with a fundamental wish to belong to their new-found community.

In times of change, the familiar templates, rituals and maps that once provided direction and filled us with a sense of security and stability are no longer appropriate. Those of us who have undergone events, such as the loss of a loved one, a house move, job or career change, redundancy or divorce, are familiar with the feelings, actions and reactions these things can cause. These events could be described as extreme, but everyday work and life abounds with change and transition, as in the example above.

Change is a constant natural phenomenon. It happens in degrees and our reactions to it are relative to our understanding of it. One of the greatest barriers to change is the understanding or misunderstanding of it. At some point, we realise that our current knowledge, skills and competencies and past experiences are inadequate or inappropriate to and for the new situation we find ourselves in. When a change needs to happen, all or some of our values, beliefs, ways of doing things and sense of community are challenged. We can no longer stay in a traditional frame of reference where the past is honoured and established values and ways of doing things are maintained. A sense of fear, loss, dissonance and anxiety prevail in these situations as we begin to seek security and stability once again.

Acceptance and understanding of what change is and brings about is an important factor if we are to cope with it and move welfare services into the 21st century. We need to give ourselves permission to be 'betwixt and between', in a place of confusion, fear and chaos and to say that it is OK to be there. Established cultures resist threats to their culture or whatever makes meaning important, until such time as an understanding is reached as to why the change has become imperative and what is needed in order to support it. The key is that what was once modern has now become traditional.

Innovations in science and technology result in new knowledge, which in turn forces a change in attitudes and values from the accepted or traditional views of reality to an ethos which is forward thinking, questioning and unaccepting of anything purportedly given; that is, it becomes modernised (Huntington 1994). According to Giddens (1994) this shift in values and attitudes from the traditional to the modern is constituted in and through reflexively applied knowledge. The reflexivity of modern life consists of the fact that social and cultural practices and values are constantly examined and reformed in the light of new incoming information. In cultures which are traditional, reflexivity is largely limited to the re-interpretation and clarification of past or existing knowledge, where to know things is accepted as reality, to know and accept that: 'that's the way things are done around here' (Braudel 1993).

Activity 15.2

Think about your own place of work. How many different cultures can you identify within your department? Talk to members of the multidisciplinary team about their professional and personal values. What values do they hold and how might these groups react if you challenged their beliefs and ways of doing things? What does this information mean with regard to how the team works together?

You may have found that all the different groups of staff have different values and that this may cause them to have different priorities to you and the group of staff to which you 'belong'. One of the greatest challenges to the clinical governance agenda is the development of mutual respect and understanding in and across teams. This process requires that we invest time and energy not just in developing robust communication systems, but also in 'getting to know' people and the part they play with regard to effective care delivery.

Understanding diversity

We hear quite a bit these days about the demographics of the workforce and have regularly come across one generation complaining about another. Familiar comments such as 'these youngsters have no sense of loyalty or responsibility these days' or 'they need to chill, maaan' abound at both ends of the age continuum. What we actually have now in many organisations is an eclectic mix of generations and we need to see this as a gift to be explored for mutual benefit. According to Weston (2001) there are four generations in the workplace today, each having their own beliefs and work ethic:

The silent generation

This group of people are aged 55 and over, and come from a background which respects authority, status, power, structure, and clear rules and guidelines. They prefer to work in hierarchical organisations which are secure and stable, and where there is a graduated career path. This generation has a strong sense of duty. They need time and plenty of direct input when learning new skills and will perform best when reassured that their perseverance will reap major benefits. Reward for this generation comes through an appreciation of their length of time and experience in the organisation, and they value obedience over individualism. The

silent generation learns best in formal, traditional settings where knowledge is communicated via formal lectures and presentations by experts. Learning for this generation needs to be directive and well structured.

The baby boomers

Baby boomers are currently the largest section of the workforce and range between the ages of 40 and 55. This group are the movers and shakers, the ones who will challenge the status quo, openly question authority and the integrity of leaders. Idealists by nature, they are guided by a higher purpose in life and have a commitment to make the world a better place in which to live and work. This group is hardworking and dedicated and is adept at balancing a busy work life with a home and family. Baby boomers prefer to work in dynamic, non-hierarchical organisations, which will support their cause and which are committed to a caring, sharing democratic culture. They perform best in an environment which values and supports life-long learning, and one which actively provides the means for them to learn interactively.

Generation X

These are the fun-loving generation, who appreciate teamwork and camaraderie, and in general are aged 39 and younger. Minimal structure and a casual, informal culture is attractive to this group. They were born into the technological age and use technology to their best advantage, particularly when it can enhance their quality of life and leisure time. They are self-directed fast learners and, as a result, they expect instant response and satisfaction from their working tools and their environment. Generation X are highly committed to their chosen careers and will constantly seek out new knowledge and skills to enhance their marketability and enable the future they desire. If they do not get it from one organisation, they will seek out another. Loyalty to one employer is not a common feature with this generation. Highly tolerant of diversity, these groups appreciate the skills that others bring, will learn from one another, and are unafraid to offer ideas and solutions to the person they think they will get results from, even if this means ignoring political sensitivities and protocols. They go out of their way to get what they need to do a job and are best left to figure things out by doing it themselves, but appreciate open, honest feedback and are very open to coaching and support.

Generation Y

Generation Y, also known as millenials and the net generation are the emergent generation who are only just coming into the workforce. They are full of optimism and faith and are attracted to meaningful work where change will be seen as part of everyday life and the daily routine. Making things happen in a fast-paced environment is second nature to this group and they will expect to be able to achieve things at the push of a button. They will balance many experiences at any given time and, as such, are predicted to adopt parallel careers. Continuous learning and a balance between work and home/social life are important value sets to this generation. In seeing life as an integrated process, i.e. an eclectic mix of work and play, they will expect future employers to adopt cooperative and flexible approaches to working practices and expectations.

Activity 15.3

Which of the above descriptors best describes you and your immediate colleagues? What impact does this have upon your team and how it works together? How might you use this information to improve teamworking, particularly when thinking about change?

Although a stereotypical approach has been used to describe the typology of the varying generations in the workforce, the primary purpose is to provide awareness to organisational leaders. Tapping into this knowledge enables the organisation to identify where each generation might best contribute to the vision and process of the everyday organisational business and what strengths they may have in a team. If we can identify what beliefs and values they hold, we are better able to identify what attractors they have to a work situation. Furthermore, we can identify how they can best be utilised in times of change, and how their talents can be mixed and matched to promote synergistic teamwork, not intergenerational conflict.

TILTING TRIANGLES – DISPELLING POPULAR MYTHS

Borders? I have never seen one. But I have heard they exist in the minds of some people.
[Thor Heyerdahl]

As the nature of health and social care is changing, we need to change our perceptions, beliefs, attitudes, behaviour and practice to keep up with it, and to see where we fit in with it. We need to challenge and change our understanding of how things are and how we can contribute. These changes apply to every person working within health and social care, from the ancillary staff to the chief executive, and to all systems at organisational, directorate, unit, team and individual levels. Not one of these areas or groups can be negated because they are all interconnected. One cannot, and does not, work in isolation from the other. In reality, there are no borders that separate one system or group from another and, consequently, no one group that should hold the control about what does and does not change.

Who 'controls' and 'decides' what happens within the service is one of the major perceptions that needs to change if the clinical governance agenda is to be successful. Prevailing thought amongst most employees is that the government of the day takes great pleasure in formulating masses of new policy which then forces staff to implement change in their working environment. This could be in the community, in a day service, at ward level, in the pharmacy, in administration, in estates, housekeeping, etc. Some would argue that all talk of change is pure rhetoric designed to get more votes in elections. It is, however, important to understand the part this plays in the macro environment that influences change and how you as a professional can work with this.

The traditional view of who is responsible for change is that it is a top-down process, initiated by government policy through bureaucratic departments, and thence passed down the hierarchy to the lower levels of the organisation. The perception at the lower levels of the organisation is that decision making in this environment is owned by 'someone at the top' and is managed by means of a command and control autocracy (see Fig. 15.1).

Whilst it is true that policy (a pre-cursor to change) is formulated at government level, the stimulus and opinions related to and for the policy change actually comes from multiple sources (see Fig. 15.2). According to Ham (1992) there are no less than seven sources of input for policy making leading to changes within the NHS:

- consumer groups and pressure groups
- health/local authorities and trusts
- parliament and the mass media
- public and professional consultation
- ministers and civil servants
- academia and research
- industry and commercial interests.

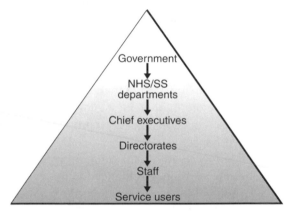

Figure 15.1 Traditional 'command and control' perceptions of ownership for change and decision making in the NHS.

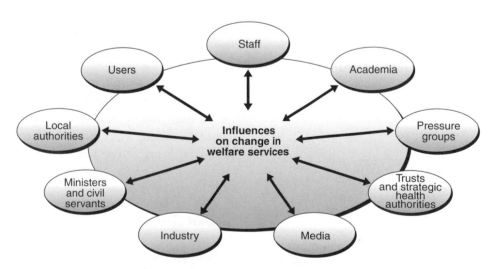

Figure 15.2 Influences of change in welfare services.

All of these groups in one way or another have an impact on what happens within the health- and social-care arena. There is interplay within the groups and policy is developed through bargaining, negotiation and accommodation (Ham 1992). In reality, every member of the public has the opportunity to influence change within the welfare services, and every employee of the NHS and social care are a member of the public. We are all users of the services, regardless of where we might sit in the above list and we all have access to the various groups so that we may have our say. This process is known as participative democracy, where interested groups are invited to contribute to the decision-making processes and where power is shared. Particular groups who previously dominated the power base have been challenged. Welfare services are now moving from a professionally driven model to one which is collectively owned and is supported by policy such as *Shifting the Balance of Power* (Department of Health 2001) and *The NHS Plan* (Department of Health 2000).

The hierarchical triangle is beginning to tilt in favour of a service that is driven by service users in collaboration with all other interested parties, and where decision making is shared and collectively owned. The myth of the omnipotent professional group, chief executive, management group or ruling political party as being the Wizard of Oz, i.e. having all the answers and the power to make all the decisions, is slowly fading into the distance.

Activity 15.4

Think about how you can influence policy making. Have you ever responded to a consultation exercise?

If you have access to the internet, go to www.doh.gov.uk and find out if any policy documents are posted for comment or contribute to a consultation exercise. What are their relevance to you and your organisation? How might you engage your team members in any relevant consultation processes?

NEW WAYS OF THINKING – INSIGHTS FROM COMPLEXITY SCIENCE

Organisational change results from changes in behaviour which can be at individual, group or organisational level, and which is supported by a variety of theories, values, strategies and techniques (Porras & Robinson 1992, p. 722: cited in Illes & Sutherland 2001). Theories and models on organisational development abound, and depict the latest ideas on how best to manage the change process to promote quality, efficiency and effectiveness. These concepts are key components of clinical governance.

The following change management strategies and techniques are ones which you can use to support this agenda:

- process re-engineering
- total-quality management
- continuous-quality improvement
- soft-systems methodology
- business-excellence model.

Whilst all of the above, and many more besides, have their worth and place, the prevailing opinion amongst change management theorists is that there is no magic bullet available for achieving change. The key to handling effective change is to realise that change programmes should not be seen as an end in themselves, and should take account of the players and the context in which they are forced to operate (Wilson 1992).

Illes and Sutherland (2001, p. 18) note that change in the NHS is a complex process. They state that:

> The NHS is a large organisation employing people with a wide range of talents, perspectives and passions. It is a complex organisation, with many different cultures and norms, arising from a number of factors including:
>
> - different socialisation processes of the professions
> - different needs and expectations of client groups
> - different histories of different institutions
> - local priorities, resource allocation and performance management.
>
> The complexity is a result of the very specialisation that has produced so many advances in healthcare. This specialisation also leads to a high degree of interdependence between practitioners and between practitioners and processes. This interdependence and continuing technical and organisational advances mean that services and organisations within the NHS are dynamic as well as complex (Illes & Sutherland 2001).

MODELS OF CHANGE

The literature on change contains a plethora of models, frameworks and approaches to change. These have developed in line with the history of management theories, which have, in turn, influenced the practice of managing change. The terms 'models', 'tools' and 'approaches' are often used interchangeably and can be confusing. To simplify matters, Taylor (1995), and Illes and Sutherland (2001) capture three types of change according to their extent and scope, and build into them three useful and cyclical models.

Planned or transitional change

This is perhaps one of the more well known types of change and has been characterised by Lewin (1951) as un-freezing-moving-re-freezing. The first stage is characterised by a realisation that something new is happening and there is a need to change – 'unfreezing'. The second stage of 'moving' involves a phase of activity, which moves the players to their planned state. The third phase of 're-freezing' occurs when the change has been internalised or fully understood to become a new way of behaving or practising. Learning and integration of the learning has taken place.

Developmental change

Taylor (1995, p. 4) describes developmental change as 'an unfolding of potential', which can be processual or planned, or may happen suddenly through a realisation that a milestone or a different way of behaving or doing something has been reached.

Transformational change

This type of change is derived from chaos theory and builds itself into systems theory and the relatively new ideas of complexity science. Transformational change suggests that we move from where we are to something which is significantly different in terms of structure, process, culture and strategy (Illes & Sutherland 2001). It is a process where continuous learning takes place through expanding people's capacity and nurturing new patterns of thinking (Miller 2000), and through supporting creativity, innovation and interaction between and amongst systems and players. As interaction takes place between the players and the systems, changes in perceptions, beliefs, behaviour and practice emerge.

Complex adaptive systems

Transformational change is ordered but not centrally controlled and passes through six phases: birth, growth, stable instability, chaos, death and emergence. Organisations which adopt transformational approaches to change are said to be 'living' or 'organic' and, according to Young-blood (1997), are characterised by openness, flexibility, responsiveness, resilience, creativity, vitality, balance and caring. That is, they are akin to nature in terms of their inter-connectedness, complexity and adaptability, the properties of which are found in 'complex adaptive systems'.

Complex adaptive systems consist of webs of interacting players and interconnected systems, which are characteristically both interdependent and independent. They have the ability and freedom to adapt to a changing environment or stimulus in diverse and unpredictable ways and are characterised by the potential for self-organisation without external or centralised control (Zimmerman et al. 1998). Complex adaptive systems border on the edge of chaos and balance on a knife-edge of 'death by equilibrium or death by dissipation' (Zimmerman et al. 1998, p. 13); this point is known as the zone of complexity (Stacey 1993).

This type of system works best in areas of boundaried instability (zone of complexity), where there is limited certainty and control of the future, e.g. the 21st century nature of care and service provision. The zone of complexity stimulates masses of creative energy and thus the emergence of innovative, yet coherent ways of seeing the world, behaving and operating within it. Plsek (2001, p. 5) defines a complex adaptive system as being:

> ... a collection of individual agents, who have the freedom to act in ways that are not always predictable and whose actions are interconnected such that one agent's actions changes the context for other agents.

Case example

A group of nurses working within an elderly mental health unit held regular team meetings in which they would discuss the welfare and care of the client group. On one particular occasion the discussion centred round a client who displayed obsessive, repetitive behaviour, which was disturbing to other clients on the residential unit and was leading to psychological crisis and behavioural difficulties in some of them. The client in question would constantly walk backwards and forwards to the door. Once there, he would rattle the door incessantly, creating as much noise as he could.

The team had tried all ways they knew to divert the clients' attention but without effect. As a result of bringing more people into the discussion of how this problem could be resolved, a diverse array of suggestions were put forward. They were guided by developing some simple parameters to the process such as:

- sedation or restraint of any kind was not an option
- keep the solution low cost
- safety was paramount.

As a team, they came up with the idea of painting a 'squiggle' maze on the floor and suggested that they paint the door to look like a book-case, but in a way which would not disguise the exit too much and cause undue danger.

The result was that the client no longer walked his familiar path to rattle a door, but wandered around the maze on the floor, which created a mental and physical diversion, which he found comforting. The rest of the clients on the unit had a more peaceful existence and the staff had changed their thinking on traditional methods of care, to one which was even more creative and which produced a previously untried and unknown, yet positive outcome.

As a result of 'telling the story' through casual dialogue, other units in the hospital have re-thought their practice in similar cases, and are adopting a more creative approach to finding solutions. Although the idea and outcome was not formally evaluated, the organisation has noted a reduction in the use of sedation on its in-patient units.

ORGANISATIONS THAT LIVE AND LEARN

If we examine the planned changes for the welfare services through the modernisation agenda, we note several key themes and recurring concepts, many of them centring on:

- inclusion and partnership
- responsiveness and ownership
- learning and innovation
- decentralised decision making and empowerment
- responsibility and accountability.

The themes and concepts suggest that the key to change within health and social care lies with the individual players and their interconnectedness as individuals and groups as complex adaptive systems. In complex, dynamic and interconnected organisations, models of change need to be flexible. They cannot be linear and adopt a cause and effect approach to change, which relies on predictability and certainty of specific and controlled outcomes. The process of changing human behaviour, values and practice is highly unpredictable, and change implemented at one level has an impact in many others.

Change should, therefore, be emergent and transformational in nature. This does not mean that it is led by out-of-control mavericks. On the contrary, the players in a living organisation are highly responsible and accountable adults and are well aware of the boundaries, which they usually set by means of negotiation and consensus. They create high levels of infectious creative energy and their environments act as magnets or attractors for change within organisations.

DEVELOPING THE ORGANIC LEARNING ORGANISATION

The reality is that welfare services cannot move to being a learning organisation overnight. Despite recent initiatives to promote a learning ethos within services, the current culture is still bogged down by blame, power play, misplaced practices of authoritarianism, bureaucracy and autocracy, backbiting and self-interest. All of these things are barriers to change, are unethical, and inhibit the spirit of inquiry, partnership building, creativity and quality, which are the central tenets of clinical governance. Although there are pockets of excellence and innovation across services, there is still a long way to go before all parties begin to understand what 'learning' is. In contrast to what currently exists in many care services, a learning organisation is characterised by its ability to learn continuously, to actively build knowledge, to facilitate decision making where the knowledge is the greatest, and to create an environment in which people can behave like responsible adults (Miller 2000). A learning organisation is a living organisation and is underpinned by five key disciplines:

- personal mastery
- systems thinking
- mental models
- building shared vision
- team learning (Senge 1990).

All of the above require:

- effort
- leadership
- self-discipline and team discipline (taking responsibility for your own actions and development needs)
- thinking (engaging in analysis and critical thinking)
- honesty and openness (all team members providing each other with effective feedback)

- interconnectedness and feedback from connectedness (systems thinking)
- interdependence (engaging in 'win–win' practices through consensus)
- inclusion (e.g. service users, all team members, groups outwith the immediate environment)
- maturity (behaving as adults)
- application (putting things into practice)
- nurturing
- an element of fun!

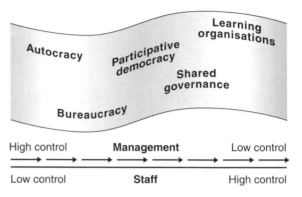

Figure 15.3 Organisational development continuum (reproduced with kind permission of Miller D and Creative Health Care Management, Inc. 2000 Leading an empowered organisation. Creative Health Care Management, Inc., Minneapolis, USA).

Activity 15.5

Using the above as a checklist, which ones do you practice well as an organisation and which ones have room for development? Think about 'having fun'; what does this mean, considering the health- and social-care services address serious business?

Senge (1990, p. 14) defines a learning organisation as one that is 'continually expanding its capacity to create its future'. He explains this idea further by saying:

Real learning gets to the heart of what it means to be human. Through learning we re-create ourselves. Through learning we become able to do something we never were able to do. Through learning we re-perceive the world and our relationship to it. Through learning we extend our capacity to create, to be part of the generative process of life. There is within each of us a deep hunger for this type of learning.

ORGANISATIONAL DEVELOPMENT CONTINUUM

The diagram in Figure 15.3 depicts the levels of managerial and staff control, which is exercised in decision-making processes in five types of organisations. As organisations move from autocratic

approaches to learning organisations, there is a change in the level of control exercised by the managers and staff, and a significant difference in quality outcomes (Miller 2000).

In autocratic organisations, managers have high control over decision making and are usually characterised by a top-down approach. Bureaucracies typically make decisions through long processes, which involve issues being moved up, down and sideways across the organisation before a decision is reached. Conversely, in organisations where there is shared governance or an empowered learning culture, staff assume, and are given, high levels of control for decision making and problem solving. Here, managers influence rather than control (Miller 2000).

In reality, we can move up and down the continuum. For instance, in the event of a local disaster, such as an explosion in a nearby chemical factory, it would be quite proper to utilise an autocratic style of leadership through direct command from the executive level, which sets in motion the major incident procedures.

Activity 15.6

Where is your department on the above continuum? Where would you like to be?

> Describe how it would feel to work in each type of organisation.

Many writers suggest that the best place for change to take place is at the local level. This is with the belief that the individuals and groups, e.g. the clinicians, at the grass roots levels of the organisation are the actual agents of change. They are aware of the needs of their clients, understand the context and, therefore, have a wealth of understanding and knowledge of what needs to change and how it can be achieved (Page et al. 1998).

The opinion of many is that if change does not happen at the local level where the knowledge is the greatest, then it does not matter where else it takes place in the organisation (Ford & Walsh 1994, Porter-O'Grady 1995, Youngblood 1995, Page et al. 1998, Chin & McNichol 2000). To support this argument, a recent study by Wallace et al. (2001), which set out to examine the organisational strategies used for influencing clinician's behaviour to implementing clinical governance and changing practice within 86 NHS trusts across the South west and the Midlands, noted that quality initiatives were most effective when applied in a localised, project-based way.

The message here is that you can have as many change strategies, models, tools and theories as you like. But, if there is no support and realisation as to the importance of the change, and the contribution of individual players in context is not seen to be valued, and if they do not feel any benefit or ownership of the change process, then they will not 'play'. Change then becomes superficial, meaningless and unsustainable.

Case example

Joan has been working as a nursing auxiliary in a GP practice for over 20 years. When the GP partners decided to introduce a system of change, which supported all members of the staff to develop their practice to meet local healthcare needs, Joan decided she was not going to play their 'game'.

She said, 'I did not feel a part of the change and could not see where I fitted into the whole thing, so I became as difficult as possible and made everybody's life a misery. I would constantly "take the mick" with sarcastic comments and trivialise their attempts to make things better. Actually, I was afraid. I felt alone and did not have a clue as to what I could do to contribute.

Eventually I saw a niche. I had been working with the practice nurses for years and seen them take blood a thousand times. I thought to myself, "I could do that with my eyes shut". I talked to the nurses and GPs about the possibility of me being properly trained to take blood. They agreed to send me for training.

I've now got a new lease of life. I take all the blood in the clinic and make sure it all goes to the right place with the right documents and labelling. If anything goes wrong, I know I am accountable and responsible. Nobody else is to blame.

By learning new things, I am not only helping the nurses by giving them more time with other patients, I am also able to utilise my skills better and really feel a part of this change and development stuff. I also have much more contact with the clients, rather than just testing urine and boring stuff like that. I understand what it is all about, and I feel supported in what I am doing. I'm a happy bunny now and so is everybody else!'

CREATING THE ENVIRONMENT

Clinical governance provides a framework for developing a client-orientated service, through continuous improvement and the use of evidence-based practice. Within this framework, innovation and creativity lie side by side with the paradox of risk and opportunity. In order for organisations to embrace clinical governance fully and to realise its maximum potential in practice, the environment in which people work must be conducive to enabling innovative practice development in line with the modernisation agenda.

Staff must be supported and facilitated to reach their full potential and function effectively together as intra-disciplinary, self-directed learning teams. In order to do this, the organisation takes on a degree of responsibility and risk, and is encouraged to demonstrate support by devolving a significant amount of control in decision making, planning and problem solving to both staff and clients. To this end, a decentralised approach to management and leadership practices is effective, where responsibility, authority and accountability are locally owned through clear communication and articulation at all levels of the organisation (Miller 2000).

Leadership

Leadership, without a doubt, is one of the most important elements in achieving change in an organisation. Leadership sets the vision, direction and tone of the organisation as a whole, and thus influences the nature and levels of energy, life and commitment in the workforce. The focus of any leader should be on the growth and development of the staff so that they can constantly 'learn to learn', create, innovate and take risks to improve their areas of practice and fulfil the commitment of clinical governance.

Most of the contemporary literature on leadership would agree that leadership is a way of being with people. It is about behaviour and relationship building. This means that what a leader actually *does* means far more than what they say, i.e. they walk the talk. A good leader treats their staff in the same way they themselves would prefer to be treated, in an adult-to-adult fashion. They will never ask their staff to do anything they would not do themselves and go out of their

way to celebrate successes and see mistakes as an opportunity to learn, not as an opportunity to wield power through punitive measures.

Leadership is about being able to ask followers, 'what is it that I need to do in order for you to succeed?' and then take affirmative action to make things happen. It is a two-way process, as leaders also need to ask themselves, 'In what ways do I need to grow and develop in order that I may help others to succeed?' In this way, leadership is a two-way process and is transformational in nature. This mature approach forms a parallel process to achieving transformational, evolutionary change.

All too often we still see transactional styles of leadership where the parent/child type of behaviour predominates. This does nothing for morale, creativity and the pursuit of quality and partnership building. An instance of this came to light quite recently when a very old friend contacted me in a state of distress. The following is Jane's story:

Jane was a week into a new role and was in a period of orientation. One of her colleagues fell critically ill and Jane had to suddenly fill in for her at a high level meeting at the last minute. Jane's job at this meeting was to present a complex new strategy. She prepared as best she could, took advice from other colleagues, took the 'bull by the horns' and got on with it.

According to Jane it went very well, and feedback from those present was very positive and appreciative. She had even finished half an hour early, at 3.30pm, much to the delight of all present. However, the organiser of the event took her to one side and reprimanded her for finishing early. Jane was told that her behaviour was unacceptable and that she was cheating the organiser out of 30 minutes of the time she had allocated to the day. The organiser reported her to her line manager with the expectation that the time delegated to this task, be re-paid in some other way.

After all of her effort Jane should have been congratulated and thanked for her adaptability, effectiveness and commitment to delivering the new strategy. As it turned out, the response centred around compliance and exchange, and was inappropriate to the situation.

Leadership in this vein is transactional and is characterised by behaviours, which at the lowest level of development serve to satisfy the personal needs of the leader and which focus around caution, rigid structure and pay back. In another situation, this style of leadership can be useful, especially when a directive, strictly controlled approach is necessary. However, it still needs to be balanced with a degree of empathy and mutual trust, and practised with a commitment to a higher purpose (Bass & Avolio 1994).

In achieving effective change, the nature of leadership within an organisation can either make it or break it. Facilitative styles of leadership are based upon an ethical commitment to the growth and development of all members of an organisation as a two-way process. In this way, we are both teacher and learner, leader and follower at any one given time. As the culture of the organisation is seen to support the development of latent talent, nurture emergent leaders and value the workforce, achieving quality through change becomes less of a battle and more of a synergistic interaction. The people that make up an organisation are its finest asset. They are the actual agents of change, but it would be wise to remember that it is good leadership that is the attractor and pillar around which a clinical governance and best value agenda can be realised in practice.

Management

Leadership cannot be seen in isolation to the role of a manager in achieving change. Management relates to the acquisition, allocation and evaluation of resources used to deliver services and care (Miller 2000). The basic role of a manager encompasses three key areas:

- personnel
- finance
- quality.

The managers' contributions to achieving effective change relies upon their ability to provide the workforce with the resources they need in order to accomplish organisational goals. Change is often stopped dead in its tracks due to underfunding, shortage of staff and a confusion around where the organisation is going and what standards it needs to achieve. These are common barriers to change and managers need to be able to find creative ways to support staff in these areas, particularly during times of pressure and 'permanent white-water', where the danger of staying in the comfort zone is at its highest. They also need to be able to convey the finer points of the mission, vision and standards of the wider organisation in a language and format that staff understand and can work with on a practical level.

The process of implementing the organisations' vision via the business plan is often placed upon managers as an organisational collective. Their job is to ensure outcomes and the achievement of targets within their own departments. These demands are then placed upon the staff in the practice areas, but what many managers forget to do is to explain the 'what' and the 'why' of the vision and purpose of the business plan to their staff. Often, the expectations are not clearly articulated at the lower levels as information is sparse and at times withheld, and the messages are mixed. In this event, misunderstanding occurs leading to a 'them and us' situation. At the practice level, staff feel divorced from the purpose of the organisation, have no sense of ownership and lack collective responsibility in achieving organisational goals. A cyclical process is then created whereby a minimalist work ethic prevails, staff adopt a self-serving, tribal attitude and clients become secondary to the primary purpose of the organisation.

Many leaders/managers are now adopting an inclusive approach to the process of creating the vision and business planning, and actively seek the views of staff and service users. A variety of strategies can be used in this consultation exercise including:

- Annual forums to which all staff and service users are invited to air their ideas and views.

- Quarterly open forums chaired by the chief executive with the primary purpose of explaining the organisational business plan, what it will entail, where the organisation is in meeting its objectives, and how all can contribute to the overall vision and direction.

- Quarterly directorate meetings where managers seek the views and ideas from staff and service users as to how the organisational business plan might translate itself into everyday practice at the local level.

- Intranet and internet sites, which are simple to use and are designed to actively seek the opinion of service users and staff on organisational goals and strategies.

- Consultation exercises with consumer and staff groups.

- Inviting units at a local level, in conjunction with service users, to submit their own mini-business plans to the organisation, which are guided by the overall vision, generic principles, national welfare policy and the explicit overall goals of the organisation.

As Useem (2001) identifies, when leaders and managers make their strategic intent abundantly clear, others know what to do without requiring myriad further instructions.

Managers and leaders, therefore, have a responsibility for being excellent communicators and creative providers of resources. If staff are given the 'what' and the 'why' in a form and language that is meaningful to their context, they will sort out the 'how' in partnership with clients. That is, providing that they are given the freedom, support and developmental opportunities, so that they continuously learn to learn and contribute significantly and visibly to the quality agenda.

PROVIDING THE FRAMEWORK FOR LEARNING AND CHANGE

A learning organisation is a collection of individuals who make up teams, which are characteristically self-directed, focused upon the principles of growth and development, and are open to change. That is, they practice the art and discipline of learning, and understand the implications of having a great deal of freedom to create, innovate, make decisions and implement change with the minimum of direction and external control.

This all sounds very complex but there are a few steps that can be taken by leaders/managers that provide a framework for learning and an environment that supports effective change.

The first step is for managers and leaders to let go of some of the responsibility for decision making, through providing clear levels of authority with associated accountability and through ensuring that staff have the competencies and capability to undertake the devolved responsibility.

Competencies

If responsibility for decision making is devolved there must be a consideration as to the competencies required in order for individuals and teams to be successful, to learn, grow and develop.

Activity 15.7

Imagine you were asked to take the lead on implementing clinical governance or best value principles in your area of work. What areas of competencies would you need to develop in order to enhance your likelihood of success in this task? How would you ensure you acquired the relevant skills? What level of authority would you need to carry out your task?

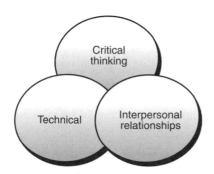

Figure 15.4 Areas of competencies.

According to del Bueno et al. (1990) there are three areas of competencies that are of importance, regardless of the role we have in an organisation (see Fig. 15.4). The areas include critical thinking, technical and interpersonal relationships. These areas overlap, and a deficiency in one area will affect another.

For instance, physiotherapists need to be *technically* competent in knowing how physical therapy equipment works so that safety is paramount and that the clients achieve optimum benefit from the equipment. *Critical thinking* comes into play for the physiotherapists during a session. They must be able to analyse the benefits of a particular therapy by using a combination of theory, experience and by monitoring the clients' responses during the sessions. They also need a high degree of competence interacting with people through the use of good *interpersonal* skills. Their patients/clients are most often physically disabled to some degree, and a caring attitude and building of a therapeutic relationship through good communication is essential to the clients' overall well-being. If a physiotherapist is not

competent in all three areas, their client will not necessarily receive the kind of support they are entitled to.

In instances where staff are asked to take on new responsibilities, consideration must be given to whether they require support in one or more areas of competence in order to be successful. As an example, the NHS is committed to utilising the benefits of information technology throughout its institutions. It would be useless to just install computers and computer systems without providing staff with the technical competence to use them. Similarly, it would be inappropriate to expect others to take on the responsibility of a budget without being able to calculate, analyse and deal with complex accounting principles, unless they have the critical thinking skills that allow them to balance the books.

Responsibility, authority and accountability

Learning cultures are effective at de-centralising decision making through a clear understanding of the meaning and processes that underpin empowerment. According to Manthey and Miller (1994) the three elements which support the empowerment process are:

- responsibility
- authority
- accountability.

The new role of the modern matron within the contemporary NHS is a good illustration for these three key elements that demonstrates their importance within this process. Although the role specification for this initiative is still ambiguous, the primary reason for introducing the modern matron was to provide service users with a highly visible authority figure, with whom they could directly communicate, and who would be seen to be responsible and accountable for general standards. Feedback from the public and the

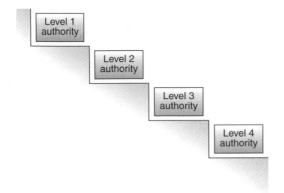

Figure 15.5 Levels of authority.

media suggested that one of the key areas that 'matron' should be responsible and accountable for was ensuring the cleanliness of the wards. Under existing arrangements this role lies with estates and housekeeping, often through external contracts.

If 'matron' is to be allocated the *responsibility* of ensuring ward cleanliness then he/she firstly needs to:

- pause and analyse what this responsibility might entail
- determine what concerns and issues may be raised, e.g. from estates
- negotiate with her managers as to what he/she needs to do to be competent and successful in taking on the responsibility, and in dealing with the issues.

Once the above needs have been met through negotiation, 'matron' then needs clarification on what level of *authority* she has to make things happen (see Fig 15.5). For instance, if the cleaning contractors are not delivering to required standards, what can 'matron' actually do about it?

- Level 1 authority would enable 'matron' to *collect information* and pass it on to a higher authority for them to deal with.

- Level 2 authority would enable 'matron' to *collect information* and *make recommendations*.
- Level 3 authority would enable 'matron' to *collect information, formulate recommendations, pause* by passing her information and recommendations by a higher authority and then act.
- Level 4 authority would enable 'matron' to *act and then inform others*.

The accountability that 'matron' holds is equivalent to the level of authority he/she is given and focuses upon the outcomes. Accountability in this sense is linked to individual ownership of outcomes, based upon the acceptance of responsibility and the awareness of the competencies needed to do the job. This process militates against the current blame culture within services, as it places the ownership of securing competency development and learning on the individual who has accepted the responsibility, and, therefore, the accountability for the outcome.

Keep the rules short and simple

The more we build up rules and regulations within an organisation the less chance there is that people will be creative. Risk is inherent with creativity, but needs to be supported at an organisational level through the creation of flexible boundaries and a non-punitive approach to mistake making through analysis and disciplined learning, not through punishment and strict boundaries that cannot be crossed. The fear of many managers and leaders is that without strict rules chaos will emerge, and the possibility for risk taking and making mistakes followed by litigation will rise. This is not typically the case with self-directed teams. As was mentioned earlier in the chapter, self-organising teams work within boundaries, guided by a clear vision and a set of simple but profound and far-reaching rules. They see risks and mistakes as learning opportunities which need to be supported at organisational level through discussion forums, dissemination of learning from risks/mistakes, and openness and honesty in the public arena. Where creativity takes place there are bound to be mistakes, particularly as organisations move along the development continuum (Fig. 15.3).

According to Plsek (2001), there are three types of simple rules under which dynamic experimentation may take place:

- direction pointing
- prohibitions
- permission providing.

In trying out new ideas, it is best to have a combination of all three. Examples of simple rules already discussed could include those outlined within the case study on the mental health unit for older people on p. 260. Other examples may include a selection from one or more of the following:

- do not harm anybody
- do nothing illegal
- be truthful, open and honest
- seek the views of clients
- keep within a stated budget/existing resources
- keep within an agreed level of authority
- keep within an agreed scope of influence
- provide something better than existed before
- provide evaluation of your innovation
- ask for what you need
- be responsible for your own learning and development needs
- work towards a win–win outcome.

PLAYING TOGETHER AS A TEAM

True teamwork is based upon 'a set of values that encourages behaviours such as listening and constructively responding to points of view expressed by others, giving others the benefit of the doubt, providing support to those who need it, and recognising the interests and achievements of others' (Katzenbach & Smith 1998, p. 21). Teamwork also needs to appreciate and actively embrace the diversity of experience and needs of the myriad of generations within an organisation. A team cannot function unless it is brought together through effective leadership, it has terms of reference or a set of principles as a guiding force, sees itself as a tool for learning and communication, and as a part of an interconnected whole.

Case example

This case example focuses upon a mental health service in Nottingham. Although the unit of practice was residential rehabilitation (mental health), the 'whole' actually consists of three multidisciplinary teams in dispersed sites in a large mental health NHS trust. Their vision is to work together as one unit to improve the experience of all those who use and work in the service and to disseminate their learning across the trust.

The team leaders stated, 'Some way into the journey, we realised we were involved in an evolutionary learning process. Our success, we came to believe, depended upon good leadership and ownership at all levels. We decided that the best framework for us was to follow a model of team learning in parallel with the practice development criteria/framework provided by the Centre (Centre for the Development of Nursing Policy and Practice 2000).

The learning model we chose was one developed by Dechant et al. (1993). This model identifies four phases to team learning:

1. fragmented learning – seeing something from a different perspective involves individuals experimenting with situations

2. pooled learning – shared learning in pockets, beginning to see things differently and crossing some boundaries, but mainly as individuals

3. synergistic learning – integrated perspectives, collective learning

4. continuous learning – collective learning is central to the practice and culture of an organisation.

As a team we see these phases as a continuum and in reality we move back and forth across the four phases, and we have done that at various times on different projects. At the beginning of the practice development unit journey we were fragmented in single teams with little cross team working. We have used different mechanisms establishing regular forums to support progress towards synergistic learning and promote a culture with collective learning as the norm. We have used this model to guide our way forward to becoming a learning organisation'.

STRUCTURES TO SUPPORT CHANGE

When implementing any change within a practice setting or organisation, one of the key destabilising factors is the uncertainty that exists within the process. Whilst it is neither possible nor necessarily desirable to control all aspects of change, it can be beneficial to create parameters and support structures in which teams can operate. This includes ensuring the following exist:

- A steering group with clear terms of reference.
- Representation on the steering group of all key stakeholders including people who use the service, those affected by the change and people who will influence the implementation process.
- Clarity about the roles of steering group members.

- A clearly articulated vision that is shared with all involved.
- The vision translated into a plan of action that guides the process of change.
- Key responsibilities for implementation clearly identified.
- Effective communication systems and structures.
- Supportive counselling systems to provide a safety net for those who may be affected by the change.
- Management support for those leading the change, particularly when resources are involved.
- Access to relevant expertise.
- A method of monitoring and evaluating the effectiveness of the change.
- Systems for acting on the information gathered from the above approaches.
- Effective strategies for disseminating outcomes and any learning that has occurred as a result of the work.

SUPPORT TO STAY OUTSIDE THE COMFORT ZONE

All organisations hold an ethical and moral responsibility to invest in the learning and developmental needs of their employees. Discovering what interests people, what values and beliefs they hold and what they need in order to succeed is a leadership imperative. This is particularly so in the case of a learning organisation where learning, change and transformation are a way of life. Organisations moving towards such a goal need to have structures and strategies in place to support people to stand outside their comfort zone and constantly learn to learn.

In recent years many organisations have sought external accreditation for strategies to support staff learning and development through initiatives such as Investors in People. Whilst there is a prevailing culture and recognition to provide opportunities for learning and continuous professional development, some initiatives are piecemeal; not openly visible or accessible to employees; or used inappropriately, e.g. clinical supervision being used as a vehicle for performance management. In addition, some areas of the workforce, which lie outside of the 'professional' realm, are often neglected.

Activity 15.8

Identify one area within your job that you want to further develop yourself. Think about all the different ways in which you might achieve this. You will need to look at *what* you might need to do as well as *who* can help you.

Learning, however, comes in many forms and can be formal and structured, informal and unstructured, serendipitous or purposeful, planned and systematic. For many years we have been led to believe that only formalised education courses can give us what we need to learn in order to improve our competencies and capabilities. Emphasis and kudos have been placed upon academic study and qualifications as the only way forward. Whilst formalised education has a vital part to play in our learning, we can also learn in less formalised ways. We can learn as we practice, and after practice. Learning can come in the form of dialogue, story telling, role play, critical incident analysis, shadowing, time out and discussion. Through such forms of discovery, we learn continuously, not only about our practice and how this can be improved, but also about ourselves. As we learn, we become more self-aware of our own learning needs, more mature in our outlook and beliefs about learning and how it contributes to quality client care. We ask ourselves the question, 'what is it that I now need to know and learn in order to be more successful in what I do and in what we provide as a team/organisation?' It is in this way that we are able to find support and the determination to remain outside the comfort zone.

The intent behind any learning is that an organisation not only builds role-related competencies, but also invests time and energy into building capacity and capability within the workforce (Fraser & Greenhalgh 2001). The role of the individual is to take up the advantages offered by the organisation to be responsible and accountable for their own learning and development. Partnerships in learning and learning alliances are then built to mutual advantage. Organisations then become the ongoing creations of the people who work in them (Flaherty 1999).

According to Clutterbuck (1998) an organisation has its own vast internal network of people who can help us to learn. Such people include:

- mentors
- coaches
- counsellors
- facilitators
- guardians.

With such a vast array of talent at our disposal we should not find it difficult to constantly learn to learn and see tangible differences in ourselves and in our practice. However, confusion arises and learning can become compromised when all these roles are intermingled, used interchangeably and, therefore, inappropriately by organisations. Labels are attached to developmental roles without clear purpose. For instance, many healthcare organisations offer internal mentorship as an opportunity to develop staff. This 'internal' approach is a contradiction in terms to the actual purpose around mentorship, which utilises personal power, focuses upon higher levels of self-awareness, career transitions and related life choices. Those best placed to provide this service need to be divorced from personal and organisational agendas, positional and resource power, and related political interests. Internal mentors can, therefore, face a conflict of interests as they try unsuccessfully to balance organisational issues and struggle with their positional power in the process of being true to the needs of the mentee. To maintain a high degree of integrity and objectivity, and to enable significant and life-changing outcomes, mentors must always come from outside the organisation.

Clinical supervision, pre-ceptorship and annual performance reviews are other types of processes which all fall under the rubric of a professional development and clinical governance strategy. Whilst the overall intent is to develop staff, improve quality and meet statutory requirements, there is a difference in the process, power base, characteristics and purpose of each of these roles (Chin & Moore forthcoming).

Clarity is, therefore, needed with respect to the added value that each role offers for achieving specific learning outcomes and will help to identify any gaps in the strategies available. There is also no guarantee that any of these developmental strategies will lead to quality improvements through actual implementation of learning into practice. Organisations need to examine what processes are in place to facilitate learning into practice and thence evaluate its impact on improving care and services.

CONCLUSION

There is no one right way to achieve change, but there are several measures which organisations can take to make it easier for themselves and their staff. The first thing is for senior executives and managers to really accept and embrace the fact that their workforce is their greatest asset, and it is the employees in conjunction with service users who actually implement clinical governance in practice. These people are the ones who will take services into the 21st century, but only if they are supported at an organisational level to do so.

Secondly, if organisations are to achieve clinical governance by embedding the idea that 'quality is everybody's business' and develop a culture where everybody in it behaves like a responsible adult, then they have to invest time, effort and leadership energy into the learning and well-being of their workforce. Similarly, the workforce must recognise that if it wants to be given more opportunities to make decisions, innovate, create, take risks and improve the quality of care and service it provides, then it must become disciplined in learning to learn, and in being accountable for the outcomes.

By its very nature, clinical governance and best value means that we must question our practice, learn from the process of questioning and discovery, and be accountable for the outcomes. In short, we can no longer do things the way we always have, behave in the ways we always have and hope somebody else will take the blame when it all goes horribly wrong. Change is a constant and so, rather than fight against it and fear it, we need to re-focus our mindset to being one in which change provides us with opportunities to learn, grow and develop. If we see welfare services as a complex adaptive system, in which everything is interconnected, and where learning and particularly feedback from learning in practice produces quality, we can begin to build a synergistic service that lives and breathes, not one that just gasps to survive.

REFERENCES

Bass BM, Avolio BJ 1994 Improving organisational effectiveness through transformational leadership. Sage, London.

Berger P, Luckmann T 1966 The social construction of reality: a treatise in the sociology of knowledge. Penguin, London.

Braudel F 1993 A history of civilisations. Penguin, London.

Carson S 1999 Organisational change. In: Hamer S, Collinson G (eds) Evidence based practice: a handbook for practitioners. Bailliére Tindall/Royal College of Nursing, London.

Centre for the Development of Nursing Policy and Practice 2000 Leadership development. University of Leeds, UK.

Chin H, McNichol E 2000 Practice development credentialling in the United Kingdom: a unique framework for providing excellence, accountability and quality in nursing and healthcare. Online Journal of Issues in Nursing 5(2): manuscript 5.

Chin H, Moore R In press Coaching: the missing link. Centre for the developing of nursing policy and practice, The University of Leeds, Leeds.

Clutterbuck D 1998 Learning alliances: tapping into talent. Institute of Personnel and Development, London.

Cowper A 2000 The future of the NHS debate; 'do not resuscitate'. British Journal of Healthcare Management 6(5): 190–192.

Cullen R, Nicholls S, Halligan A 2000 Reviewing a service-discovering the unwritten rules. British Journal of Clinical Governance 5(4): 233–239.

Dahlan HM 1992 What is changing? In: Sabah, traces of change. Universiti Kebagsaan, Malaysia.

Dechant K, Marsick VJ, Kasl E 1993 Towards a model of team learning. Studies in Continuing Education 15: 1–14.

del Bueno D, Griffin LR, Burke SM, Foley MA 1990 The clinical teacher: A critical link in competence development. Journal of Nursing Staff Development 6: 135–138.

Department of Health 1998 A first class service, quality in the NHS. London, HMSO.

Department of Health 2000 The NHS plan. London, HMSO.

Department of Health 2001 Shifting the balance of power. London HMSO.

Douglas M 1966 Purity and danger: An analysis of the concepts of pollution and taboo. Routledge, London.

Flaherty J 1999 Coaching: evoking excellence in others. Butterworth-Heinemann, London.

Ford M, Walsh P 1994 New rituals for old: nursing through the looking glass. Butterworth-Heinemann, London.

Fraser SW, Greenhalgh T 2001 Coping with complexity: educating for capability. British Medical Journal 323: 799–803.

Geertz C 1993 The interpretation of cultures. Basic Books, New York.

Giddens A 1994 Institutional reflexivity and modernity. In: The polity reader in social theory. Polity Press, London.

Ham C 1992 Health policy in Britain: the politics and organisation of the National Health Service. Macmillan, London.

Harrison D 1988 The sociology of modernisation and development. Routledge, London.

Huntington S 1994 The clash of civilisations. Foreign Affairs 72(3): 22–49.

Illes V, Sutherland K 2001 Managing change in the NHS. Organisational change: a review for healthcare managers, professionals and researchers. National Co-ordinating Centre for NHS Service Delivery and Organisation R&D.

Katzenbach JR, Smith DK 1998 The wisdom of teams: creating the high performance organisation. McGraw-Hill, London.

Lewin K 1951 Field theory in social science. Harper Row, New York.

Louis MR 1980 Surprise and sense making: what newcomers experience in entering unfamiliar organisational settings. Administrative Science Quarterly 25: 226–251.

Manthey M, Miller D 1994 Empowerment through levels of authority. Journal of Nursing Administration 24: 7/8 July/August.

Miller D, Creative Health Care Management, Inc. 2000 Leading an empowered organisation. Creative Health Care Management, Inc., Minneapolis, USA.

Page S, Allsopp D, Casley S 1998 The practice development unit: an experiment in multi-disciplinary innovation. Whurr, London.

Plsek PE 2001 Redesigning healthcare with insights from the science of complex adaptive systems. In: Institute of medicine (IOM) Committee on quality of healthcare in America. Crossing the quality chasm: a new health system for the 21st century. National Academy Press, USA.

Porras J, Robertson P 1992 Organisation development. In: Dunnette M, Hough L (eds) Handbook of industrial and organisational psychology 3: 719–822. Consulting Psychologists Press.

Porter O'Grady T, Kruegar Wilson K 1995 The leadership revolution in healthcare: altering systems, changing behaviours. Aspen, USA.

Senge PM 1990 The fifth discipline: The art and practice of the learning organisation. Century Business, London.

Stacey RD 1993 Strategic management and organisational dynamics. Pitman, London.

Taylor B 1995 Helping people change. Oasis Publications, Boston Spa, West Yorkshire.

Turner V 1967 The forest of symbols. Cornell University Press, USA.

Turner V 1982 From ritual to theatre: the human seriousness of play. PAJ Publications, New York.

Useem M 2001 The leadership lessons of Mount Everest. Harvard Business Review. October issue 2001.

Wallace LM, Freeman T, Latham L, Walshe K, Spurgeon P 2001 Organisational strategies for changing clinical practice: how trusts are meeting the challenges of clinical governance. Quality in Healthcare 10: 76–82.

Weick KE, Quinn RE 1999 Organisational change and development. Annual Review of Psychology 50: 361–386.

Weston M 2001 Coaching generations in the workplace. Nursing Administration Quarterly 25(2): 11–21.

Wilson DC 1992 A strategy of change: concepts and controversies in the management of change. Routledge, London.

Youngblood MD 1997 Life at the edge of chaos: creating the quantum organisation. Perceval Publishing, USA.

Zimmerman B, Lindberg C, Plsek P 1998 Edgeware: insights from complexity science for healthcare leaders. VHA Inc. Texas, USA.

FURTHER READING

Buzan T 2000 Head first: 10 ways to tap into your natural genius. Thorsons, London.

Covey SR 1989 The 7 habits of highly effective people: powerful lessons in personal change. Simon and Schuster, London.

O'Connor J, McDermott I 1997 The art of systems thinking: essential skills for creativity and problem solving. Harper Collins, London.

Page S, Allsopp D, Casley S 1998 The practice development unit: an experiment in multi-disciplinary innovation. Whurr, London.

Plsek PE 2001 Crossing the Quality Chasm: A New Health System for the 21st Century. Committee on Quality of Health Care in America, Institute of Medicine, National Academy Press, Washington, DC, USA.

Senge P 1994 The fifth discipline fieldbook: strategies and tools for building a learning organisation. Nicholas Brealey Publishing, London.

Youngblood MD 1997 Life at the edge of chaos: creating the quantum organisation. Perceval Publishing, USA.

16

Towards sustainable change and improvement

Thinking globally, acting locally

Phil Glanfield

KEY ISSUES

◆ Why doesn't improvement last?

◆ Why is it so difficult to sustain our
  achievements?

◆ Why don't good ideas spread?

◆ Thinking globally – two different ways of
  understanding organisations, change
  and sustainability.

◆ Acting locally – ideas for action, so what
  can you do to encourage sustainability?

INTRODUCTION

The pressure for improvement in health services is enormous and yet change management programmes have such a poor record. The first section describes two different ways of seeing organisations: one is mechanical, scientific and engineered; the other is complex, participative, emergent and dynamic. It is not a question of which one is right, but how we 'see' organisations; the beliefs, values and assumptions we hold. How we see organisations informs and guides when and how we act. Creating a sustainable organisational environment is active, not passive. It happens in the detail of day-to-day action and interaction, in the relationships between individuals. As such, the second section describes a framework for sustainability and a number of practical ideas for action.

THE CHALLENGE OF SUSTAINABILITY

What are we trying to sustain?

There at least three possible answers to this question:

1. A particular set of (changed and improved) working practices – how things are done.
2. The attainment of a particular set of (measurable) improvement outcomes – what is achieved.
3. A way of doing things that results in continuous improvement – a 'learning organisation'.

Clinical governance is firmly rooted in the notion of continuous improvement and it is tempting to assume that (3) is the 'right' answer. But, in any specific context either (1) or (2) could be a legitimate, significant and more realistic goal. So what is the relationship between these answers? Does (1) + (2) = (3)? Are (1) and (2) both sufficient and necessary to achieve (3)? These relationships will be explored in this chapter.

Clinical governance and best value are part of a much wider picture in which pressure for the sustainable improvement of welfare services has never been greater. This is a worldwide challenge that has very different manifestations. For some, the challenge is the provision of basic hygiene and physical care, and for others it is access to the latest treatments and therapies to prolong and improve the quality of life. This chapter takes a narrow view by focusing on the most developed services, particularly in the UK.

However, placing sustainability in a global context highlights the highly connected and interdependent nature of the world we inhabit. In ecological terms we expect the link between cause and effect to be contested – is there global warming and if so what is causing it? We are not surprised when one country places its interests higher than another's; for example, 'we cannot allow control of emissions to harm our industry'. We also recognise the deep complexity of global warming and the hazardous nature of potential solutions which often, unintentionally, make things worse, not better. So it is with organisational change and improvement, although we often behave as if it were much more straightforward. In practice, the causes of a particular pattern of behaviour are contested; it depends who you are and where you are. Every potential solution has it supporters and detractors and seems to have as many disadvantages as advantages. What is more, we cannot predict the outcome of any particular course of action with any certainty, but we know from our experience that things never turn out exactly as planned. However, 'it's all too difficult' is an unconvincing strategy and so this chapter uses the ecological maxim, 'think globally, act locally' to explore sustainable improvement. We need to be aware of the wider context and the importance of the moment, the 'here and now' detail of what we do and how.

When focusing upon sustainable change, a number of questions present themselves:

- Why doesn't improvement last?
- Why is it so difficult to sustain our achievements?
- Why don't good ideas spread?

In considering these questions, this chapter explores two areas:

- Thinking globally – two different ways of understanding organisations, change and sustainability.

- Acting locally – ideas for action; so what can you do to encourage sustainability?

Management makes it worse: the improvement paradox

One of the inherent difficulties with change management is that '... the bulk of the research evidence points to either the outright failure or ambivalent success of ... change journeys ...' (Pettigrew 1997). How many times have you heard it said that 'things get done around here in spite of the management' or 'if only I didn't have to go to this meeting or fill in this form or write this report I could get on with my job'. Frustration with the bureaucracy of organisations is everywhere. We seem to spend so much time and effort auditing what we do, counting it, reporting it and being checked up on that we have little time or energy to do what we want to do and do best. So we initiate a change programme to improve the service, eliminate waste, drive out bureaucracy, streamline the system, improve the services. A project team and manager are appointed, the initiative is launched, enthusiasm is encouraged and cynicism is derided. Training workshops are held, a vision is described, tools and techniques are introduced, changes are made, some things improve, some things get worse, doubts are expressed, the project manager is promoted and the cynics pronounce that they told you so. Then a little while later a new initiative is launched, a project manager is appointed ... and so on.

Is it any wonder that we are tired of change programmes? It seems the harder we push the further away we get. Over the years we have become used to the language of, and prescriptions for, change, such as:

- articulate a clear vision
- ensure top management commitment
- focus on a few measurable improvements
- implement effective project management.

These change prescriptions equate to '10 Ways to Get Rich/Find Happiness/Improve Your Life' that shout at us from magazines and books. The things to do are obvious and yet they seem irrelevant or unrealistic. We know that drinking too much or eating a fatty diet can cause health problems, but telling someone with an alcohol dependency to 'stop drinking' or a weight problem to 'eat less' is ineffective. Somehow we cannot find the resources, incentives or motivation to 'make it happen'. Perhaps there is something more complex happening to do with the internal world – how we see ourselves – and the external world, the environment as a whole in which we live, and the interaction between the two.

So what goes wrong, why can't we 'do change' better?

If this is the case with individual improvement, then how do we understand and appreciate the world of organisational change? The literature contains some recurring explanations: some of the most common major reasons for failed change programmes (Pettigrew 1997, Axelrod 2001) include:

- Change programmes being managed through parallel and exclusive organisations that define the rest of the world as 'resistant to change'.
- Oversimplification: promoting standardised solutions and short term re-design rather than cultural change.
- Treating everything as a project when it is obvious that some things are long term and continuous.
- Not connecting the change programme to the business or political interests, and ignoring the contextual and embedded nature of human systems.
- Following exclusive and over-zealous consultants (who move on) and over reliance on project teams which break up.

THINK GLOBAL: TWO DIFFERENT PERSPECTIVES ON ORGANISATIONS AND CHANGE

Picking up these themes let us consider two contrasting views of organisation. Of course there are multiple images of organisation (Morgan 1986) and we all have our own preferred models that we apply in practical ways. The purpose in describing two models is not to suggest that we have a straight choice, but that both models operate all the time and simultaneously. By becoming more aware of the beliefs, assumptions and values that underpin our mental model of organisations, we can make more deliberate choices about how we act and place our local action in the context of our global understanding.

Model 1: the mechanical organisation

This is the model of classical, western, scientific management which pervades our thinking and can be traced to Taylor (1947) in the USA and Fayol (1949) in western Europe. Management, even improvement, is a discrete science through which processes can be standardised, optimised and improved. Management is the process of forecasting, planning, organising, co-ordinating and controlling. The organisation is seen as a machine in which inputs can be measured against outputs and it is possible to stand outside that machine and change it, using scientific principles. Over time this mechanistic view of organisations was challenged by, and adapted through, the application of systems theory. Here the interest is not in the parts of an organisation, but in the interaction between the parts and how that interaction creates a whole that is more than the sum of its parts. Systems' thinking extends the mechanistic model of organisation, but holds onto an engineering perspective of organisation that has underpinned most recent approaches. Re-engineering, re-design, total quality management and clinical governance are based in systems thinking. Stand back, step outside the

process, benchmark the performance, measure and monitor it, adapt and improve it. The results that a system achieves are seen to be the property of the system itself. Every system is designed to achieve the (intentional and unintentional) results that it achieves and so it is a deterministic view of organisation.

In this model, organisational culture is seen as traits, characteristics or variable properties of an organisation. These properties can be described, measured, manipulated and changed. In effect, the change leader is seen as standing outside of the organisation culture and re-engineering it. This thinking has spawned a multitude of linear change management models, usually derived from Lewin's unfreeze–change–refreeze (Lewin 1951).

Model 2: the complex, organic organisation

This model begins with our personal experience of organisations and accepts that we find them hard to understand, constantly moving, stable and unstable, informal and formal, complex and unpredictable with multiple reporting relationships. In the detail of the day-to-day working life, we are constantly finding ways to work around the system, because 'the system' won't quite do what we judge to be appropriate in any given particular circumstance. Work gets done in spite of the systems and processes for managing it.

The model draws on the so called 'new science' of chaos and complexity to describe organisations as complex adaptive systems (Capra 1997, Wheatley 1999) or complex responsive processes (Stacey 2001). This perspective helps us to understand our experience of organisations as messy. Organisations are seen as a massive bundle of dynamic relationships, a living system that has boundaries, but they are blurred, personal and changing. In this model:

- Continual creativity is a natural state, things are stable and unstable at the same time, life and death are in constant tension.

- Small changes can have big effects and big changes can have small effects. Some things 'take off', other things die.
- The whole shapes the parts and the parts shape the whole; all the parts participate (actively or passively) all the time and action by any part affects the whole.
- All the parts of the system can act independently and all the parts are intimately connected, and the relationships between them matter.
- The systems self organise – patterns of order emerge from the independent and interdependent actions of the parts and without central control.
- Complex patterns and outcomes can result from a few simple rules that may be explicit but are often implicit.
- Redundancy, or spare capacity, is a natural state and is necessary for innovation. Without redundancy the system degrades and dies.
- Accurate prediction is not possible, but consistent patterns can be identified.

Contrasting the mechanical and the complex

As can be seen from Box 16.1, these two models have quite different foundations and implications.

Ralph Stacey (1992, 2001) is one of the most challenging and creative writers on organisation, change and innovation. Using insights from complexity science, Stacey describes the relationship between order and chaos. The alternative to order is not chaos but there is a zone of complexity between order and chaos, which is both stable and unstable at the same time. When we know what to do and how to do it (we agree and are certain), then we can plan and control what we do and there is a good chance it will work. But the further away we are from agreement and certainty about what to do and how, the closer we are to the 'edge of chaos'. It is at the 'edge of chaos' that the conditions for innovation, change and improvement exist. In this zone there is the opportunity to test and experiment. Information moves around freely, there is a high level of connection between participants and a high level of diversity, so that ideas are contested and argued. This is not a comfortable state; the 'edge of chaos' is an anxious place which is why we

Box 16.1

Assumption	Model 1 thinking	Model 2 thinking
Scientific foundation	Newtonian	Quantum
Time is	Monochronic – one thing at a time	Polychronic – many things at once
Understand by	Dissecting into parts	Seeing in terms of the whole
Information is	Ultimately knowable	Infinite and unbounded
Growth is	Linear, managed	Organic, chaotic
Managing means	Controlling, predicting	Insight, participation
Workers are	Specialised, segmented	Multi-faceted, always learning
Motivation from	External forces and influence	Intrinsic, creativity
Knowledge is	Individual	Collective
Organisation is	By design	Emergent
Life thrives on	Competition	Cooperation
Change is	Something to worry about	All there is

Reproduced from Allee V 1997 The knowledge evolution: expanding organisational intelligence. Butterworth-Heinemann, Boston, MA, with kind permission.

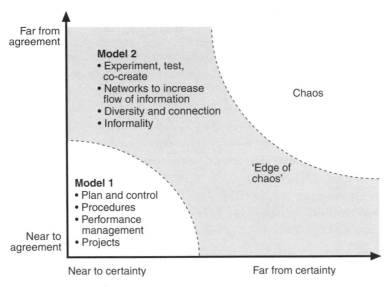

Figure 16.1 Stacey curve.

are often much more comfortable with order and control.

This gets us to the heart of the question – 'what is it we are trying to sustain?' If it is a particular set of improved, proven working practices that are agreed, then model 1 is the type of organisation that would plan, control and sustain the improvement (see Fig. 16.1). However, if new, innovative and creative ways of doing things are needed, then model 2 is much more likely to find innovative solutions. The attainment of a particular set of (measurable) improvement outcome (externally set) targets seems to fit better with model 1 (although it may lead to sub-optimisation because the best that can be achieved is that the targets are hit). In model 2 there is the possibility of higher, better and different results being achieved, as new, internally generated targets are set along the way. Learning is part of both models, but the nature of the learning is different. In model 1 systems are in place for measuring and identifying best practice and spreading best practice by pushing it at underperforming parts of the organisation. In model 2 learning is through collective enquiry where the experience of all is engaged in solving a problem or creating new possibilities.

So what?

How we 'see' organisations, how we conceive them in our minds eye and the assumptions we make about how they work directly affects the action that we take. Some ideas for action are explored in the second half of this chapter. Before moving on, and to balance the reasons for failure cited earlier, what general statements can be made about change, improvement and sustainability? At the risk of sounding like yet another change prescription here are a few suggestions:

- See change as a long journey, not a short term episode.
- Promote coherence across the (inevitably) multi-faceted change agenda – you cannot avoid 'doing everything at once'.
- Emphasise what will *not* change and create zones of continuity and comfort.

- Promote customisation – local solutions for local people – let go of the solution, concern yourself with the intended outcome.
- Find opportunities for leaders to marry top-down pressures with bottom-up concerns.
- See change as a political process, operate inclusive and voluntary principles and create conditions for self organisation. This means:
  - widening the circle of involvement
  - connecting people to each other and their ideas
  - creating communities for action
  - embracing democratic principles
  - letting go of figuring it all out from the top.

ACT LOCALLY: IDEAS FOR ACTION

Thinking globally is all very well, but what does this mean in practice? What do we do? Is model 2 right and model 1 wrong? Should we abandon objectives, targets and project management in favour of a few loose intentions; let it go, do nothing, see what emerges?

Doing everything at the same time

In practice we have to hold onto both models. This is particularly important in public and personal services where the policy is set by elected politicians. 'Let's see what emerges' is not a mandate that is likely to win elections, whereas improvement targets in education, transport or health are food and drink to politicians. Externally imposed, measurable targets are here to stay. Prominent or senior leaders (political and otherwise) are likely to describe change and improvement in terms of large scale vision, strategy and intended results. However, what really matters in implementing any improvement successfully is the detail. Not only the detail of what is to be done, but also the detail of how it is to be done. Change and improvement may sound sexy, exciting,

big and strategic, but the reality of implementation is day to day, moment by moment, in which every step and every interaction matters. Therefore, it takes time, there are no 'silver bullets', small actions are more significant than grand designs, good relationships between individuals and groups are more significant than the slickest of systems and processes.

Geometry of sustainability

Hence the ideas that are in this section. They are drawn from a wide range of sources and mostly from the personal experience of people seeking to improve health services. The ideas are rooted in people's experience of the world and have proved to be useful in certain circumstances (but not in others). The ideas are not original, some are rooted in model 1, others in model 2. It is not the idea itself that matters so much as the way in which it is applied. They represent an attempt to pay attention to the whole thing, to the detail and to the interaction between the different details.

Figure 16.2 develops further a framework from the University of Birmingham (Bate 2002) and describes a way of thinking about the whole thing, i.e. implementing targeted, specific, measurable improvement projects within a particular context. It has three dimensions: method, implementation and context. Each dimension has a polarity (based on models 1 and 2), although, again, these dimensions are not 'either/or' choices but 'both/and'. Figure 16.1 summarises the ideas into a neat framework – with all the limitations of all 'neat frameworks'. Organisational life cannot be described or contained within a triangle, but setting it out in this way helps communication and emphasises that the whole thing, including the interaction of the different dimensions, is of more significance than the parts.

The framework has been built up from the experience of many people involved in specific improvement efforts. The overriding consideration

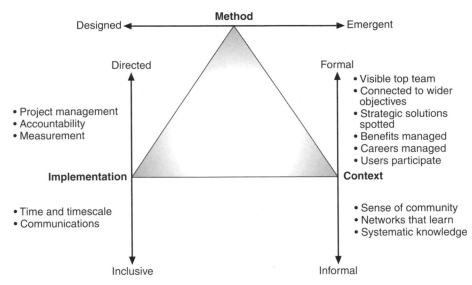

Figure 16.2 Key elements for achieving sustainable change.

is that of the particular circumstances that apply in any given situation; only you can judge what needs to be done. Therefore, the ideas for action are often in the form of good questions to ask or things to think about rather than actions to take.

Let us consider method, implementation and context in turn.

Method

This refers to the particular approach to improvement to be employed. The ends of the methodology spectrum are:

- Designed changes originate in model 1 where improvements are conceived and designed, often externally or by senior management, and implemented as part of a planned process, often with the use of experts. The improvements can be incremental as in continuous improvement methodologies, such as total quality management of which clinical governance is a subset. However, if a costly new investment is to be made, or if something major has gone wrong, a more radical (and risky) approach may be

attempted such as process re-engineering (Iles & Sutherland 2001). Designed approaches to change are often the subject of fashion or fad.

- Emergent approaches have their root in model 2: human beings are constantly and intuitively finding new and better ways to do things, particularly since the systems and processes we design can never foresee every eventuality. Our daily experience is of working round, rather than through management systems. The approach here is to find ways of recognising, supporting, getting out of the way of the innovation and creativity that is inherent in every organisation.

So how to choose?

Our managerial habit is to start with designed change, but in an important sense you do not have a choice! Whichever starting point you choose, in each and every situation, intentional design and emergence will be operating. This is because learning is at the centre of change, and without it there can be no adaptation or transformation.

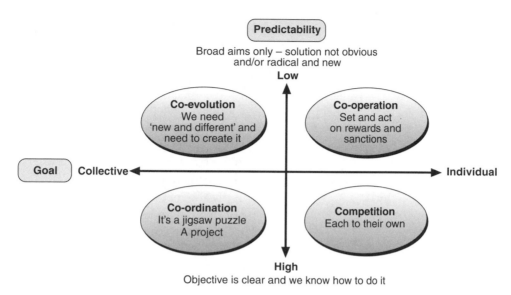

Figure 16.3 Predictability and goals (adapted from Pratt et al. 1999 with kind permission of The King's Fund, London)

Learning is a social process, dynamic and uncontrollable. Individual and group learning happen at the same time, they are not separate. So even in the most designed and managed of processes there must be learning and, therefore, emergence. However, there are some helpful distinctions to be drawn as summarised in Figure 16.3.

This is an extension of the Stacey curve in Figure 16.1 and helps to identify what approach to take. The axes are:

- Predictability – do we know clearly what we are trying to do and how to do it? Has it been done elsewhere; is there good evidence (however defined) and experience? If so predictability is high, if not then it is low.

- Goal – does the goal that we are trying to achieve have many interdependencies and does it require high levels of cooperation between a number of people and groups? Is it a collective goal? Or, can individuals implement it on their own?

The interaction of these two attributes produces four possible approaches:

- Competition – if it is clear what needs to be done and how it is to be done and interdependence is low, then individuals can be left to get on with it in their own way.

- Coordination – if, however, it is clear what needs to be done and how it is to be done but interdependence is high, then you need to coordinate the interconnected players via a project.

- Cooperation – if it is not clear what needs to be done nor how it is to be done and interdependence is low, then since there is no right answer, many solutions are possible, but solutions that do serious damage to another are undesirable. So people can be encouraged to get on with it by rewards or incentives, and discouraged from harming others with sanctions.

- Co-creation – if it is not clear what needs to be done nor how it is to be done and interdependence is high, then it is important to engage all those who have an interest in the problem in finding potential solutions.

This will lead to a wider range of ideas as well as increasing the ownership of the solution. Eventually, this may turn into a project but be careful about stifling co-creation with target driven project management.

Implementation

Whatever the methodology, it should be well executed. The distinction here is between:

- Directed – in this context, managed means 'hard' direction setting and project management: the objectives, measures to be used, plans and milestones, resources available, plus the skills and tools thought to be necessary.
- Inclusive – refers to the 'soft' or hard to measure aspects of implementation, such as the inclusion of staff, patients and stakeholders. Of course real inclusion means a willingness on the part of the 'hard' management system to adapt its objectives, measures etc. in the light of what emerges.

The theme of this chapter is sustainable change, and this includes the take up, spread or adoption of improvement ideas within and between organisations. Rogers (1995) identified five characteristics of change that are most likely to be more widely adopted:

- There is a clear advantage or benefit compared to the current way of doing things.
- The change is compatible with the current systems and its values.
- The change is relatively simple and it is relatively easy to implement.
- It is possible to try out the new way of doing things and relatively easy to fall back to the old way if it doesn't work.

- It is easy to see that the change has been made and that it has made a difference.

Directed implementation

Project management. This is an important discipline with its own body of knowledge. The more critical systems that are being changed, the greater the need for project control; but project management is an overhead, so it is important to apply the methodology to an appropriate level – not over or under doing it. This includes ensuring that the Project Manager has time to carry out the role. More commonly a 'good' member of staff is asked to take on a project when their time is fully committed! (see below)

Project-management knowledge, skills, tools and techniques are important and can be taught. Of greater importance is the choice of project manager. Finding someone who is known, trusted and respected is critical. The project will rely on their knowledge of the organisation, their personal networks and strong relationships with key people as well as their capacity to influence and motivate more widely. No surprise, therefore, that this person is already busy. However, often an individual organisation is taking part in a wider, regional or national change effort. This affords the opportunity to balance the external 'expert' project manager with the local project manager who knows the people and the patch.

Accountability. Usually there are a number of individuals and organisations who have an interest in a change effort. The Trust, or at least a part of it, might be a member of a specialty specific clinical network, the project might be part of a wider local, regional or national programme, external support from management consultants or an agency might be involved. Questions to ask include:

- Are we all trying to achieve the same thing? Not a simple question as specific interests and timescales may well be different.

- Who is accountable for what and who is holding it all together? Another challenging question to explore openly with the wider team.

- Critically, from the perspective of sustainability, who is accountable for and interested in longer term improvement, not just this short term project?

Measurement. In the world of model 1, what matters is what can be measured, and what gets measured gets done. Those investing in improvement will want to see a return, and there may well be performance targets to hit that have been set externally. How benefits are realised and measured is discussed later; the issue here is that measurement for improvement is often different from measurement for performance. For improvement you may want to set an ambitious or 'stretch' target that challenges the organisation. An external target may well have been set with other intentions, perhaps political, and therefore may be more modest. Not only are performance targets and measures likely to be different from improvement targets and measures, but also the data gathered are used in different ways. Those involved in the improvement effort must be able to trust each other and the measurement system. Therefore it is important to be clear about:

- What is being measured for which purpose?
- How will the data be gathered and handled?
- How will reports be compiled, who will have access to them and for what purpose?
- How will we gather data on unexpected benefits? (see below)

Inclusive implementation

This relates to the earlier point about emergent methodology – in each and every situation, intentional design and emergence will be operating. If model 1 is deeply embedded in your psyche you may not like this idea, but it is fundamental to human existence and evolution so you may as well get used to it, and why not try to embrace it? This means:

- Seeing yourself as a participant in the organisation you are trying to improve along with all the other interested parties. Not a someone who stands outside the system trying to change it from one design to another.

- Seeing yourself as a partner in an enquiry about improvement, not as someone who holds special knowledge or has better motivation than anyone else. Of course your knowledge and motivation are special and different, unique to you. But then the same must be true of all the others.

- Letting go of your ideas; the harder you push the further away you get. You may be confident in your solution but if you insist on it, implementation will be superficial. On paper you will have your designed change, but emergence will ensure that it is adapted, or ignored and degrades rapidly. If the outcome is more important than the process then accept that those who know most about it can improve the process. This is not about winners, losers, or managing resistance, it is about letting go of personal power and notions of optimisation in favour of something that will work in the particular context.

- Telling the truth so that 'letting go' does not mean doing nothing or compromising on everything for the sake of a quiet life. It means:
  - openly recognising power differentials and working to change them

– expecting and encouraging emotional and irrational responses, and being open about your own feelings and irrational ideas – this is where creativity and innovation thrive
– working with confrontation and competition as it arises.

In embracing inclusivity and emergence you are likely to face some particular challenges including:

Time and timescale. There is a double challenge and paradox here. Often the areas of service that are in most need of improvement are the ones where the staff are most hard pressed and may feel 'nothing can be done'. All the more reason for their active engagement, but finding time to improve the service becomes yet another thing to do: there are no easy answers. From model 2 we can see that for a change effort to take hold inclusion and engagement must be real, but this takes time. Without creating capacity, opportunity and 'headroom' change cannot be initiated or sustained.

There is a further paradox. Usually, externally set targets and their associated timescales are set around average performance, so those organisations who are already doing well have the least to do. This is the major problem with national targets, for some they are unrealistic, for others they are too modest. As discussed above, local improvement measures that challenge the current position are needed.

Communication. Constantly widening the circle of engagement is important and so is wider awareness raising to stimulate readiness and interest in related parts of the organisation or health community. Finding ways to keep everybody up to date and maintaining specific, open communication channels with key players is very challenging. Sarah Fraser (2002) has a useful way of describing a wide range of communication methods, shown in Box 16.2.

Box 16.2

Share information		Shape behaviour	
Publications	Personal invitation	Interactive	Face to face
Flyers	Letters	Telephone	Mentoring
Newsletters	Reports	Email	Coaching
Videos	Postcards	Visits	Secondment
Articles		Seminars	Shadowing
Posters			Learning set

Context

This means working with the formal and the informal. Again, this is not a matter about which you have a choice and it is not either/or. Both are in operation all the time. The formal relates closely to model 1 and systematic management. It includes the chief executive and top team, and the alignment of project objectives to the overall business plan. Most importantly, the institutionalisation of improvements that work through sanctions, rewards and harvesting benefits, and deploying them elsewhere. The informal context is closely connected to model 2 and emergence and inclusivity. It includes developing a sense of community and shared purpose, nurturing informal networks, and encouraging the growth and spread of knowledge.

Formal context

Be visible as a top team. Senior managers may not be in control to the extent that model 1 would suggest, but what they do makes a difference.

Develop a script. 'Joining things up', being coherent and consistent, help others see how individual projects fit with your organisation and its wider goals. Use plain English to describe its objectives and importance. Consider the following:

• This programme/project is about…
• It is important for us because…

- The advantages of this work are …
- I expect the impact to be …
- We can support our team by …

Consider politics and power. Fortunately not everybody has to agree with everything for a change to be implemented effectively. But organisations are bundles of politics and power (positional, personal, professional), and it matters. Often it is helpful to understand the position of key individuals and opinion formers, for example:

- Who will make this happen?
- Who must let it happen?
- Who can stop it happening?

You can even use a table to be explicit about where you see people now and where you think they need to be. But beware of your own prejudices and assumptions when carrying out an exercise like this. Other people might see the world quite differently – so include them in this process – and don't forget to include yourself too!

Connect improvement projects to wider (organisational) objectives. Map the connections: because of the size of the agenda and the multiple initiatives within any one organisation, it is hard to see how it all joins up with core organisational objectives.

- Starting with your current strategic goals and operational objectives, work at a high level and include ALL goals and objectives, not just the ones that are most obviously connected to change and improvement. On a piece of paper record the goal or objective on the left hand side and, on the right hand side, record the ways in which the particular initiative supports the goals/objectives.
- This is not a desk-top exercise for one individual. Different people will have different views on how the objectives and the initiatives connect: some connections may not

be obvious immediately and, as the initiative progresses, further connections will become apparent.

Make and maintain connections. Often project teams become separated from the organisation and are seen as special or elite. This weakens their ability to have an impact beyond the project itself and contributes to project failure. Whether you are within a project team or part of a senior management group, it is important to see the bigger picture. How is the project team perceived by the organisation as a whole and how well is it connected to other initiatives? Within your team and, more importantly, with other teams and key individuals, consider the following:

- How is this project seen at the moment by the organisation – marginal or mainstream, part of the organisation or separate and elite?
- Are there signs of elitism and how can this be challenged constructively?
- How is the project team communicating with the wider organisation? Are they communicating in ways that connect their project to wider organisational concerns and objectives?
- Which groups (inside or outside, staff or patient) would be interested in the project? How can you widen the circle of engagement and understanding?
- How involved are staff and patients? How can you move from 'telling and consulting' to 'engaging and co-creating'?
- What connections can you see between this project and other things that are happening in your organisation? Which groups, led by whom? What opportunities are there for connecting different groups and building a community of interest?
- What else is going on in your health community? Are there connections and alliances to be made?

Strategic solutions spotted and implemented. Change and improvement activity at a local level often involves multiple, small scale, trail and error changes. This works well in finding out what works and building momentum. However, sometimes the small changes are not sustainable in the long term because the overheads (e.g. paper-based data collection and the time it takes) are too high. The IT industry calls this 'scalability' – can a small-scale solution be 'scaled-up' to work organisation-wide. For example, registers are very helpful in monitoring for a number of patient conditions. However, separate systems are not sustainable and there is a need to integrate registers into daily working practice and core patient data via the patient management computer.

In other words, for some projects the transition from small-scale pilot to 'the way things are done around here' requires integration with mainstream operational systems. But how do you know which ones? This is where the link to knowledge and communities of practice is critical (see below). Finally, if a solution is strategic and system wide, then it must be implemented and policed. For example, once the computer system for ordering radiology is in place, take the cards away from the wards, and if one or two find their way through, send them back.

Benefits reaped and re-used. When an improvement is made, either a local operational improvement or a strategic solution, the systematic follow-through of improvement benefits is important. Firstly, benefits often go unnoticed and unrecognised. We tend to monitor and count only those benefits that we originally intend to achieve. In practice, improvement efforts produce all sorts of unintended and unexpected benefits which are just as valuable as the original intention. This is more likely to be the case if the implementation is inclusive as described above. Secondly, benefits (expected and unexpected) can easily be diverted. For example, improvements in

surgery may mean a reduction in length of stay with the intention of using the increased capacity to reduce waiting lists and times. However, often this extra bed capacity is used for medical emergencies. So what can you do?

- Be realistic from the start about the costs and benefits of your improvement effort – avoid natural tendency to overestimate benefits and underestimate costs.
- Treat improvement activity as a long term investment, not just a cost.
- Expect, identify and value qualitative as well as quantitative benefits.
- Keep looking, keep identifying benefits – count them, particularly if they are not ones that you anticipated when you started.
- Where investment is being made, be clear with the directorate or team the basis on which it is being made. 'What we expect in return is …'
- Be rigorous and systematic about harvesting planned benefits when they are realised. Identify the improvements in other systems that are necessary to achieve this, e.g. protecting bed capacity.
- Be clear with the directorate or team what will happen to any financial benefits that are realised, e.g. 50/50 split between directorate, to be used at the directorate's discretion, and the Trust to be used for re-investment in improvement elsewhere.
- Consider creating a local improvement fund that directorate teams can 'borrow' from to test and develop improvement ideas.

Users and patients participate. Quality and safety matter to everybody, particularly the patient and their family, but so often they are the last to be asked. In the world of model 1 the user or patient is consulted and kept at a distance; improvement is seen as an activity for experts.

In model 2 the patient is an equal participant and the question of power imbalance between professionals and patients is addressed. Patients and professionals are involved together from the start, not when the professionals are ready. This has a number of effects:

- The things that matter are addressed, i.e. the things that matter to patients/clients.
- Perspectives are altered – clinicians and professionals.
- Accountability is real – for all staff, but particularly for front line staff accountability to patients is much more powerful and important than any performance management system.

Manage careers. Often staff who are instrumental in bringing about improvements do so on short, fixed term contracts or secondment. They find the work challenging, stimulating and developmental. But what happens at the end of the project? As we have seen, the personality and the relationships that the project manager holds can make or break the project. Change and improvement takes time, but secondments are short term. Often when the project manager moves on the project falters. Helping people to manage their careers so that personal and organisational objectives are met is important.

Informal context

Develop a sense of community. This is not a romantic notion about promoting harmony – often change and improvement results from conflict, and always from difference and diversity. Without difference and diversity, challenge and question, learning, change and improvement are not possible. But often in organisational life one section or another dominates a group. For example, the Kennedy Report (The Stationery Office 2001) highlighted 'paternalism and a club culture' as one of the major factors that led to children being

'failed by the system that was supposed to make them well'. Such situations do not arise overnight, but are created moment by moment. It is not enough to have the intention of listening to a patient or service user. It means shutting up in every encounter and listening attentively. It is not enough to have multi-disciplinary team meetings if only the senior doctors talk and there is no meaningful conversation and participation. In these micro-moments our sense of organisation and community are formed.

The next sections describe networks that learn and the creation of knowledge. Wenger (1996) links these things to the notion of community of practice: 'Communities of practice are not just places where local activities are organised, but also where the meaning of belonging to broader organisations is negotiated and experienced. In healthcare practice the tension between the local and the global is a daily experience. Protocols, regulations, procedures and professional standards must be interpreted locally and translated into a practice that addresses the specifics of clinical cases'. Community creates learning, learning creates improvement, and improvement creates learning that creates community.

Support and nurture networks that learn. If we are trying to sustain a way of doing things that results in continuous improvement – a 'learning organisation' – then we have to 'learn about learning' and 'improve the way we improve'. Within every organisation and health- and social-care community, there are many people engaged in improvement activity, but often they are disconnected. Model 2 thinking has given greater insight into how knowledge is created and moves around, typically through informal networks. This is a natural, rather than a mechanical process and should not be overmanaged. Rather than trying to establish something new, it may be better to seek out and support informal networks that are already happening. Here are some key points for encouraging networks that learn (Bessant & Tsekouras 2000). The suggestion is not that the following need to be decided in advance of establishing the network, rather that those who are enthusiastic should be encouraged to consider these issues.

- Purpose – a clearly defined shared purpose with a focused and measurable learning target is most viable. Success measure might include number of members as well as examples of knowledge being applied to achieve improvement.

- Participants – who are the members and what is the basis of membership? Defining boundaries helps to create commitment, focus and coherence.

- Type of learning and network structure – is the purpose the acquisition and absorption of explicit codified data (model 1) or is it creating new knowledge and releasing tacit knowledge by challenging assumptions and re-framing problems (model 2)? If the former then it will need a coordinating centre; if the latter then a more distributed member-to-member structure is appropriate.

- Coordinator and facilitator roles – networks need them. The emphasis is on someone with process skills who can facilitate learning, not necessarily to have expert knowledge of the particular subject.

- Methods to be used – how will all the different stages of the learning cycle be addressed? What approaches to use: face-to-face meetings, workshops, site visits, website, mailing lists, newsletters? Meetings: how often, how long, when and where?

- Pump-priming, initiating – how will people find out about it? What will attract them to join?

- Resources – what does the network have at its disposal and how are resources deployed?

Create, grow and apply knowledge. We have become more and more aware of the value and importance of knowledge, particularly its role in supporting change and improvement. In model 1 thinking we talk about 'spreading best practice', but somehow it is elusive; the more you try to pin knowledge down the more it slips away. It seems that knowledge (adapted from Allee 1997):

- is messy – everything is connected
- is self-organising – around a group, identity or purpose
- seeks community – lives in social interaction
- travels on language – is created in conversation as we seek new ways to describe our experience
- is temporal – does not grow forever: some things die; unlearning and letting go are necessary.

So it is not simple or straightforward, but research into organisations that are perceived to value knowledge suggests the following patterns. Knowledge is:

- strategically valued and future oriented
- created with patients, users, consumers and stakeholders
- more people centred than technology centred
- measured in innovative ways
- supported with flexible technology, including easily communicated maps or frameworks to orient people towards it
- encouraged to expand and connect across all modes.

CONCLUSION

This chapter has tried to demonstrate that how we see organisations, our values and belief assumptions, matter because it informs how we act. Organisational theory allows us to develop abstract models of organisation so that we can increase our awareness of our own belief system.

Change and improvement happens in the detail of day-to-day action and relationships. What we do matters more than what we say we do. Therefore, it is important for all the participants in a change process to pay attention to the detail of their interactions and the various ideas that have been put forward. These ideas are held together by a triangular framework of method, implementation and context. The context is the most important dimension because it holds the conditions for success and failure.

ACKNOWLEDGEMENTS

I take responsibility for the ideas expressed which were developed in conversation with a number of people, particularly my erstwhile colleagues Anne Lacey and Neil Riley.

REFERENCES

Allee V 1997 The knowledge evolution: expanding organisational intelligence. Butterworth-Heinemann, Boston, MA.

Axelrod RH 2001 Why change management needs changing Reflections – Society for Organizational Learning 2(3): 46–57.

Bate P, Robert G, Hardacre J, Locock L 2002 Evaluating the effectiveness of the mental health collaborative in Trent and Northern and Yorkshire Regions Health Services Management Centre, University of Birmingham.

Bessant J, Tsekouras G 2001 Developing learning networks. AI and Society 15(1/2): 82–98.

Capra F 1997 The web of life: a new synthesis of mind and matter. Flamingo, London.

Fayol H 1949 General and industrial management. Pitman, London.

Fraser S 2002 Accelerating the spread of good practice. Kingsham Press, West Sussex.

Iles V, Sutherland K 2001 Organisational change. The National Co-ordinating Centre for NHS Service Delivery & Organisation R&D, Department of Health, London.

Lewin K 1951 Field theory in social science. Harper & Row, New York.

Morgan G 1986 Images of organisation. Sage, London.

Pettigrew A 1997 Success and failure in corporate transformation initiatives pp. 271–289. In: Galliers RD, Baets WRJ (eds) Information technology and organizational transformation: innovation for the 21st century organization. John Wiley, Chichester.

Pratt J, Gordon P, Pampling D 1999 Working whole systems. The King's Fund, London.

Rogers EM 1995 Diffusion of Innovations, 4th edn. Free Press, New York.

Stacey R 1992 Managing the unknowable: strategic boundaries between order & chaos in organisations. Jossey-Bass Inc, San Francisco.

Stacey R 2001 Complex responsive processes in organisations: learning and knowledge creation. Routledge, London & New York.

Taylor FW 1947 Scientific management. Harper & Row, New York.

The Report of the Public Inquiry into children's heart surgery at the Bristol Royal Infirmary 1984–1995: Learning from Bristol (Cm 5207). The Stationery Office, July 2001.

Wenger E 1996 Communities of practice the social fabric of a learning organisation. Healthcare Forum Journal July/August 1996.

Wheatley 1999 Leadership & the new science. Berrett-Koehler, San Francisco.

Index